D1758307

Miklós Szendrői · Franklin H. Sim (Eds.)

Color Atlas of Clinical Orthopedics

Miklós Szendrői · Franklin H. Sim (Eds.)

Color Atlas
of Clinical Orthopedics

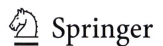 Springer

Miklós Szendrői

Department of Orthopedics
Semmelweis University Budapest
1113 Budapest
Hungary

Franklin Sim

Mayo Clinic
200 First Street SW
Rochester, MN 55905
USA

ISBN 978-3-540-85560-6   e-ISBN 978-3-540-85561-3
DOI 10.1007/978-3-540-85561-3

Springer Dordrecht Heidelberg London New York

Library of Congress Control Number: 2009926318

Cover design: Frido Steinen-Broo, eStudio Calamar, Spain

Printed on acid-free paper

Springer is part of Springer Science+Business Media (www.springer.com)

Preface

The evaluation of musculoskeletal disorders is often problematic because of the variety of diseases and diagnostic complexity. This is compounded by the increasing specialization in this field. While a variety of recent textbooks give comprehensive coverage of these disorders, this color atlas is intended to provide a succinct guide to evaluation and treatment. The atlas is organized into sections according to diagnosis. The text is brief and gives concise information on the clinical features, radiographic characteristics and pathological features that are important for the diagnosis. The reader will appreciate the many illustrations demonstrating the characteristic features of musculoskeletal disorders. The atlas includes more than 600 clinical photographs of patients, 710 radiographs, 272 MRI and CT illustrations, 128 intra-operative and surgical photographs, and 73 microphotographs which help to understand the basic characteristics of more than 250 orthopedic disorders.

This atlas offers a starting point for orthopedic, radiology, and pathology residents. Furthermore, it emphasizes a team approach and should be attractive to the clinician, the rheumatologist, the radiologist, and pathologist and offer them the opportunity to familiarize themselves with and enhance their diagnostic acumen of these musculoskeletal conditions.

This atlas of clinical orthopedics is a joint effort from two large institutions, the Orthopedic Department of Semmelweis University (Hungary) and the musculoskeletal tumor center of Mayo Clinic (USA), both of which have extensive experience in the different areas of musculoskeletal diseases.

It is the hope of the authors that this atlas will prove educational and be a resource that will assist doctors in the care of their patients.

Miklós Szendrői
Franklin H. Sim

Acknowledgments

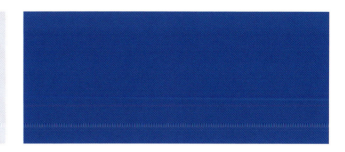

I wish to express my gratitude to the colleagues and medical staff of the Orthopaedic Department of the Semmelweis University who contributed to the material of this Atlas with their own case presentations, excellent photographs and radiographs. My debt of gratitude goes to Dr. András Vajda for the translation of the text from Hungarian to English. My special thanks for the efforts and skillful help of our medical photographer Mr. Péter Kovács, who made the great majority of the excellent gross photographs and reproduced the radiographs and photomicrographs. The final preparation of the manuscript was made possible by the invaluable work of Mrs J. Daróczi and Miss M. Alexa.

I owe a special acknowledgment to the editors of the Semmelweis and Medicina publisher companies for granting permission to reproduce some illustrative material from my books published by them earlier.

I am also greatly indebted to the staff members and publishers of Springer for their careful attention to this Atlas, especially to Mrs G. Schröder, Mrs I. Bohn, Mr. C.-D. Bachem and Mr. T. Reichenthaler for their untiring efforts.

Miklós Szendrői

Contents

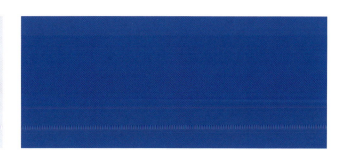

List of Contributors

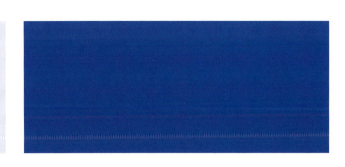

Lajos Bartha
Department of Orthopedics
Semmelweis University Budapest
1113 Budapest, Karolina út 27
Hungary

Zoltán Bejek
Department of Orthopedics
Semmelweis University Budapest
1113 Budapest, Karolina út 27
Hungary

István Böröcz
Department of Orthopedics
Semmelweis University Budapest
1113 Budapest, Karolina út 27
Hungary

Anikó Deli
Department of Orthopedics
Semmelweis University Budapest
1113 Budapest, Karolina út 27
Hungary

Robert Esther
Department of Orthopedics
University of North Carolina
100 Mason Farm Road
3155 Bioinformatics Building CB# 7055
Chapel Hill, NC 27599
USA

Gergely Holnapy
Department of Orthopedics
Semmelweis University Budapest
1113 Budapest, Karolina út 27
Hungary

Jenő Kiss
Department of Orthopedics
St. John Hospital Budapest
1125 Budapest, Diós árok 1–3
Hungary

Sándor Kiss
Department of Orthopedics
Semmelweis University, Budapest
1113 Budapest Karolina út 27
Hungary

Katalin Köllő
Department of Orthopedics
Semmelweis University Budapest
1113 Budapest, Karolina út 27
Hungary

József Lakatos
Department of Orthopedics
Semmelweis University Budapest
1113 Budapest, Karolina út 27
Hungary

Ferenc Mády
Department of Orthopedics
Semmelweis University Budapest
1113 Budapest, Karolina út 27
Hungary

János Rupnik
Department of Orthopedics
Semmelweis University Budapest
1113 Budapest, Karolina út 27
Hungary

Franklin Sim
Mayo Clinic
200 First Street SW
Rochester, MN 55905
USA

Gábor Skaliczki
Department of Orthopedics
Semmelweis University Budapest
1113 Budapest, Karolina út 27
Hungary

László Sólyom
Department of Orthopedics
Semmelweis University Budapest
1113 Budapest, Karolina út 27
Hungary

Péter Somogyi
Department of Orthopedics
Semmelweis University Budapest
1113 Budapest, Karolina út 27
Hungary

Zsuzsa Süth
Department of Orthopedics
Semmelweis University Budapest
1113 Budapest, Karolina út 27
Hungary

Miklós Szendrői
Head of Orthopaedic Department
Semmelweis University Budapest
1113 Budapest, Karolina út 27
Hungary

György Szőke
Department of Orthopedics
Semmelweis University Budapest
1113 Budapest, Karolina út 27
Hungary

Tamás Terebessy
Department of Orthopedics
Semmelweis University Budapest
1113 Budapest, Karolina út 27
Hungary

Tibor Vízkelety
Department of Orthopedics
Semmelweis University Budapest
1113 Budapest, Karolina út 27
Hungary

Doris E. Wenger
Mayo Clinic
200 First Street SW
Rochester, MN 55905
USA

Ákos Zahár
Department of Orthopedics
Semmelweis University Budapest
1113 Budapest, Karolina út 27
Hungary

Chapter 1

Common Bone Dysplasias and Malformations

Contents

Chapter 1

Common Bone Dysplasias and Malformations

S. Kiss, T. Vízkelety, K. Köllő, T. Terebessy,
G. Holnapy, G. Szőke

1.1 Skeletal Dysplasias with Predominantly Epiphyseal Involvement

1.1.1 Multiple Epiphyseal Dysplasia

Multiple epiphyseal dysplasia (MED) is characterized by the disturbance of enchondral ossification involving numerous epiphyses. MED is usually transmitted in an autosomal dominant manner, although autosomal recessive transmission has also been reported. Different levels of deformities may be present in one patient. Usually lower extremity joint pain with decreased range of motions and limping are the main complaints. Dominantly hips, knees, and ankles are affected. Irregular, fragmented epiphyses and flat articular surfaces with normal metaphyses and mild shortening of the tubular bones can be observed. Upper extremity involvement may differ from minimal to severe with significant deformities (Figs. 1.1–1.8).

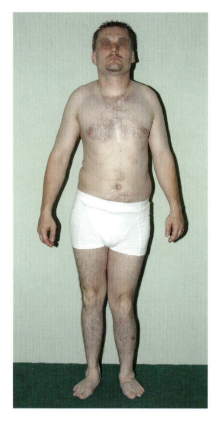

Fig. 1.1 Normal or moderately short height with normal proportions

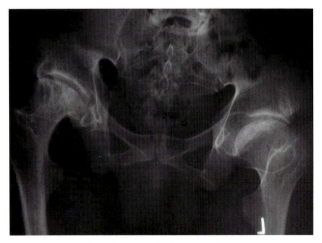

Fig. 1.2 Severely affected right hip with fragmentation of the epiphysis and flattening joint surfaces

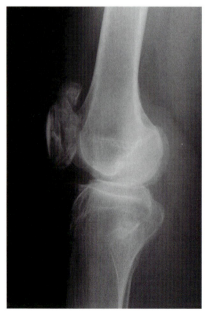

Fig. 1.3 Normally developed knee joint with fragmentation and moderate deformity of the patella

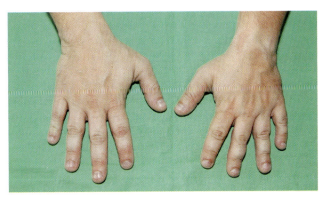

Fig. 1.4 Fingers are equally shortened

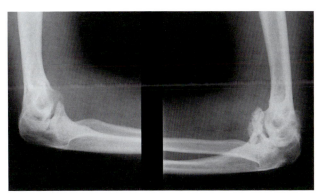

Fig. 1.7 Bilateral irregular distal humeral epiphyses with deformity of the trochlea

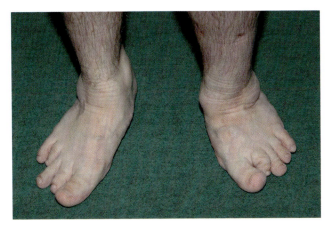

Fig. 1.5 Toes are variably shortened

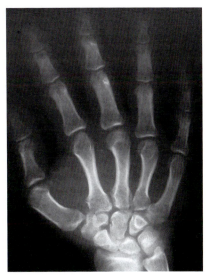

Fig. 1.8 The short tubular bones of the hand are shortened without any significant deformity

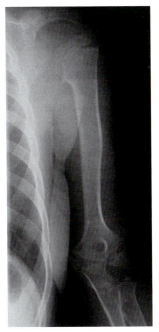

Fig. 1.6 Irregular proximal humeral epiphysis with large, flat articular surface

1.2 Skeletal Dysplasias with Predominantly Metaphyseal Involvement

1.2.1 Achondroplasia

Achondroplasia is a disproportionate short-limb dwarfism, by far the most common of the human chondrodysplasias. It occurs in three of 100,000 live births. Achondroplasia is inherited in an autosomal dominant manner. Over 80% of individuals with achondroplasia have parents with normal stature and have achondroplasia as the result of a "de novo" mutation of a gene, localized to the distal short arm of chromosome 4.

In infancy, hypotonia is typical, and acquisition of developmental motor milestones is often delayed. Intelligence and life span are usually normal. Compression of the spinal cord and upper airway obstruction increase the risk of death in infancy.

Mean adult height in males is 131 ± 5.6 cm, and in females 124 ± 5.9 cm (Figs. 1.9–1.16).

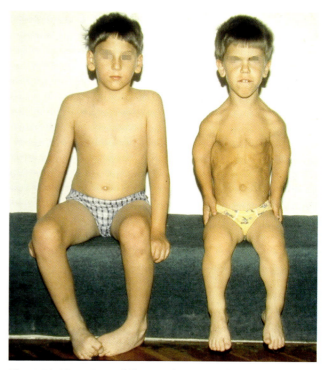

Fig. 1.10 There is no difference between them in the height of the trunk; however, the chest and shoulders are narrower in achondroplasia

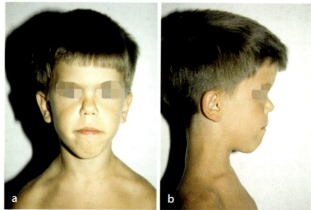

Fig. 1.11 a, b The head is disproportionately large in relation to height, the forehead is prominent, and nasal bridge is broadened and depressed

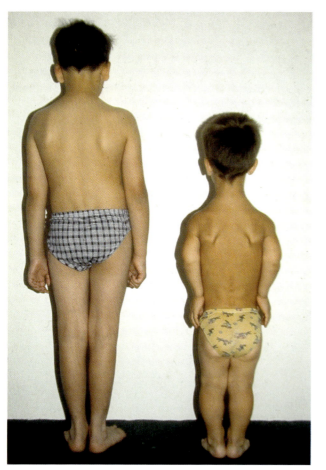

Fig. 1.9 Two 8-year-old boys. Normal body proportion is on the left. Characteristically rhizomelic (proximal) shortening of the arms and legs, which cause the disproportionate short-limb dwarfism on the right

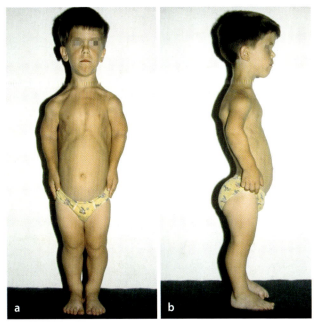

Fig. 1.12 a, b Exaggerated lumbar lordosis, limitation of elbow extension and rotation, genu varum, hyperextension of the knees and most other joints is common

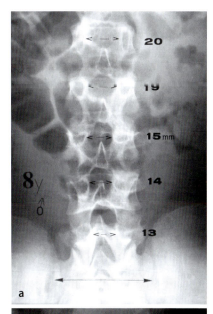

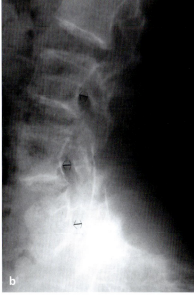

Fig. 1.14 a, b The interpediculate distance decreases from upper to lower lumbar spine (**a**). Characteristic short pedicles are seen on the lateral view (**b**)

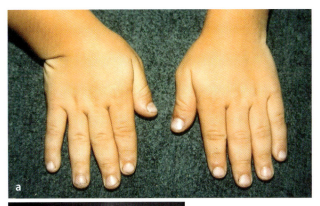

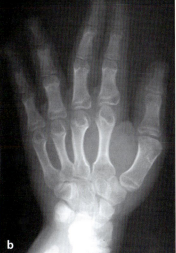

Fig. 1.13 a, b The fingers in achondroplasia are not as short as in many other short-limb dwarfism

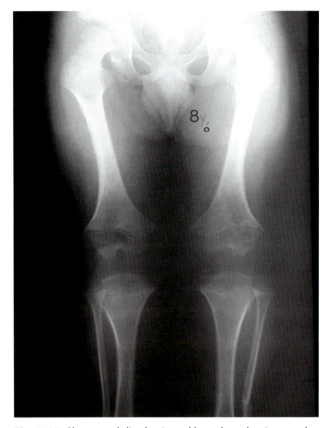

Fig. 1.15 Shortened diaphysis and broadened epi-metaphyses of femur with typical oval radiolucent areas are seen at the age of eight

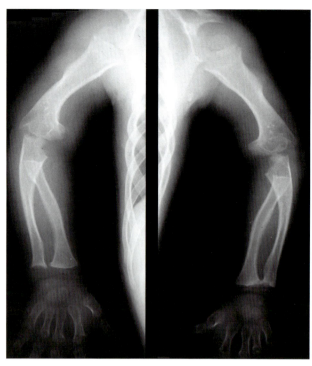

Fig. 1.16 Rhizomelic shortening of upper extremities. There is a characteristic prominence of muscle attachment of the humerus

1.2.2 Hypophosphatasia (Congenital)

The congenital form of hypophosphatasia is a rare error of metabolism characterized by defective bone and teeth mineralization. The birth prevalence is 1/100,000. The mutation in the ALPL gene results in reduced activity of tissue nonspecific alkaline phosphatase. The severity of hypophosphatasia is highly variable, ranging from intrauterine death due to the defective skeletal mineralization to premature loss of teeth only (odontohypophosphatasia). Fractures and pseudo-fractures are common. Spinal deformity such as scoliosis and prominent scapula have also been described. Depending on the age of diagnosis, clinical forms are the following:

- The lethal perinatal form with intrauterine impaired mineralization;
- The infantile form with respiratory complications because of rachitic chest wall deformities;
- The childhood form with doliocephalic skull, enlarged joints and delay in ambulation, short stature and waddling gait;
- The adult form includes primarily autosomal dominant inheritance with foot and thigh pain, stress fractures of metatarsal bones, and femoral pseudo-fractures (Figs. 1.17–1.19).

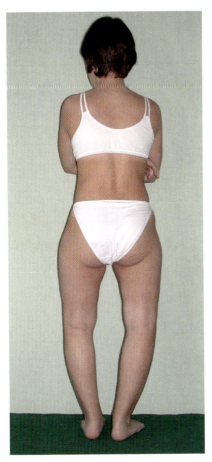

Fig. 1.17 Varus knee deformity of lower limbs in hypophosphatasia of a female patient

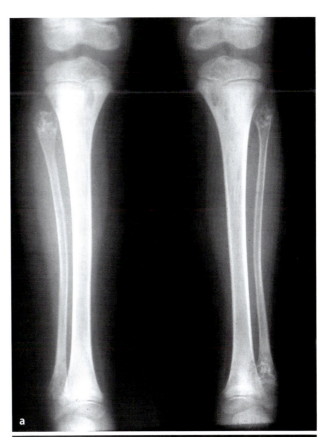

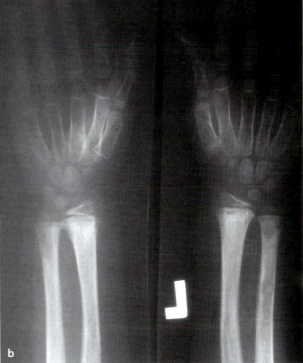

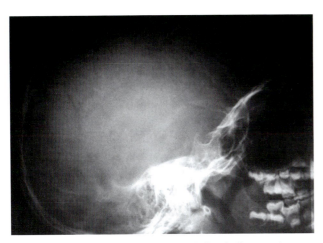

Fig. 1.19 Radiographs of a doliocephalic skull. Lateral view

Fig. 1.18 a, b Radiographs of a 12-year-old boy. Enlarged knee joints, bowed fibulas, and impaired mineralization at epi-metaphyseal region of both tibias (**a**). Impaired mineralization of radius and ulna, with bowing (**b**)

1.2.3 Chondroectodermal Dysplasia (Ellis–Van Creveld's Syndrome)

Ellis-van Creveld's syndrome is characterized by short stature, disproportionate dwarfism, short limbs, polydactyly, and congenital heart disease due to ventricular septal defect. But variable oral findings such as fusion of upper lip to the gingival margin, multiple frenula, abnormally shaped and microdontic teeth, or congenital missing teeth, malocclusion, neonatal teeth, and notching of the lower alveolar process also play an important role in the diagnosis of this syndrome. Absence of clavicles, narrow chest, hypoplastic maxilla, urinary tract anomalies, ichthyoids, plantar keratoderma, and anomalies of hair are associated with this disease.

This syndrome is an autosomal recessive, mainly a generalized disorder of the maturation of enchondral ossification. The link of the Ellis-van Creveld's syndrome gene to marker HOX7 in a region proximal to the FGFR3 gene is responsible for the achondroplasia phenotype (Figs. 1.20–1.23).

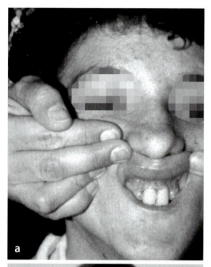

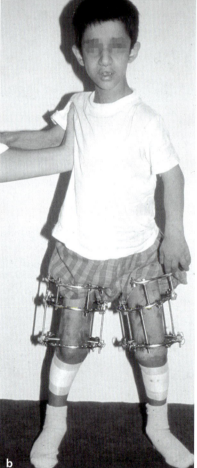

Fig. 1.20 a, b Archive photographs present fusion of upper lip to the gingival margin (**a**), and short stature, disproportionate dwarfism, characteristic for Ellis-van Creveld's syndrome (**b**)

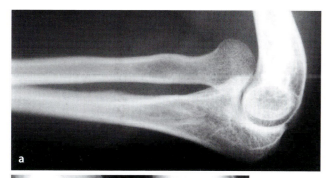

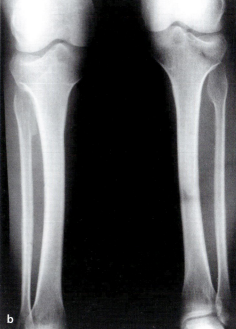

Fig. 1.21 a, b Lateral view of the elbow (a) and both tibias and fibulas (b). The tubular bones are short and thick

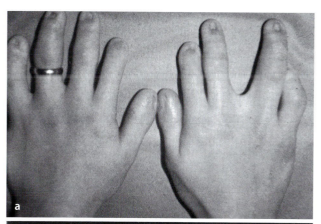

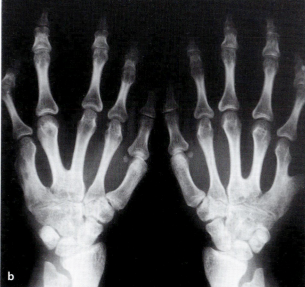

Fig. 1.22 a, b The hands after the resection of bilateral postaxial polydactyly presenting dystrophic nails. Postaxial polydactyly and dystrophic nails (a), and shortening of the digits on radiograph of the hands (b). Note the partial fusion of the metacarpal bases

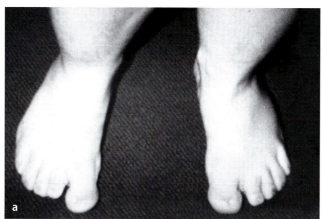

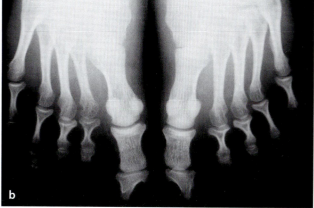

Fig. 1.23 a, b Shortening of the digits of the toes and feet (a) and radiograph of the short tubular bones (b)

1.2.4 Metaphyseal Dysplasia (McKusick Type)

Metaphyseal dysplasia is characterized by typical radiographical changes in the metaphyses of the short- and long tubular bones, with normal epiphyses. The disease frequently associates with malabsorption, neutropenia and recurrent infections in younger children.

Schmid-type is transmitted in autosomal dominant manner, and presents later than other types of metaphyseal dysplasia. Upper extremity involvement is mild, evidenced by wrist swelling and flexion contractures of the elbows. The decreased standing height is due to a greater involvement of lower extremities. Varus deformity of the ankles and knees is present with bowing of tibia and femur, with characteristic coxa vara.

McKusick type also called cartilage-hair hypoplasia, is transmitted as an autosomal recessive trait. In Amish population the incidence is 1/1,000 live births, but in other populations it is less frequent than the Schmidt type. Disproportionate short stature is characteristic,

with genu varum and varus ankle deformity due to distal fibular overgrowth. Short and pudgy hands and feet are the typical deformities. Chest-wall involvement with enlargement of costochondral junctions causes "rachitic rosary" (Figs. 1.24–1.26).

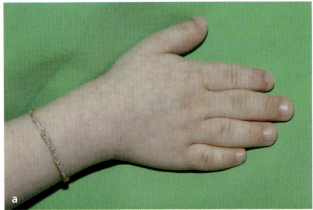

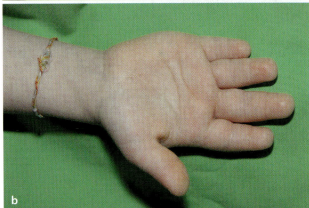

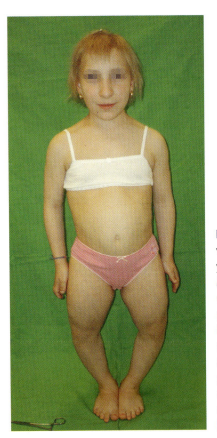

Fig. 1.24 Anterior view of a 17-year-old girl with McKusick type of metaphyseal dysplasia with typical light-coloured and sparse hair. Note also the disproportionate short stature and varus deformity of the lower extremity

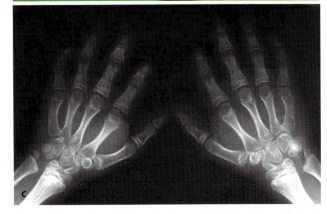

Fig. 1.25 a–c Dorsal (**a**) and palmar (**b**) clinical view of short and puffy hands of the same patient. Anteroposterior radiograph (**c**) of both hands. Note the metaphyseal shortening of the metacarpals and phalanges

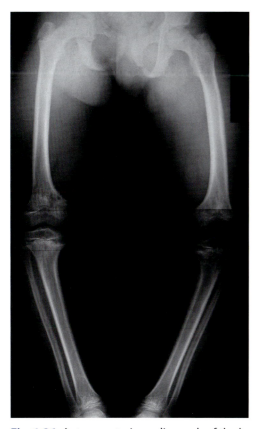

Fig. 1.26 Anteroposterior radiograph of the lower extremities: in hip with mild coxa vara and with varus deformity of the knee of the same patient. Note the scars in longitudinal trabeculae in metaphyseal region of the femur

1.3 Skeletal Dysplasias with Major Involvement of the Spine

1.3.1 Spondyloepiphyseal Dysplasia Congenita, Tarda

Congenital spondyloepiphyseal dysplasia is an inherited chondrodysplasia with short stature, which is associated with a short trunk due to a growth disorder of the spine and epiphysis of the limbs. Platyspondyly, os odontoideum with or without atlantoaxial instability and epiphyseal dysplasia of the femoral head are also common. This deformity occurs through a mutation in the COL2A1 gene encoding type II procollagen.

Spondyloepiphyseal dysplasia tarda is an X-linked recessive progressive osteochondrodysplasia that is characterized by defective growth and "champagne bottle" shaped vertebrae. The disorder manifests in childhood with disproportionate short stature, short neck and trunk and a broad chest. Heterozygous carrier females are generally clinically and radiographically normal; the disease affects males only. It can associate with progressive arthropathy (Figs. 1.27–1.36).

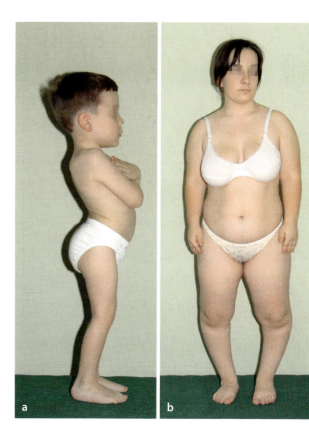

Fig. 1.27 a, b Characteristic view from lateral of an 8-year-old boy (**a**) and an anterior view of a 28-year-old female (**b**). Both of them short statured due to congenital spondyloepiphyseal dysplasia

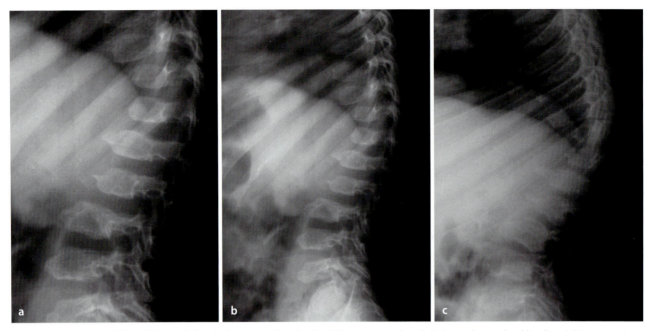

Fig. 1.28 a–c Spondyloepiphyseal dysplasia congenita: Typical "champagne-bottle" shaped vertebral bodies (**a**) Progressive dorsolumbar kyphosis with platyspondyly and deformed vertebras at a boy age of 5 (**b**), and 17 (**c**)

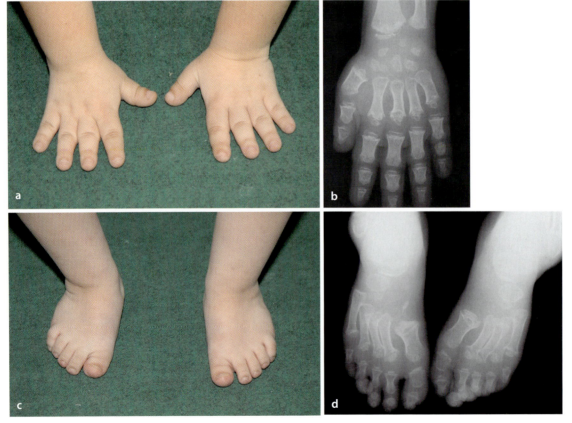

Fig. 1.29 a–d Short small tubular bones: clinical view of the hand of a girl (**a**) and radiograph of the hand (**b**) of the same patient. Broad feet (**c**) of a 28-year-old female, and radiograph of the feet of a young patient (**d**)

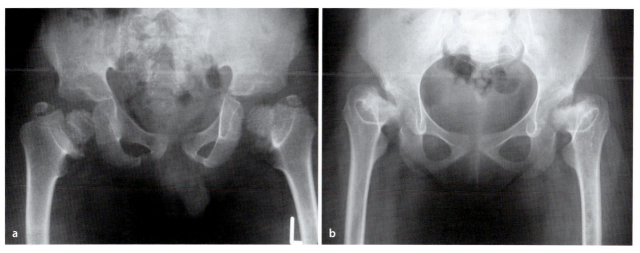

Fig. 1.30 a, b Retarded ossification of the proximal femur on radiograph of a young patient (**a**), which is usually accompanied by coxa vara in elderly period as seen on the radiograph of a 28-year-old female (**b**)

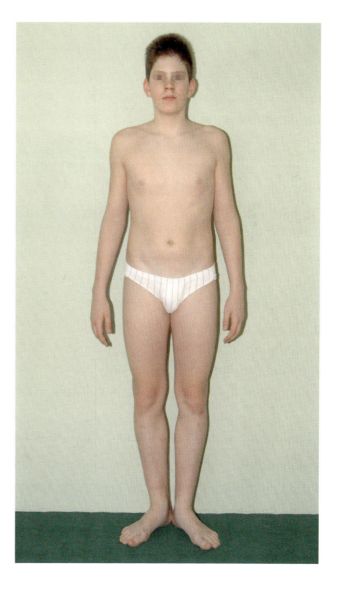

Fig. 1.31 Spondyloepiphyseal dysplasia tarda. Normal stature of a 13-year-old boy

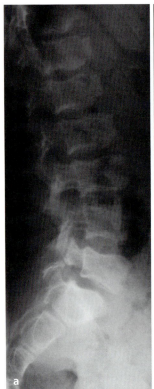

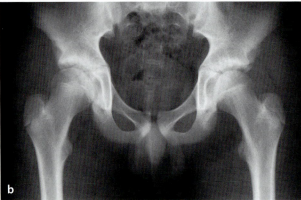

Fig. 1.32 a, b Moderate deformities of the thoracolumbar spine (**a**) and hip and pelvis (**b**) of the same patient

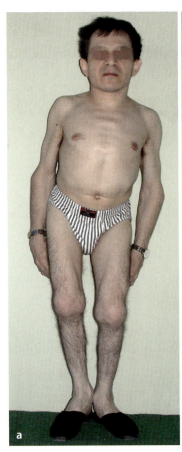

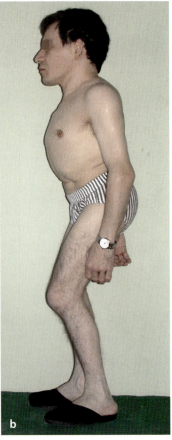

Fig. 1.33 a, b Late form of spondyloepiphyseal dysplasia congenita: Short stature of a 39-year-old male

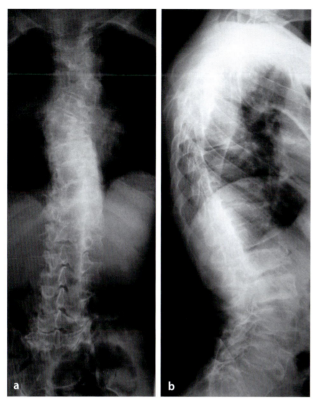

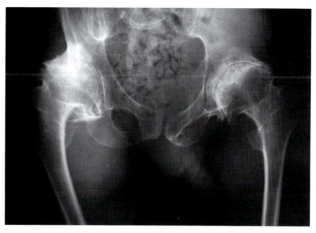

Fig. 1.35 Late form of spondyloepiphyseal dysplasia congenita: Severe bilateral coxarthrosis

Fig. 1.34 a, b Platyspondyly and narrow disc spaces on anteroposterior (**a**) and lateral (**b**) thoracolumbar spine radiographs. Characteristic "champagne-bottle" shaped vertebras of the lower thoracic spine can be observed

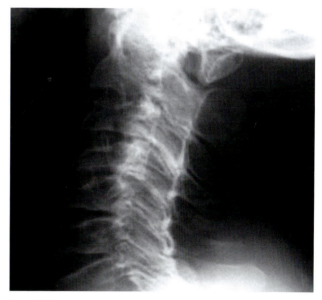

Fig. 1.36 Severe cervical spondylosis causing myelopathy

1.4 Mucopolysaccharidoses

The mucopolysaccharidosis (MPS) is a rare lysosomal storage disease with autosomal recessive inheritance. It is caused when a hydrolase enzyme deficiency creates an accumulation of mucopolysaccharides. Diagnosis is made using urine analysis for glycosaminoglycan, tissue samples, and leukocyte enzyme analysis. These patients are characterized by coarsening of the face, epiphyseal deformation with restricted motion of the joints (particularly in the elbow), corneal clouding, deafness, mental deterioration and cardiac disease. Most patients become symptomatic in early childhood and the life span is variably shortened. At least six different types of MPS had been described. The Hurler syndrome (MPS type I.) is the most common and Morquio syndrome (MPS type IV.) is the most severe MPS (Figs. 1.37–1.43).

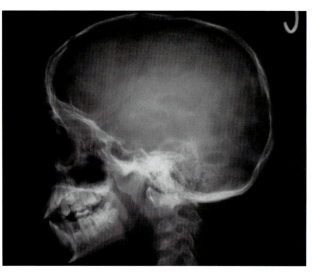

Fig. 1.38 Hypoplasia of the odontoid process (dens axis) is the most problematic finding in Morquio syndrome since together with ligamentous laxity atlanto-axial instability may occur. Cervical spine fusion is recommended in almost every case

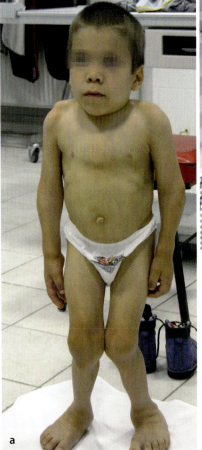

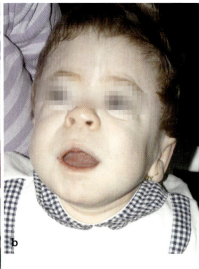

Fig. 1.37 a, b In Hurler type (courtesy of Gy. Fekete, Semmelweis University, Budapest) of MPS the patient develops a short body trunk and a maximum stature of less than 4 ft. The valgus knee deformity is not rare in this mucopolysaccharidosis (**a**). The distinct facial features including flat face, depressed nasal bridge, flared nostrils, widely spaced, prominent eyes, thick lips with open mouth and bulging forehead become more evident in the second year (**b**)

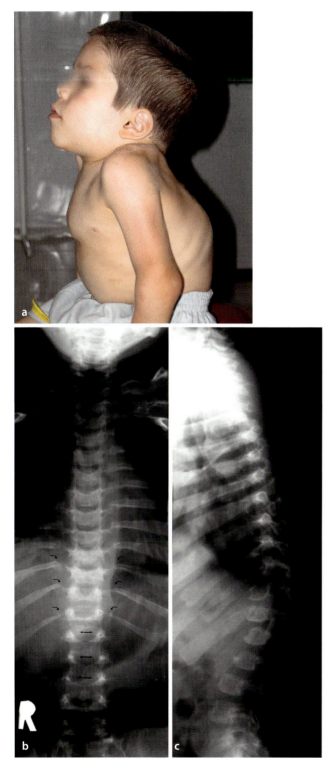

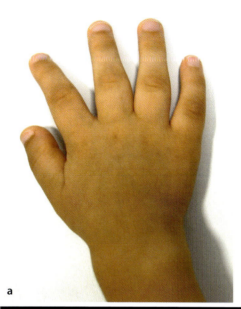

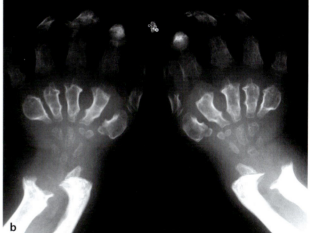

Fig. 1.40 a, b The hand is relatively small but wide, the fingers are shortened (**a**). Widening of the proximal part of the phalanges and pointing of the proximal part of the 2–5 metacarpal bones together with claw hand can be observed on radiograph (**b**) in Hurler disease

Fig. 1.39 a–c Characteristic features for Hurler syndrome are the dorsal kyphosis (**a**), widening the lateral portion of the ribs and ossification defect on the vertebral bodies (**b**) with the very typical dorsolumbar gibbus (**c**)

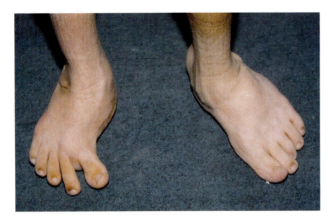

Fig. 1.41 Toe axis deformity and flatfeet can be observed due to generalized ligamentous laxity in Morquio disease

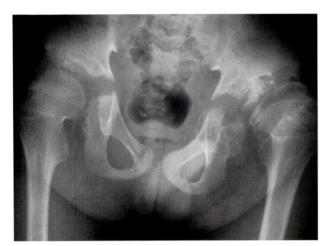

Fig. 1.42 Coxa valga, dysplasia of the femoral head and the acetabulum are very frequent in MPS IV

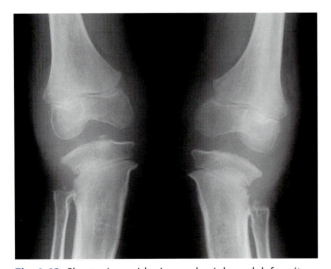

Fig. 1.43 Shortening, widening and epiphyseal deformity of the femur and tibia in MPS I

1.5 Skeletal Dysplasias due to Anarchic Development of Bone Constituents

1.5.1 Dysplasia Epiphysealis Hemimelica

Dysplasia epiphysealis hemimelica (DEH) is a rare skeletal developmental disorder affecting the epiphyses in young children. The etiology of DEH is still unknown. The incidence is 1 in 1,000,000. Males are affected twice as frequently as females. The age of onset is usually between 2 and 14 years. The presence of a mass with the consistency of bone, deformity, aching pains and limited range of motion are the most common presenting symptoms. It occurs usually in the lower limb, with the distal femur, distal tibia and talus being most commonly affected. Upper limb involvement is extremely rare. Characteristically the involvement is hemimelic, i.e. the medial or lateral epiphysealis side is involved. These lesions show on radiographs asymmetric epiphyseal enlargement with multiple ossification centers. Histologically the lesion is similar to osteochondroma, but osteochondroma arises from the meta or diaphysis, whereas DEH arises from the epiphysis (Figs. 1.44–1.49).

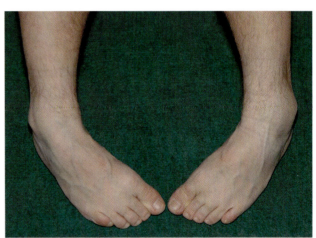

Fig. 1.44 Moderate, painless, bone-hard swelling at the lateral side of the left ankle

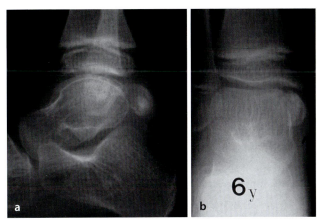

Fig. 1.45 a, b Lateral (**a**) and anteroposterior (**b**) radiographs of the left ankle showing an irregular calcified mass on the postero-medial side of the talus

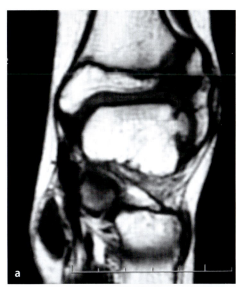

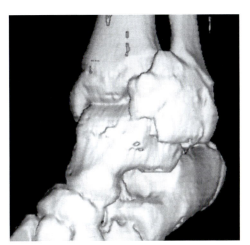

Fig. 1.46 3D CT scan shows an "exostosis" on the lateral side of the talus

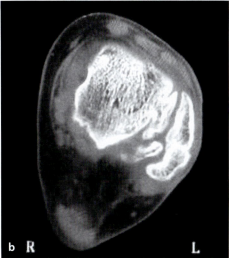

Fig. 1.48 a, b DEH localized on the lateral side of the talus: MRI frontal plane (**a**) and CT (**b**) slides

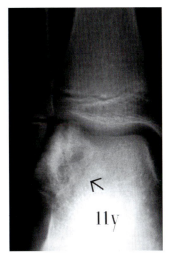

Fig. 1.47 Anteroposterior radiograph of the talus with DEH, protruding from the bone. In other cases DEH could be destructive, enlarged bony mass

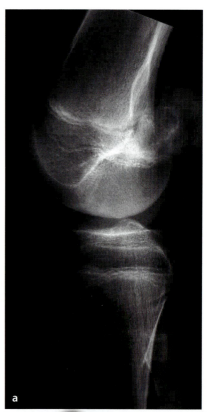

Fig. 1.49 a, b Lateral radiograph of the knee joint with DEH (**a**) and MRI slide in sagittal plane of the same joint with protruding bone mass from the distal femoral epiphysis to the popliteal fossa (**b**)

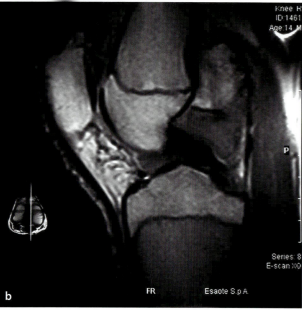

1.5.2 Multiple Exostoses

Hereditary multiple exostosis is an autosomal dominant disorder (mutation in EXT1 or the EXT2 gene) manifested by the presence of multiple osteochondromas, multiple projections of bone, mainly at the metaphyses of long bones at the extremities. The risk of malignant transformation of the cartilaginous portion of the exostoses, is up to 2%.

Most common deformities include short stature, limb length discrepancies, valgus deformities of the knee and ankle, bowing of the radius with ulnar deviation of the wrist, and subluxation of the radiocarpal joint, asymmetry of the pectoral and pelvic girdles. In rare cases associated nail deformity appear also (Figs. 1.50–1.57).

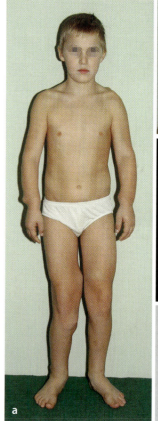

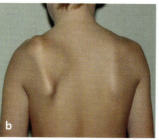

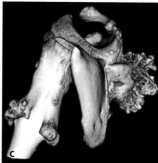

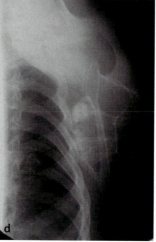

Fig. 1.50 a–d Photograph of a 11-year-old boy. Note the seriously deformed legs (**a**) due to the numerous osteochondromas. One of the largest tumor is developed from the inner surface of the scapula as presented on photograph (**b**), 3D CT picture (**c**) and radiograph (**d**)

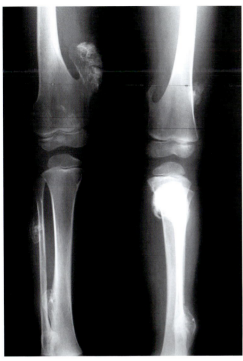

Fig. 1.51 Large tibial, fibular, and femoral osteochondromas, with deformity of the extremities

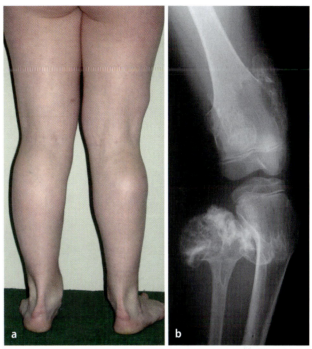

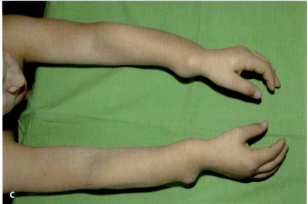

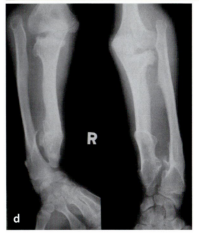

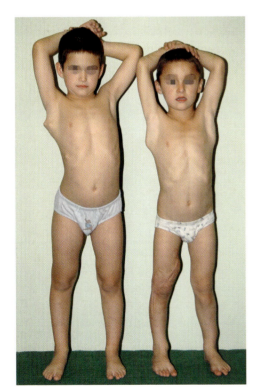

Fig. 1.52 Deformed lower extremities and chest due to multiple osteochondromas. The boys are cousins, 4 and 6 years, both of them have osteochondroma developing from the right scapula

Fig. 1.53 a–d Osteochondroma around the knee joint can lead to malalignment of axis, as in this case, where valgus deformity of the knees developed (**a, b**). Severe deformation of forearms is seen (**c**) with bilateral elbow dislocation on radiographs (**d**)

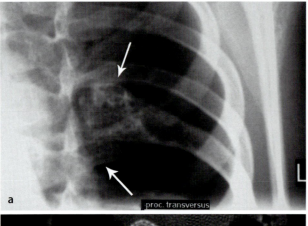

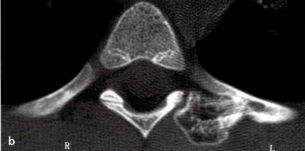

Fig. 1.54 a, b Radiograph of a 16-year-old girl with rib exostosis at left side (**a**) and CT scan of the same patient (**b**)

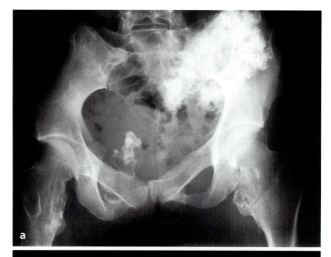

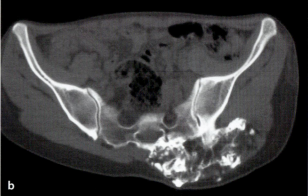

Fig. 1.56 a, b Malignant transformation of an osteochondroma of the iliac wing. Anteroposterior radiograph (**a**) and CT (**b**)

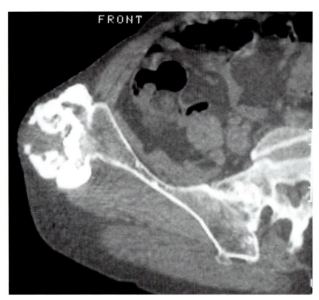

Fig. 1.55 Osteochondroma of the iliac bone (CT)

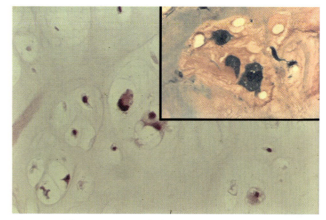

Fig. 1.57 Photomicrograph demonstrates a typical secondary low grade chondrosarcoma, developed from a previous osteochondroma

1.5.3 Enchondromatosis
(Ollier's Disease, Maffucci's Disease)

Enchondromatosis also known as dyschondroplasia or Ollier's disease is characterized by multiple enchondromas within the metaphyseal region of tubular bones and also within the scapula and pelvis. In about 50% of the cases the lesions occur unilaterally. Normal contours of the tubular bones are lost when the lesions develop and significant shortening or bowing can be observed. The limb length discrepancy often needs elongation procedure. Pathological fractures also occur frequently. Malignant transformation of the lesions to chondrosarcoma is not rare; furthermore, the patients face a higher risk of developing other nonskeletal malignant tumors. In case multiple enchondromas occur together with multiple cutaneous and soft tissue hemangiomas (Maffucci's syndrome), the risk for malignant transformation is close to 100% (Figs. 1.58–1.62).

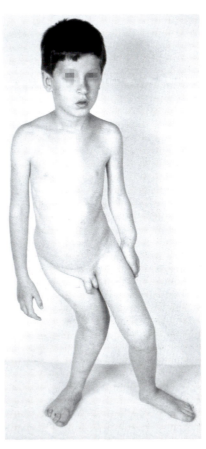

Fig. 1.59 Archive photograph taken from a 9-year-old boy with enchondromatosis. Note the significant shortening and bowing of the right femur and the left radius

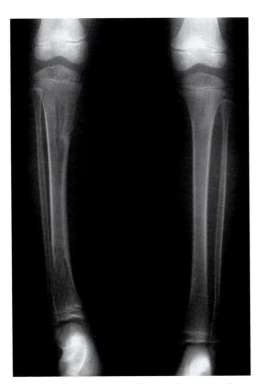

Fig. 1.58 Early stage of Ollier's disease in the proximal and distal part of the tibia. The cartilage masses show stippled calcification and extend linearly from the physis to the metaphysis. Epiphysis is not affected. There is a shortening of the right leg as consequence of the process

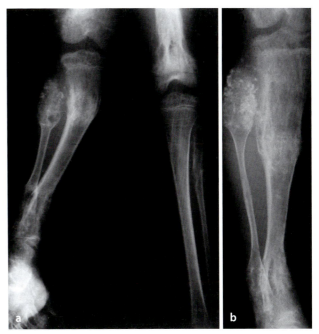

Fig. 1.60 a, b Lesions of the right tibia and fibula resulted a 7 cm shortening and bowing of the leg (**a**). The same extremity after correction of axial deformity (**b**)

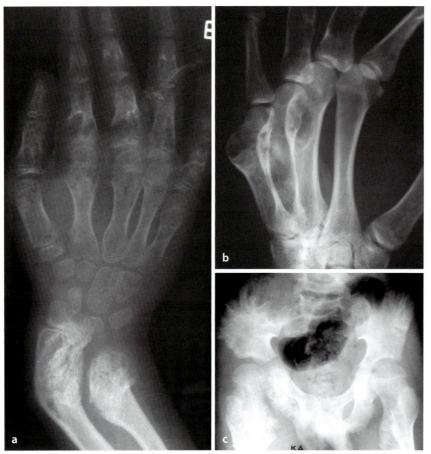

Fig. 1.61 a–c Ollier's disease: Enchondromas in the short tubular bones and in pelvis. Radiograph of the hand of an 8-year-old boy (note the deformed axis of the forehand) (**a**) and a 25-year-old patient (**b**). Multiplex enchondromas also seen in pelvic region (**c**)

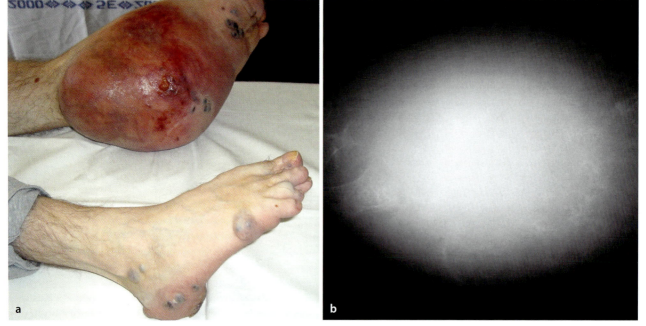

Fig. 1.62 a, b Enchondromas appear together with cutan and soft tissue hemangiomas in Maffucci's syndrome. Clinical view (**a**) and radiograph (**b**) of a patient at the age of 25 with Maffucci's syndrome. Note the cutan haemangiomas on both leg. Huge secondary chondrosarcoma developed from the previous chondroma of the distal tibia, which destroys the entire ankle and foot

1.6 Skeletal Dysplasias with Predominant Involvement of Single Sites of Segments

1.6.1 Mesomelic Dwarfism (Nievergelt and Langer Type)

Mesomelic dwarfism is a rare mesomelic chondrodysplasia with an elective defect of the mesial segments of the limbs. This disease is high penetrating autosomal dominant with pleiotropic expression syndrome of the upper and lower limbs with atypical clubfeet, radio-ulnar and tibio-fibular and intertarsal synostosis, and deformities of the elbow joints, caused by mutations in the SHOX gene.

Acro–coxo–mesomelic dwarfism described as autosomal recessive dwarfism, with hip dislocation, clubhand and foot, short malformed fingers, reduced articular mobility of elbows, clinodactyly, brachyrhizophalangia.

Types of mesomelic dwarfism are: Nievergelt's (Campailla and Martinelli) type, Langer (Reinhard and Pfeffer's) and Robinow's type (1.63–1.66).

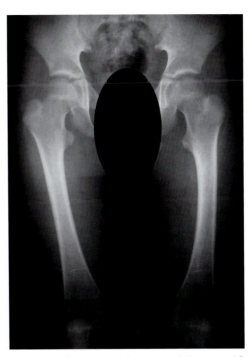

Fig. 1.64 Short femoral neck, and shortened femur in mesomelic dwarfism of a 14-year-old patient (Langer type)

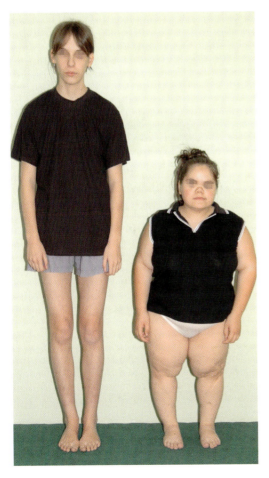

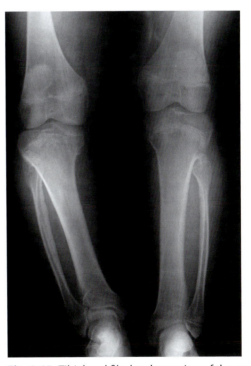

Fig. 1.65 Tibial and fibular shortening of the same patient

Fig. 1.63 Thirteen-year-old mesomelic dwarf beside a same aged girl with normal growth

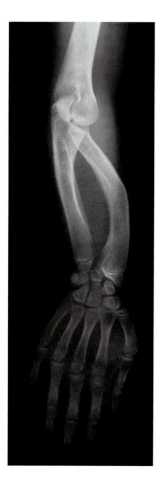

Fig. 1.66 Typical shortening and deformity of the ulna and radius with subluxation of the radial head and deficient supination capacity of the forearm. Radio-ulnar synostosis is common also

1.6.2 Larsen's Syndrome

Larsen's syndrome is characterized by the association of congenital knee, hip, and elbow dislocations, joint hyperlaxity, facial abnormalities and other inconstant malformations as a result of connective tissue maldevelopment during gestation. One-third of the patients die in early childhood.

Spinal deformities are present as flattening of the vertebrae, abnormal segmentation, vertebra plana, cervical kyphosis and thoracolumbar kypho-scoliosis, cervical spine instability or atlanto–axial subluxation.

Larsen's syndrome has got an autosomal dominant transmission with varying levels of expression, but autosomal recessive and familial mode of inheritance is also described (1.67–1.70).

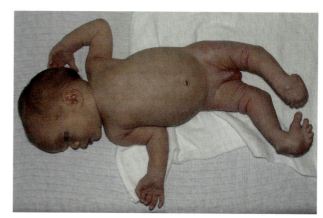

Fig. 1.67 Anterior dislocations of both knees with severe clubfoot deformity. Hip dislocations can also occur

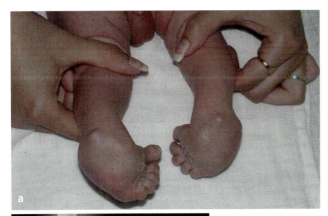

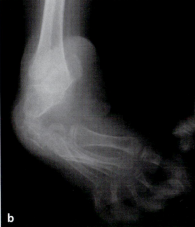

Fig. 1.68 a, b Rigid clubfoot with shortened metatarsals (shortened metacarpals especially laterally can appear) in a newborn (**a**) and severe deformed symptomatic clubfoot at 5-year-old boy (**b**)

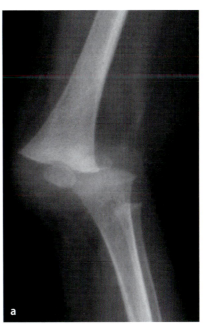

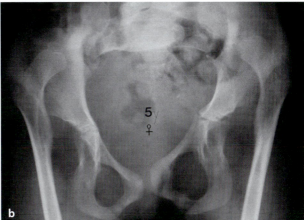

Fig. 1.70 a, b Radiograph of congenital knee dislocation and hyperlaxity in a 1-year-old child (**a**) and bilateral high dislocation of the hip in elder age in Larsen syndrome (**b**)

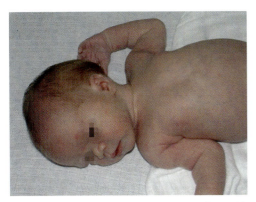

Fig. 1.69 Elbow dislocation, depressed nasal bridge

1.6.3 Cleidocranial Dysplasia

Cleidocranial dysplasia (CCD) is a rare disorder of autosomal dominant inheritance that causes disturbances in the growth of bones of the cranial vault, the clavicles, the maxilla, the nasal and lacrimal bones and the pelvis. Mild shortening of stature may be seen. Oral findings include a high-arched palate with delayed eruption of poorly formed and supernumerary teeth. The ability to approximate the shoulders anteriorly is related to clavicle hypoplasia, and is the classic diagnostic sign of this disorder. Hearing loss is common owing to abnormalities of the ossicles. Genu valgum and short fingers can be seen (1.71–1.74).

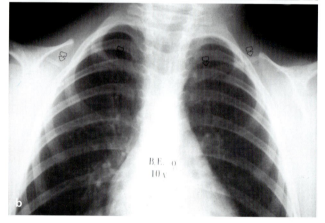

Fig. 1.72 a, b Anteroposterior chest radiograph of the patient shows bilateral clavicular hypoplasia at the lateral side of the clavicles (**a**) and a girl with almost clavicular aplasia (**b**). Just a small part of the lateral clavicle is visible on radiograph

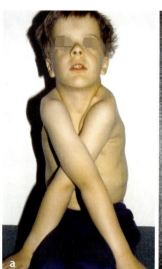
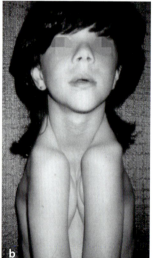

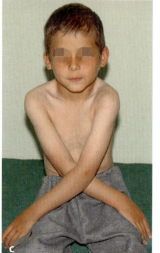

Fig. 1.71 a–c Typical cranial deformities are as follows: the head is large and brachycephalic, with a small face and bossing of the frontal, parietal, and occipital bones. The skull sutures are wide, and their closure is delayed. An increased interorbital distance may occur, with the bridge of the nose appearing wide and flat. Note the abnormal ability of an 8-year-old child (**a**) and a 10-year-old girl ((**b**), from our archives) with cleidocranial dysplasia to approximate the shoulders anteriorly. An 8-year-old healthy child with forced attempt to approximate his shoulders (**c**)

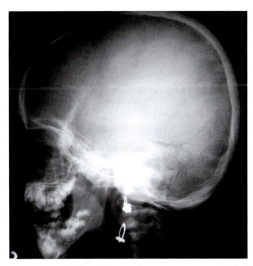

Fig. 1.73 Skull radiograph in a 10-year-old child demonstrates wide sutures and bossing of the frontal, parietal, and occipital bone. Note the basilar impression and the "wormian bones" visible especially on occipital region

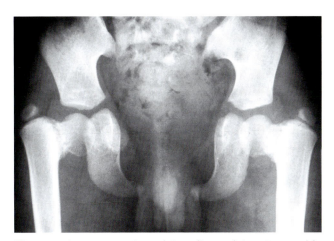

Fig. 1.74 Anteroposterior pelvic radiograph in a 5-year-old child shows delayed ossification of pubic bones and the development of idiopathic coxa vara. This type of CCD called also pelvico–cranial dysostosis

1.6.4 Osteo–Onycho–Dysostosis (Nail Patella Syndrome)

Osteo–onycho–dysostosis, an autosomal dominant disorder, is also called "nail-patella syndrome" (NPS). The etiology is still not known. Clinical manifestations are most frequently seen in the second and third decades of life. It has a prevalence of 2/100,000 live births. Age of onset and degree of severity cannot be predicted. Males and females are equally affected. Limited ROM in the elbows, decreased pronation or supination of the elbows, appearing unilaterally or bilaterally are frequent. On radiographs, the head of the radius is underdeveloped and displaced posteriorly. In the knee, absence or hypoplasia of the fibula and patella, with hypoplasia of the lateral condyle. Abnormalities of the pelvis consist of dysplasia of the iliac wings and the presence of "posterior iliac horns". Soft tissue alterations include flexion contractures of the hip, knee, elbow, fingers, and quadriceps hypoplasia (Figs. 1.75–1.80).

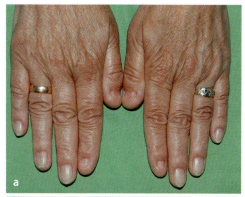
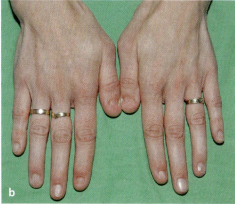

Fig. 1.75 a, b Nails of a 59-year-old woman (**a**) and her 32-year-old daughter (**b**). Absent or dysplastic nails are the most common nail findings, nonspecific changes include discoloration, longitudinal ridging, and poorly formed lunulae. You may note the splitting of the nails, specially in the thumb and in the second digit of both hands. Other nails may be less fragile. Nails are progressively less affected toward the fifth digit. Note the nails of first and second digits of both patients at both sides

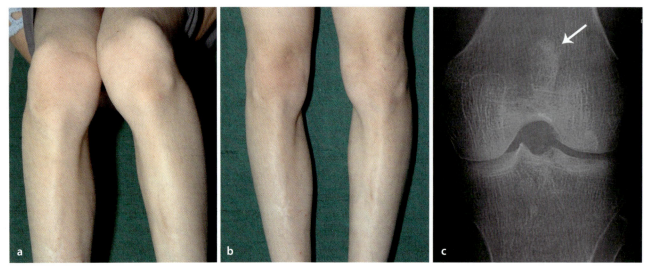

Fig. 1.76 a–c The younger patient in sitting (**a**) and standing position (**b**). Skeletal deformities include patellar hypoplasia with dislocation, which may decrease flexion.

Anteroposterior radiograph of the knee joint shows the laterally placed, very hypoplastic patella (*arrow*) (**c**). Osteoarthritis, and knee effusions are associated complications

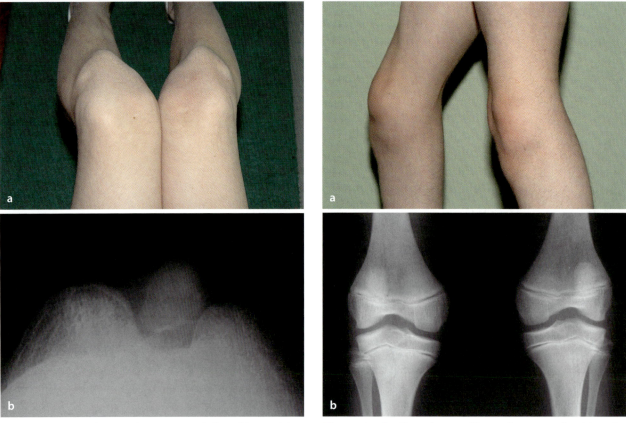

Fig. 1.77 a, b Axial view of a patient with flexed knees (**a**), and axial radiograph of right hypoplastic patella (**b**)

Fig. 1.78 a, b Clinical view of hypoplastic patellae (**a**) and anteroposterior knee radiograph (**b**) of a 13-year-old child. Both patellae are hypoplastic and lateralized

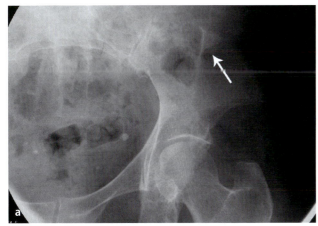

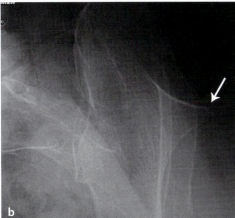

Fig. 1.79 a, b Pelvic ap (**a**) and oblique (**b**) radiographs show the characteristic posterior iliac horns (*arrow*)

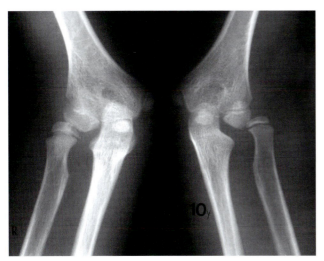

Fig. 1.80 Associated bilateral luxation of elbows, due to arthrodysplasia of the elbows

1.6.5 Tricho–Rhino–Phalangeal Dysplasia (Giedion I), TRP Type 1

Associated with submicroscopic deletion of chromosome band 8q24. Autosomal dominant or recessive inheritance is described.

Symptoms in infancy: short stature, sparse hair, pear-shaped nose, and brachydactily. Described in 1966 (Giedion) differentiated from TRPS II (Langer-Giedion syndrome 1974) by lack of multiple cartilaginous exostoses (Figs. 1.81–1.87).

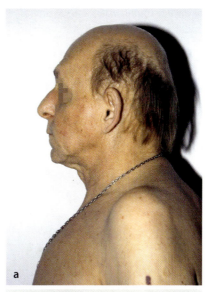

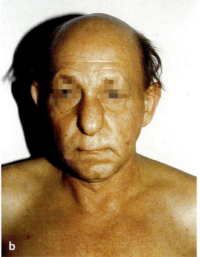

Fig. 1.81 a, b Symptoms on the face (**a, b**): sparse hair, hypoplastic pinnae, prominent forehead, bulbous nose, long philtrum, small jaw, thin upper lip, and micrognathia, occlusion disturbances

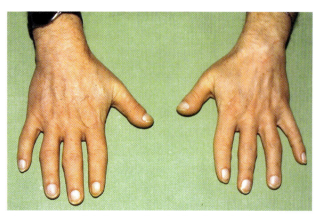

Fig. 1.82 Hand deformity: brachydactily with shortening of one or more phalanges and/or metacarpals, lateral deviation of fingers, and sometimes abnormal nails can appear

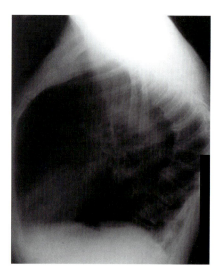

Fig. 1.84 Radiograph reveals kyphosis and severe osteochondrosis and secondary spondylosis of the dorsal spine

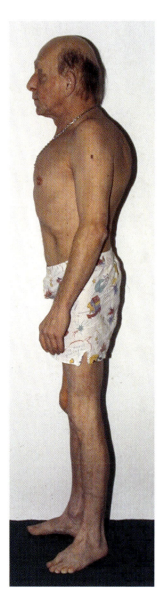

Fig. 1.83 Deformities of the trunk: short stature, pectus carinatum (pigeon chest), scoliosis, sometimes winged scapulae (Sprengel's -deformity)

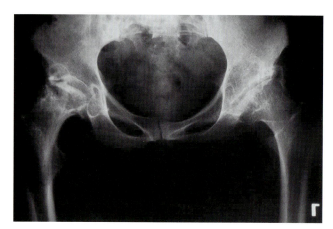

Fig. 1.85 Radiograph shows the signs of epiphyseal dysplasia. The entity belongs to the "Perthes-like diseases." Flattening of the femoral heads and shallow acetabulae without subluxation of the joint. Small capital femoral epiphysis can be also observed

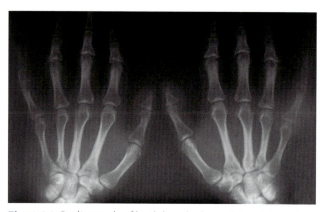

Fig. 1.86 Radiograph of both hands shows lateral deviation of the long fingers

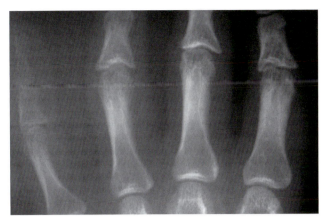

Fig. 1.87 Cone-shaped epiphyses on the middle-phalanges are typical symptoms

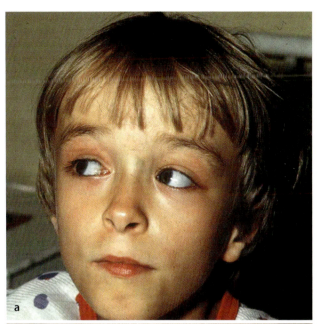

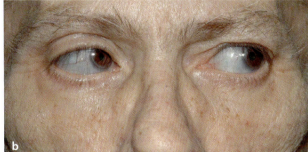

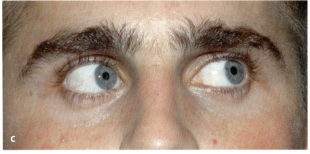

Fig. 1.88 a–c Osteogenesis imperfecta, type I. Mis-shaped skull with triangular face and blue sclerae of 9-year-old boy (**a**). Comparing the blue sclerae of a 54-year-old patient with osteogenesis imperfecta (type I) (**b**) with the normal sclerae (**c**)

1.7 Skeletal Dysplasias with Abnormalities of Bone Density and/or Modeling Defect

1.7.1 Osteogenesis Imperfecta

Osteogenesis imperfecta is a heritable disorder of the connective tissue (affecting both bone and soft tissue) with decreased bone density that is characterized by bone fragility, short stature and scoliosis, blue sclera and dentinogenesis imperfecta with soft, translucent and brownish deciduous or permanent teeth.

This disease is heterogeneous both clinically and biomechanically. In patients of type I the collagen is usually abnormal as a result of mutations in the COL1A1 and COL1A2 genes. Nonskeletal abnormalities can develop too, as deafness, blue-colored tympanic membrane, cackling laugh and squeaky voice. Cardiac manifestations such as vascular fragility with arterial or aortic dissection are also known.

Types: (according to Sillence)

- Autosomal dominant; bone fragility with fracture onset after birth; blue sclerae; without (type A) or with dentinogenesis imperfecta (type B)
- Autosomal recessive; death before or after birth; intrauterine curved and multiplex fractured long bones; beaded ribs; blue sclera
- Autosomal recessive; fractures at birth; progressive deformity; normal sclerae and hearing
- Autosomal dominant with X-linked inheritance; bone fragility; normal sclerae and hearing; without (type A) or with dentinogenesis imperfecta (type B) (Figs. 1.88–1.97)

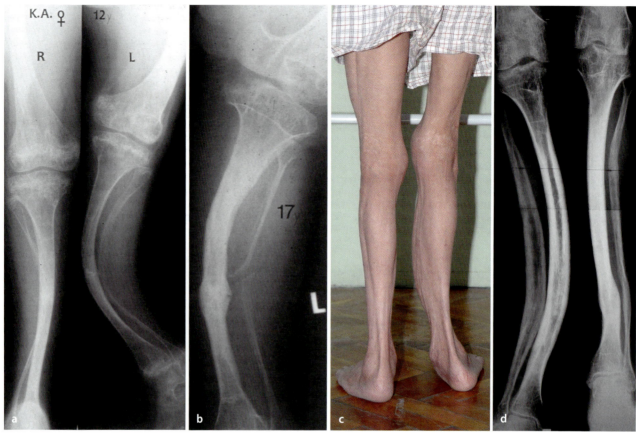

Fig. 1.89 a–d Osteogenesis imperfecta type I. Radiographs of a female patient: Bowing of both tibias (**a**) at age 12, and after fracture healing with hyperplastic callus formation on left tibia (**b**) at the age of 17. Posterior clinical view of the lower extremities of a 54-year-old patient (**c**), and anteroposterior radiographs of the extremities of the same patient (**d**)

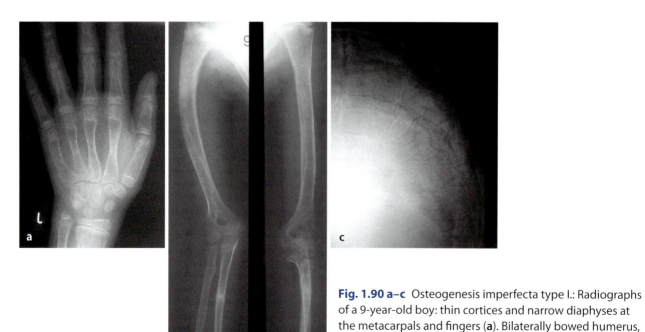

Fig. 1.90 a–c Osteogenesis imperfecta type I.: Radiographs of a 9-year-old boy: thin cortices and narrow diaphyses at the metacarpals and fingers (**a**). Bilaterally bowed humerus, also with thin cortices (**b**). On scull radiograph "wormian bones" are also visible (**c**)

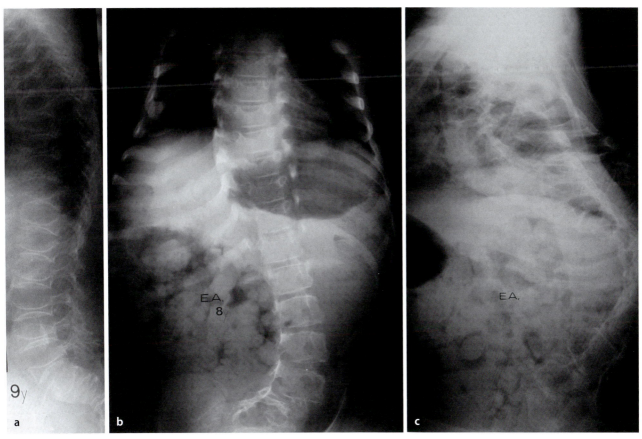

Fig. 1.91 a–c Osteogenesis imperfecta type I. Thoracolumbar X-ray of a girl. Platyspondyly of the thoracolumbar spine at the age of 9 years (**a**). In more severe cases progressive scoliosis develops (**b, c**)

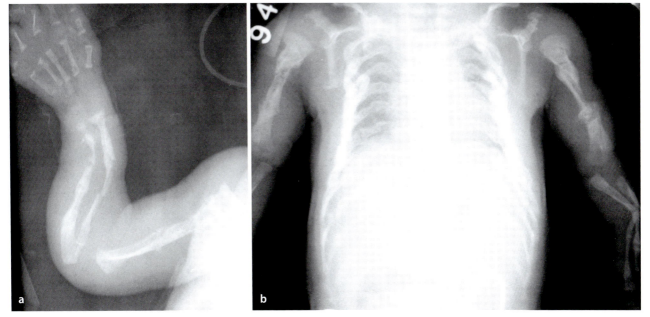

Fig. 1.92 a, b Osteogenesis imperfecta type II. Archive radiographs of a patient with lethal form of OI; intrauterine curved and multiplex fractured long bones on the upper extremity (**a**). Beaded ribs are also visible (**b**)

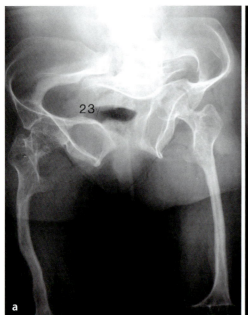
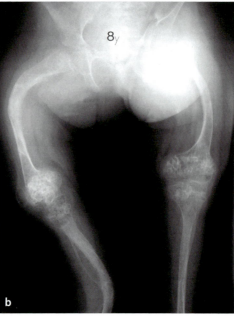

Fig. 1.93 a, b Osteogenesis imperfecta, type III. Acetabular protrusion with "trefoil" shape pelvis of a 23-year-old male (**a**). Bowing and fractured long bones of an 8-year-old girl (**b**). In other cases hyperelastic joints and luxation or subluxation of joints are also common

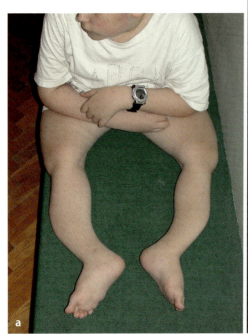
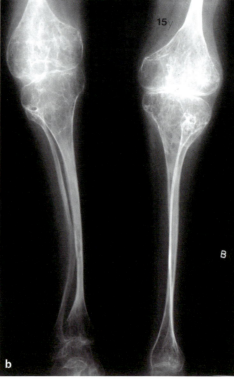

Fig. 1.94 a, b Osteogenesis imperfecta, type III. Clinical view of an 11-year-old boy with bilateral bowing of lower extremities (**a**). Radiograph of cystic and "trumpet" shaped metaphysis of femur and moderate bowing of tibia of a 15-year-old boy (**b**)

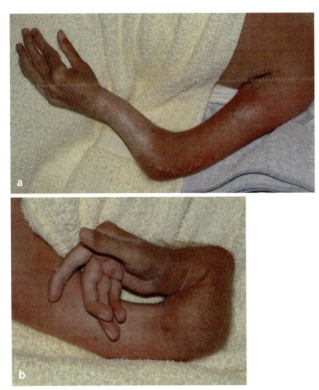

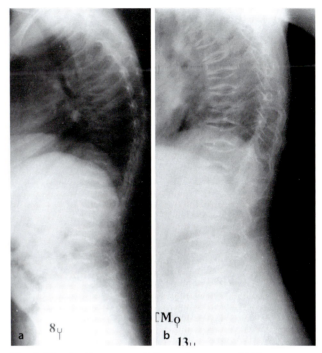

Fig. 1.95 a, b Osteogenesis imperfecta, type III. Severely deformed forearms with thin and distensible skin on left (**a**) and right (**b**) side of a patient

Fig. 1.96 a, b Osteogenesis imperfecta type IV. Thoracolumbar radiograph of a girl at age of 8 (**a**) and 13 (**b**), presenting platyspondyly of the thoracolumbar spine

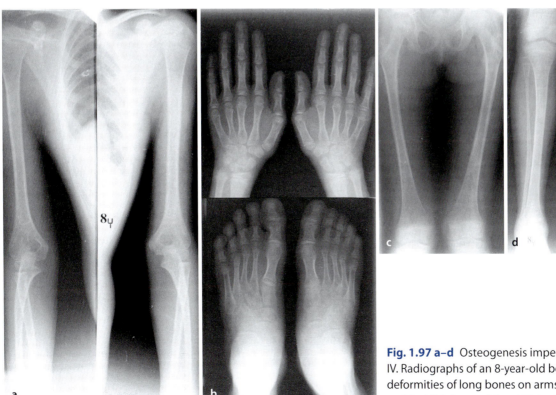

Fig. 1.97 a–d Osteogenesis imperfecta type IV. Radiographs of an 8-year-old boy. Moderate deformities of long bones on arms (**a**), hands and feet (**b**), femurs (**c**) and tibias (**d**)

1.7.2 Marfan's Syndrome

Marfan's syndrome is a relatively common (1/10,000) autosomal dominant hereditary disorder of connective tissue with typical skeletal, ocular, and cardiovascular manifestations.

Most significantly symmetrical elongation of bones especially in hands (arachnodactyly) is visible. Atrophic muscles, joint stiffness, scoliosis, kyphosis, and acetabular protrusion are common. Pectus excavatum can develop due to longitudinal overgrowth of the ribs. Ectopia lentis and congenital cataracts represent the ocular manifestations.

High penetrance but variable expressivity of this disease caused by the mutation in gene encoding the microfibrillar protein FBN-1 and mutations in the gene encoding transforming growth factor-β receptor 2 (TGFBR2).

Cardiovascular changes as acute aortic dissection or progressive dilatation of ascending aorta, bicuspid valve prolapse are frequently leading causes of death (1.98–1.103).

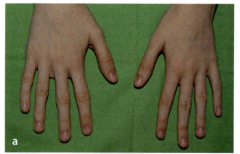
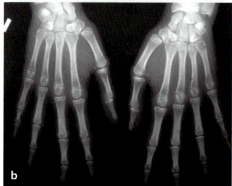

Fig. 1.99 a, b Clinical view (**a**) and radiograph (**b**) of arachnodactyly of hands. Note the symmetrical elongation of small tubular bones

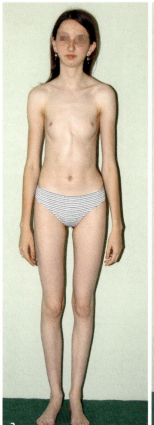
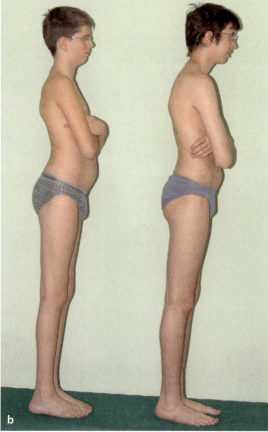

Fig. 1.98 a, b Anterior view of a 13-year-old girl (**a**) and lateral view of a 12 and 14-year-old brothers (**b**) with typical signs of Marfan's syndrome

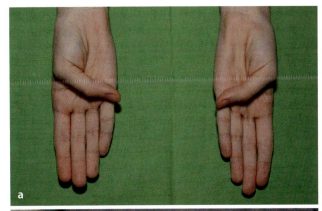

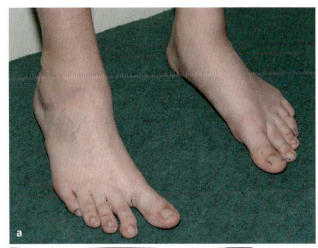

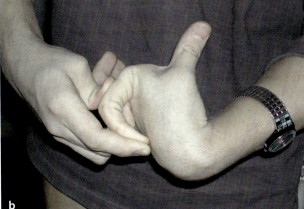

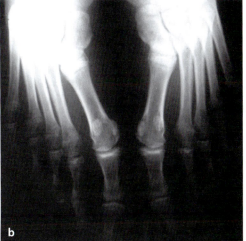

Fig. 1.101 a, b Clinical view (**a**) and radiograph (**b**) of arachnodactyly of the foot. Symmetrical elongation of bones and pes planus

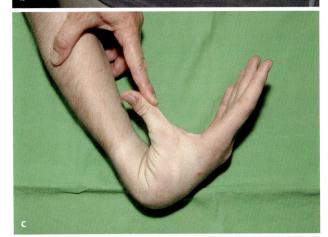

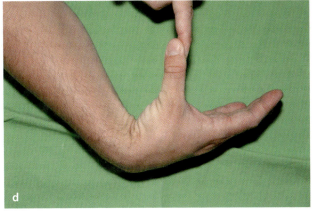

Fig. 1.100 a–d Hyperlaxity of joints in Marfan's syndrome (**a, b**). Comparing the laxity of the wrist and the first carpometacarpal joint of a patient with Marfan's syndrome (**c**) with a normal joint laxity (**d**)

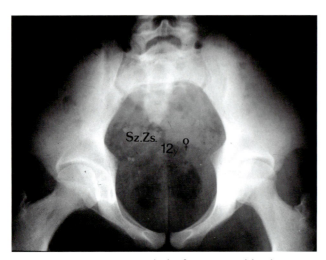

Fig. 1.102 Protrusion acetabuli of a 12-year-old girl

1.7.3 Down Syndrome (Mongolism)

The most frequent chromosomal anomaly, trisomy 21 is associated with numerous orthopedic abnormalities. Although congenital heart disease (most commonly atrioventricular canal defect) is the main cause of morbidity in mongolism, effective cardiac surgical techniques decreased the mortality of Down syndrome children and doing so increased the importance of their orthopedic problems such as dislocation of the hip, habitual luxation of the patella, genu valgum, flatfoot, atlanto–axial instability and scoliosis. The most probable origin of these problems is generalized ligamentous laxity which occurs in almost every Down syndrome patient (Figs. 1.104–1.108).

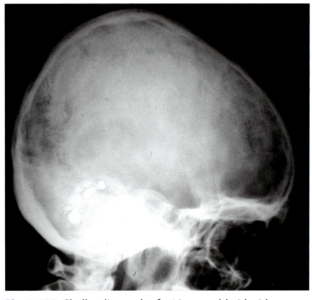

Fig. 1.103 Skull radiograph of a 13-year-old girl with Marfan's syndrome

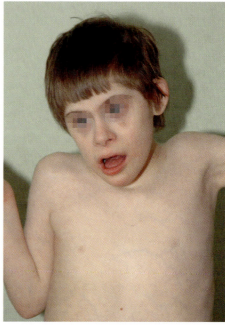

Fig. 1.104 The clinical phenotype of Down syndrome includes microbrachycephaly, low-set ears, up-slanted eyes, epicanthic folds, protruding tongue, short neck and lax skin

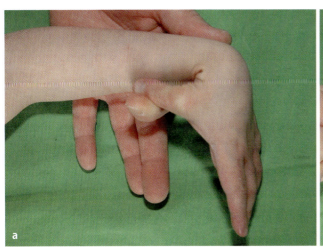

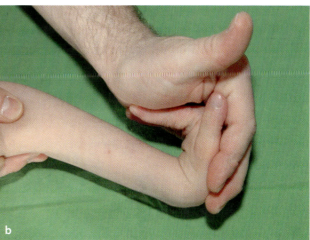

Fig. 1.105 a, b Generalized ligamentous laxity. According to Carter and Wilkinson the diagnosis of generalized joint laxity can be set if more than two of the following tests are positive: (1) passive apposition of the thumb to the flexor aspect of the forearm, (2) passive hyperextension of the fin- gers so that they lay parallel with the extensor aspect of the forearm, (3) ability to hyperextend the elbow more than 10°, (4) ability to hyperextend the knee more than 10°; excessive range of passive dorsiflexion of the ankle end eversion of the foot

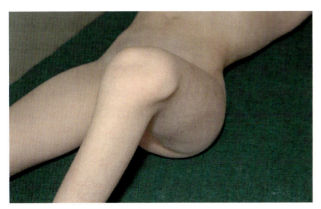

Fig. 1.106 Recurrent or habitual luxation of the patella is a frequent finding in patients with Down syndrome

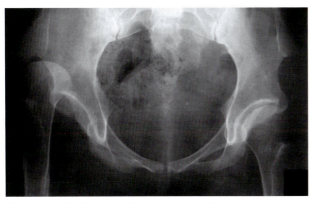

Fig. 1.107 Children (5–30%) with trisomy 21 develop spon- taneous dislocation of the hip. Ligamentous laxity but not acetabular dysplasia is the cause of acute dislocation of the hip

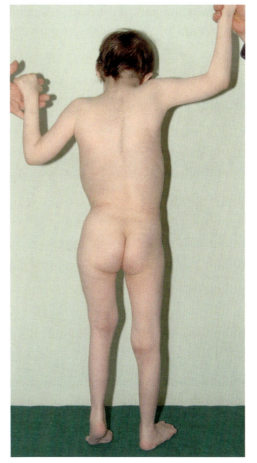

Fig. 1.108 Recurrent hip luxations may result fixed disloca- tion in untreated cases, like this patient with the prominent leg length discrepancy

1.7.4 Osteopetrosis (Albers-Schönberg's Disease, Generalized Congenital Osteosclerosis, Ivory Bones, Marble Bones, Osteosclerosis Fragilis Generalisata)

Osteopetrosis has two forms. The autosomal recessive form is manifest in early age; anemia, hepato-splenomegaly, hypocalcaemia, hypophosphataemia are the concomitant symptoms.

The autosomal dominant form present in the second decade, after puberty, is more benign; 30% of cases are anemic with progressive hepato-splenomegaly.

Osteosclerosis is visible in all bones, the increased density is homogenous. Corticomedullar and trabecular structure decreases. The structure of the bone metaphyses is damaged.

Possible symptoms are macrocephaly, brain nerve dysfunctions (disturbed vision, hearing, facial nerve paresis), hydrocephaly, bone pain, series of bone fractures). The fractures are transverse and not comminuted. Common complication is maxillar and mandibular osteomyelitis (Figs. 1.109–1.113).

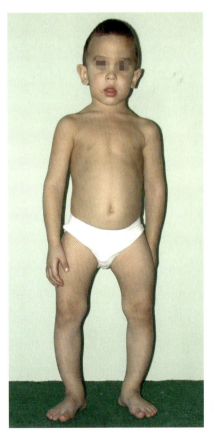

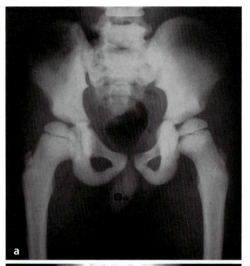

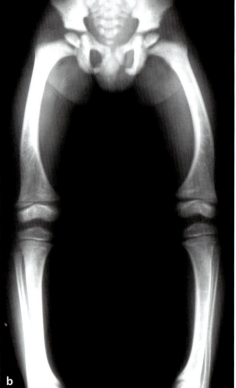

Fig. 1.110 a, b Radiograph of the pelvis (**a**) and lower extremity (**b**) of a boy – seen in previous picture. Sclerotic bony structure also observed. Note the narrow medullar cavity and widened metaphyses in this early form

Fig. 1.109 The short stature of a 5-year-old boy with macrocephaly and with bilateral varus deformity of the knee and leg

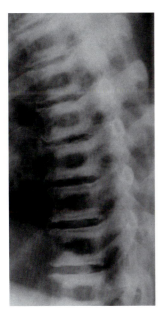

Fig. 1.111 Radiograph of characteristic "'sandwich vertebrae," with diffuse sclerosis accentuated near to vertebral endplates

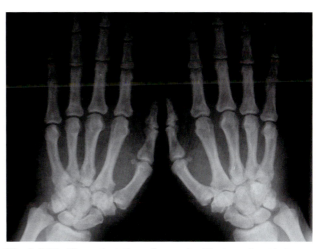

Fig. 1.112 Characteristic radiograph of "osteosclerotic ivory bones" on hands

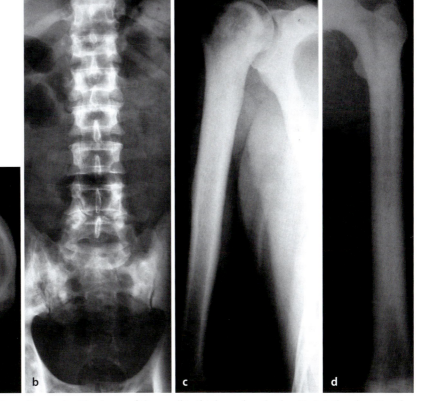

Fig. 1.113 a–d Late form of osteopetrosis in radiographs: The base of the scull is thickened and sclerotic (**a**), the density of bones like vertebral bodies (**b**) are less increased, the medullar cavity is narrowed but present in the humerus (**c**) and in distal femur (**d**)

1.7.5 Osteopoikilosis (Osteopathia Condensans Disseminata, Ostitis Condensans Generalisata, Osteosclerosis Disseminata)

Osteopoikilosis usually appears in the third decade. It causes joint pain in 30% of the cases. Sometimes skin lesions are observed: slightly protruding, white–yellow lentiform fibro–collagenous infiltrations (dermatofibrosis lenticularis disseminata). Intensive, small patchy sclerosis (compact bony islands) is visible on bones, the patches sometimes are confluent. The structural changes of bones are frequently located near joints, in children even in epiphyses. Osteopoikilosis is transmitted in an autosomal dominant manner. Pubertas praecox, short stature in women are also possible symptoms (Figs. 1.114–1.116).

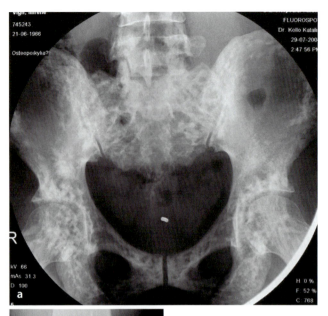

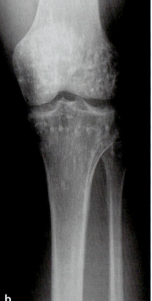

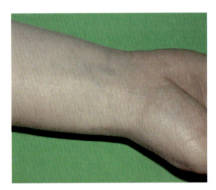

Fig. 1.114
Forearm and wrist of a female patient: small, lentiform whitish-yellowish skin lesions

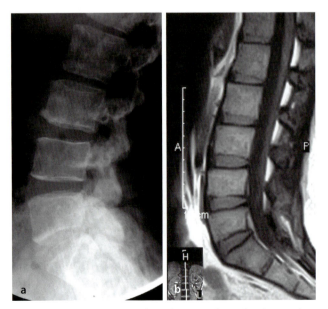

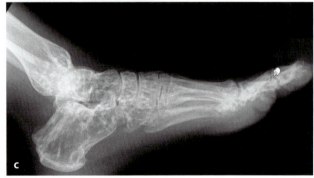

Fig. 1.116 a, b Small patchy sclerosis in lateral radiograph of lumbar spine and sacrum (**a**). Respective signal intensity changes on sagittal MRI images (**b**)

Fig. 1.115 a–c Small patchy sclerosis is visible on radiographs of pelvis (**a**), knee (**b**), ankle and foot (**c**). (Similar structural changes of bones are visible on both children of this patient)

1.7.6 Melorheostosis

Melorheostosis appears at young age. The symptoms include soft tissue contractures involving one or more joints or palmar, plantar fascia. Bowing of the limbs and length discrepancy may also be present. Pain and occasional swelling may occur at the joints involved, with tense, shiny, erythematous skin, subcutaneous edema. Muscular atrophy may also occur. On long tubular bones in children, calcifications are present along the bony axis. In adults, ectopic periosteal and endosteal sclerosis, so-called "candle dripping," are visible. The disease appears in monostotic, monomelic, and polyostotic form (Figs. 1.117 and 1.118).

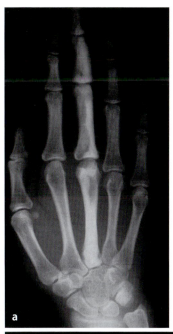

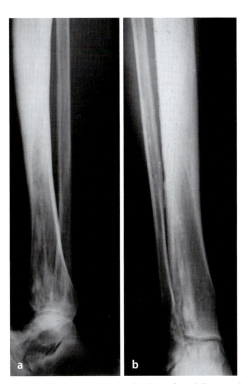

Fig. 1.117 a, b Tibia and talus of middle aged man: longitudinal calcifications are presented along the bony axis, '"candle dripping" ectopic periosteal calcification is seen at the lateral part of tibia on lateral (**a**) and anteroposterior (**b**) view

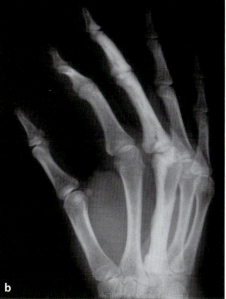

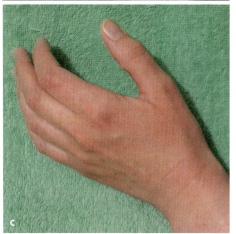

Fig. 1.118 a–c Characteristic longitudinal calcifications on the third ray of the hand of a young female on anteroposterior (**a**) and lateral (**b**) radiograph. Clinical view (**c**) of the same patient's hand, with moderate joint contracture of the third metacarpophalangeal joint

1.7.7 Progressive Diaphyseal Dysplasia – Camurati–Engelmann Disease

Progressive diaphyseal dysplasia, also known as Camu-rati–Engelmann disease, is an autosomal dominant dis-order involving the diaphyses of the long bones, skull base, and clavicles. The most frequent symptoms are: limb pain, muscle weakness, waddling gait, and some-times deafness. The radiography shows a periosteal and endosteal sclerosis and thickening of the diaphysis of the long bones (Figs. 1.119–1.122).

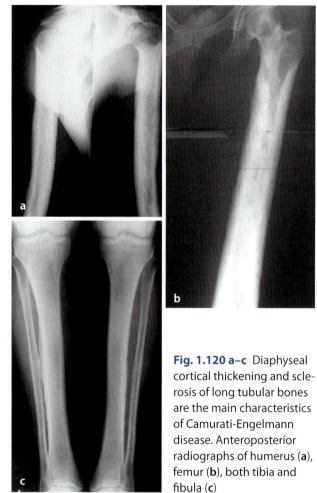

Fig. 1.120 a–c Diaphyseal cortical thickening and scle-rosis of long tubular bones are the main characteristics of Camurati-Engelmann disease. Anteroposterior radiographs of humerus (**a**), femur (**b**), both tibia and fibula (**c**)

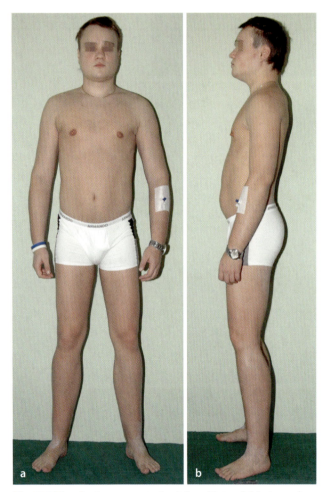

Fig. 1.119 a, b Anteroposterior (**a**) and lateral (**b**) view of a 24-year-old male. No special deformities of the body are revealing for diaphyseal dysplasia. Sometimes decreased muscle and subcutaneous fat mass and thin habitus with columnar shaped extremities occur

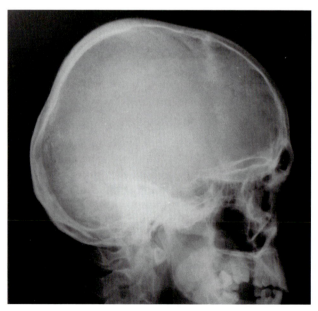

Fig. 1.121 Sclerosis and thickening also can be observed at the base of the skull

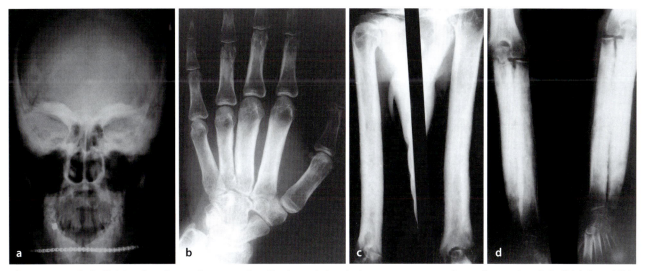

Fig. 1.122 a–d Definitive, late form of progressive diaphyseal dysplasia on anteroposterior radiographs of skull (**a**), hand (**b**), arm (**c**), forearm (**d**) (radiographs from our archives)

1.7.8 Infantile Cortical Hyperostosis (Caffey's Disease)

Infantile cortical hyperostosis occurs in children younger than 5 months. This disease may be present at birth in familial form –which is inherited in an autosomal dominant manner–, or shortly thereafter –sporadic occurrence. Clinically it is characterized by soft-tissue swelling, hyperirritability, fever may occur also and characteristic radiographic changes of cortical hyperostosis as thickening or bony expansion. All races and sex are equally affected. The tibia is the most frequently involved bone, but the disease has been described in any bones. The appearance is often multifocal and asymmetric. In case of serious mandibular involvement, babies may refuse to eat. Radiography is the most valuable diagnostic study in infantile cortical hyperostosis. Contrary to the significant osseous alterations the general condition of the baby is good. Until the age 2, a spontaneous remodeling of the bones occur and the typical X-ray appearance disappears (Figs. 1.123–1.127).

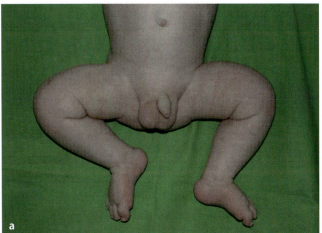
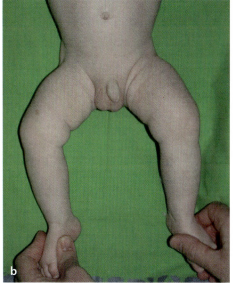

Fig. 1.123 a, b A 4-month-old boy with Caffey's disease. Note the soft-tissue swelling especially on left lower extremity. It causes flexion contracture of the knee also

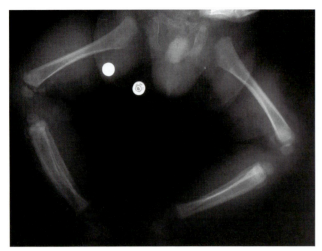

Fig. 1.124 Anteroposterior radiograph of both lower extremities of the same child. Both limbs are affected, but the left side is more severe. Note that the periosteum remains thickened and subperiostal immature lamellar bone is observed. The adjacent fascia, muscles, and connective tissues are also involved causing soft-tissue swelling

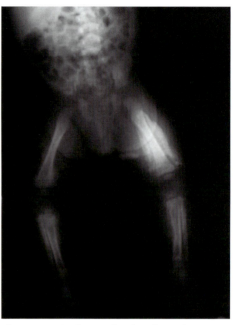

Fig. 1.126 Radiograph taken from the same patient 2 weeks later: changes can be observed at the ipsilateral femur, with rapid radiological progression

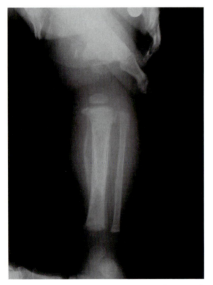

Fig. 1.125 Anteroposterior radiograph of the left tibia of the same child, the possible onset of this disease: periosteal new bone is observed engulfing the diaphysis of the bone, causing an increase in diameter of the bone

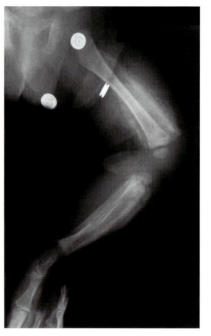

Fig. 1.127 Some months later the periosteal new bone density increases, becoming homogenous with the underlying cortex

1.7.9 Neurofibromatosis

The neurofibromatosis is one of the most frequent inheritable disorders, with autosomal dominant transmission. It is called also von Recklinghausen's disease, and the frequency is approximately 33/100,000. Both genders are affected with equal severity. Type I. is known especially for peripheral involvement: cutaneous fibromata, "café au lait" pigmentation disorders, pigmented iris hamartomes – called also Lish's nodule –, scoliosis, and thin long bones. Type II is characterized by the central involvement as neurinomes of acoustic nerve, cataract and it may compress the spinal cord, giving the typical picture of spinal cord tumor (Figs. 1.128–1.132).

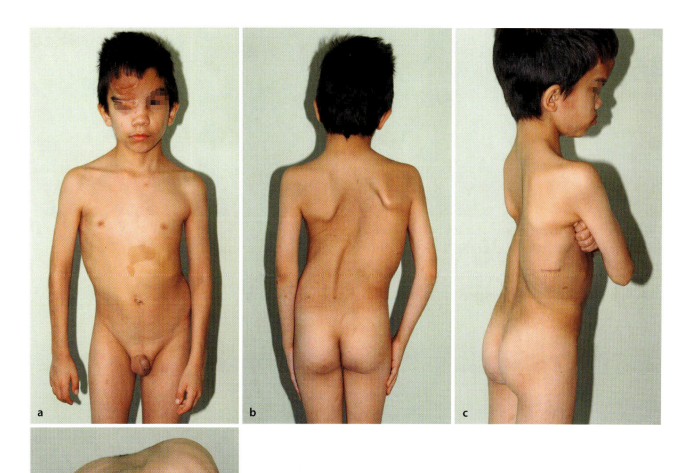

a   b   c   d

Fig. 1.128 a–d Early onset of structural scoliosis of a 9-year-old boy with neurofibromatosis (**b–d**). Typical café-au-lait spot is visible on the trunk, and huge neurofibromatic node on the forehead (**a**)

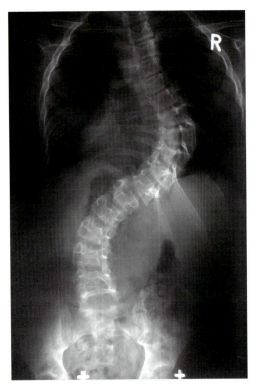

Fig. 1.129 Radiograph of the same patient with type I of neurofibromatosis with rapidly progressing secondary juvenile scoliosis. The typical signs of dystrophic vertebras with hypoplastic or missing pedicles are the thin spinous and transversal processes, scooped vertebral bodies

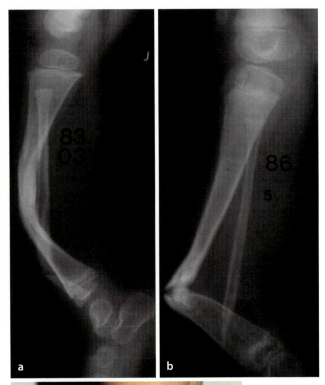

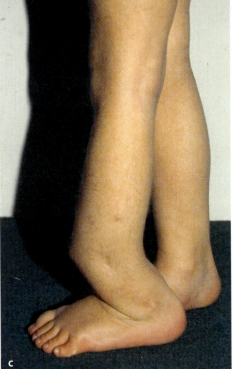

Fig. 1.130 a–c Neurofibromatosis develops in early childhood with various deformity of the lower extremity. In this patient the disease started with an angulation of the tibia at age 2 (**a**). Three years later a typical pseudoarthrosis developed at the same site of the tibia (**b, c**)

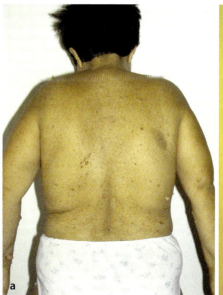
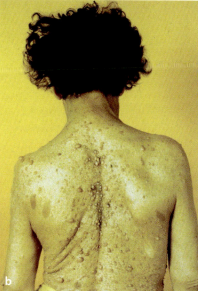
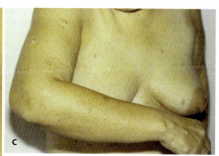

Fig. 1.131 a–c Typical cutaneous findings: Posterior clinical view of two female patients with moderate (**a**) and severe (**b**) cutaneous fibromas and "Café au lait" pigmentation (**c**)

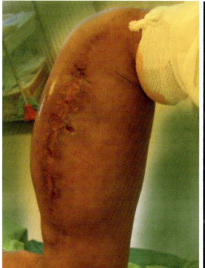
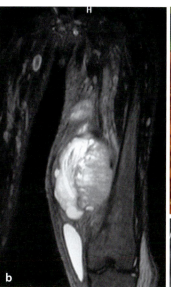
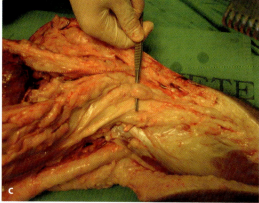
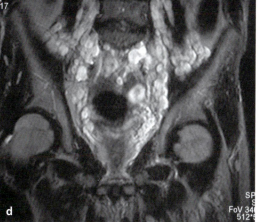

Fig. 1.132 a–d In adult life the lesions often undergo malignant transformation and malignant schwannoma develops, as in this case. Preoperative photograph from the thigh of a 18-year-old male patient (**a**) and the MRI picture (**b**) present a huge malignant schwannoma. The forceps points to a neurofibroma of the enlarged peroneal nerve in the amputated specimen (**c**). MRI picture of the pelvis (**d**) reveals neurofibromata on the enlarged nerves. Between 3 and 13% of patients with von Recklinghausen's disease will develop a malignant schwannoma

Chapter 2

Infection

Contents

Infection

Á. Zahár and K. Köllő

2.1 Bacterial Osteomyelitis

2.1.1 Acute Hematogenous Pyogenic Osteomyelitis (Figs. 2.1–2.6)

Osteomyelitis is a complex disease, which is often associated with high morbidity and considerable health care costs. Bacteriaemia, contiguous focusses of infection, penetrating trauma or surgery are the major predisposing factors for this infection. Acute hematogenous osteomyelitis may occur in newborn, infant, childhood and adult ages (in 75% at childhood and adolescents). The course of the disease depends on the age of the patient, on the virulence of the causative agent, on the immunological state of the host, on the localization and on the blood supply.

Bone necrosis and bone destruction occur early in the course of osteomyelitis, leading to a chronic process and eliminating the host's ability to eradicate the pathogens. The pathogens are in 90% of all cases *Staphylococcus aureus* colonies. The presence of poorly vascularized tissues, the adherence to bone structures and implants and a slow bacterial replication rate are recognized as important factors for the persistence of the infection.

Bone necrosis begins early, limiting the possibility of eradicating the pathogens, and leading to a chronic condition. Chronic pain and recurrence of infection still remain possible even when the acute symptoms of osteomyelitis have been resolved.

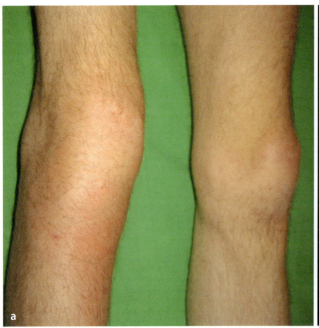

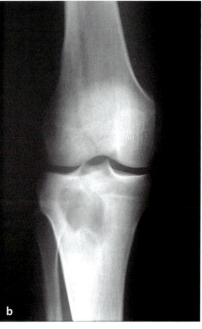

Fig. 2.1 a, b The photograph (**a**) shows the knee of a patient with osteomyelitis: the skin is red, the leg is swollen. The radiograph (**b**) reveals a well-defined lytic lesion in the proximal metaphysis of the right tibia: no sclerotic margin is observed. Biopsy proved osteomyelitis

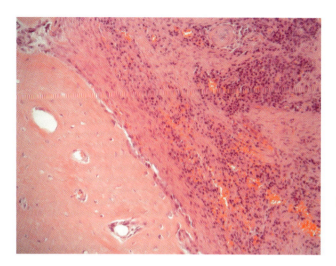

Fig. 2.2 The histological picture of acute hematogenous osteomyelitis. The bone trabeculae are partly necrotic, the marrow cells in the medullar cavity are replaced by inflammatory cells, edema and fibrin

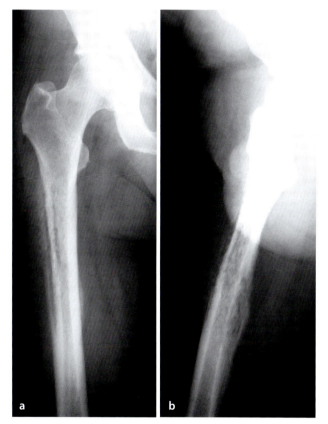

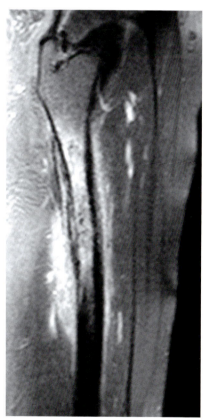

Fig. 2.3 a, b Plain radiographs of an acute hematogenous femoral osteomyelitis caused by *Lactococcus*: the lesion has a permeative radiographic appearance with "onion peel"-like periosteal reaction, which is also seen in malignant bone tumors (e.g. Ewing's sarcoma)

Fig. 2.4 MR image of the same femoral *Lactococcus*-osteomyelitis: edema and pus formation in the bone marrow and perifocal edema in the surrounding soft tissues

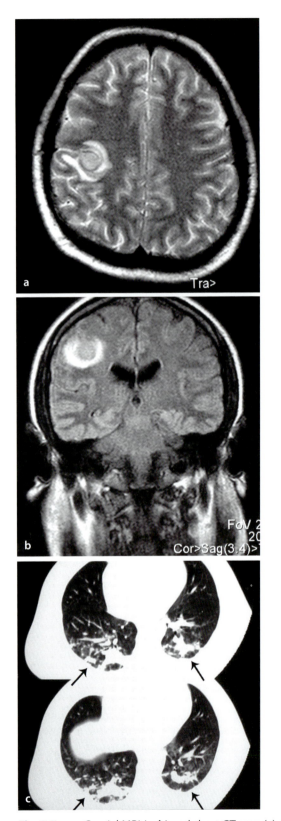

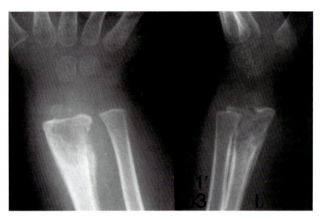

Fig. 2.6 Radiographs showing the acute bacterial osteomyelitis of the left distal radius of a child: permeative destruction with ill-defined border and marked periosteal reaction is present

Fig. 2.5 a–c Cranial MRI (**a, b**) and chest CT scan (**c**) of the same patient with *Lactococcus*-osteomyelitis: metastatic purulent foci are present in the brain and the lung (*arrows*), causing a life threatening condition

2.1.2 The Newborn's Coxitis/"Säuglings Coxitis"

In newborns and in infants under the age of 1 year, osteomyelitis affects the epiphyses and the joints, and it is associated with arthritis, which may result in articular destruction (epiphyseal osteomyelitis).

S. aureus and *Haemophilus influenzae* are the most common bacteria causing coxitis in newborns. The bacteria are transmitted hematogenously, and the primary infection is mostly in a discharging ("wet") umbilicus, bacterial skin inflammation or otitis. The metaphyseal vessels of the femur contain bacteria, which may penetrate into the epiphysis and the hip joint, thus the metaphysis is localized intra-articular.

High fever, flexion–abduction–external rotation of newborn's hip, painful hip movement (crying baby), limited range of motion, lymphadenomegaly are characteristic of the condition. Newborn's coxitis is at highly septic condition, and the lab tests show high Westergreen and white blood cell levels and a left shift in the qualitative blood test (Figs. 2.7–2.12).

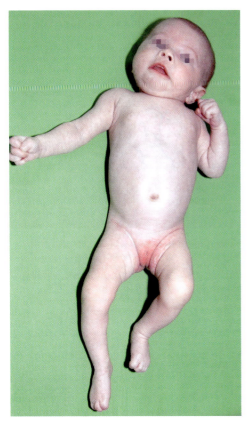

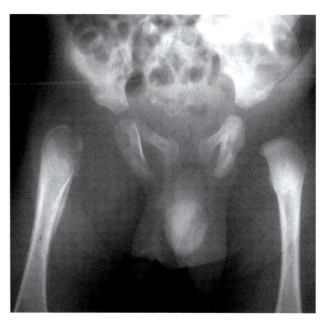

Fig. 2.9 Another young patient with bacterial coxitis: the right hip is dislocated and metaphyseal involvement is seen. Because of pus formation in the hip joint, subluxation or complete dislocation of the femoral head may occur

Fig. 2.7 One-month-young baby with septic coxitis of the left hip (so called "Säuglings-coxitis"). Note the abduction–flexion–external rotation position of the left hip, which is painful when moved passively

Fig. 2.8 a, b Bilateral ultrasound image of the hips in the same baby (Fig. 2.7): (**a**) in the left hip joint the capsule is dilated (*arrow*); below a less echo dense area (*tip of arrow*), which indicates a thick fluid formation, femoral head is dislocated (1), the cartilaginous acetabulum is lifted (2), the osseous acetabulum is intact (3), the greater trochanter is in high position (4). In the right hip (**b**) normal findings are detectable: femoral head (1), cartilage of acetabulum (2), osseous socket (3) and greater trochanter (4)

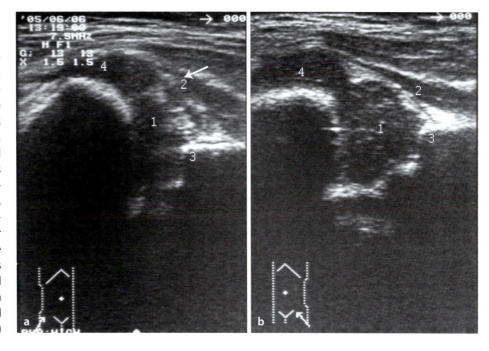

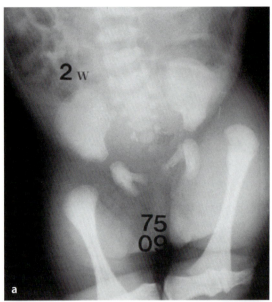

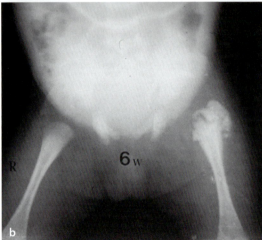

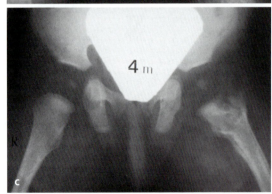

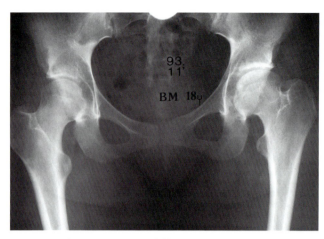

Fig. 2.11 The same patient following the successful antibiotic treatment at the age of 18 years: almost full recovery with slight signs of secondary osteoarthritis of the left hip, moderate leg length shortening

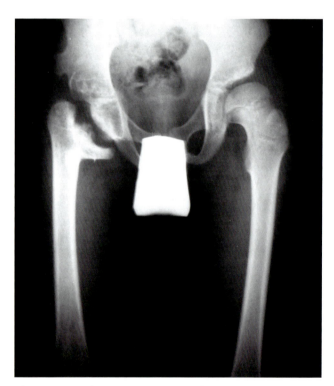

Fig. 2.10 a–c Series of radiographs: patient with coxitis at newborn age (**a**), at 6 weeks (**b**) and at 4 months (**c**), respectively. In small children osteomyelitis is a bone producing process, resulting in condensed, sclerotic bones, sometimes in overgrowth of the affected bone (**b**). Sequester is a lytic site inside the sclerotic zone, which is filled with pus, when surgically opened. Diagnostic tools are plain radiographs, fistulography and CT scans

Fig. 2.12 Another young patient with a similar history of coxitis at newborn's age, but the outcome is different: the right femoral head and the neck are destroyed as a consequence of the newborn's coxitis. The protruded lesser trochanter supports the deteriorated acetabulum. Severe hip deformity is already present at adolescent age

2.1.3 Chronic Bacterial Osteomyelitis

Chronic osteomyelitis may occur, if the treated acute form turns to be chronic, or the acute osteomyelitis is be- ing reactivated even after years or decades and becomes chronic, or the acute phase has a subclinical appearance and the chronic form becomes manifest.

Chronic osteomyelitis is not a life threatening con- dition: it is much more a steady state between the bone inflammation and the resistance of the host's organism. In the cancellous bone, inactive bacteria may become virulent again, and the osteomyelitis process may be ac- tivated.

Bacterial cultures can be negative in up to 50–70% of the cases, but the same *Staphylococci* are responsible for the disease, as in acute osteomyelitis.

The site of the infection may be swollen, the skin is often red, and fluid formation may be detectable. A dis- charging sinus may be developed, pus and necrotic mass is running out of the bone. Fever may be higher, but is not characteristic (Figs. 2.13–2.20).

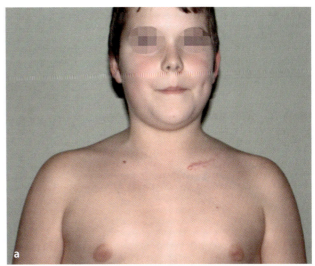
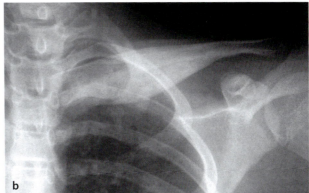
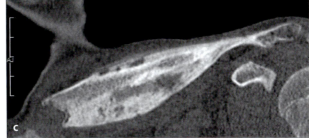
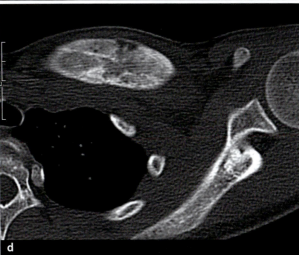

Fig. 2.13 a–d Chronic bacterial osteomyelitis of the left clavicle in an adolescent boy. The photograph of the patient illustrates a protuberant clavicle and scar refers to previous biopsy (**a**). The plain radiograph (**b**), 3D CT reconstruction (**c**) and CT cross section (**d**) demonstrate a condense and fusiform enlarged clavicle

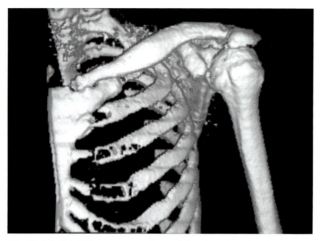

Fig. 2.14 3D CT reconstruction of the shoulder in chronic bacterial osteomyelitis of the left clavicle: the bone is thickened and condensed

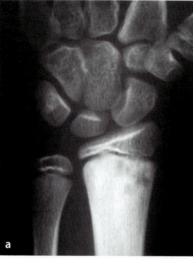

a

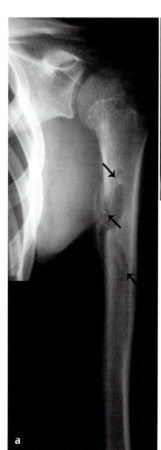

a

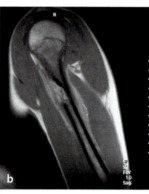

b

Fig. 2.15 a, b Radiograph (**a**) and MR image (**b**) of chronic bacterial osteomyelitis of the left humerus with sequester formation (*arrows*), cortical destruction and periosteal reaction in an adolescent girl. The process with the ill-defined border can mimic malignant bone tumor

Fig. 2.16 a, b AP radiograph (**a**) of chronic bacterial osteomyelitis of the left distal radius in a young girl: note the confluent lytic areas in the sclerotic metaphysis. Bone scan (**b**) shows an enhanced isotope uptake in this area

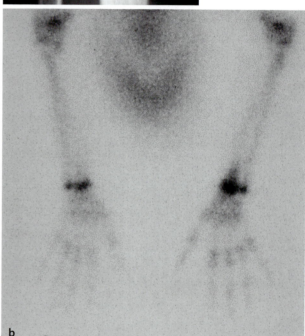

b

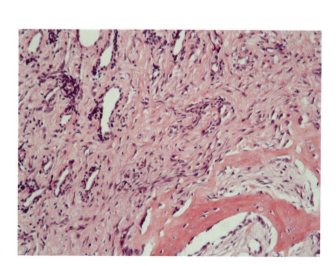

Fig. 2.17 Chronic osteomyelitis: remnants of bone trabeculae, the medullar cavity is filled by loose connective tissue rich in vessels, which are surrounded by chronic inflammatory cells

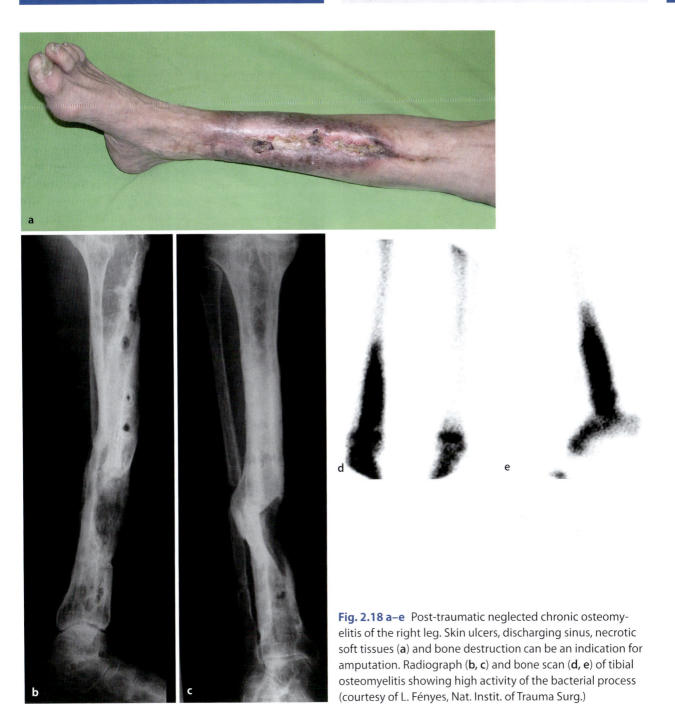

Fig. 2.18 a–e Post-traumatic neglected chronic osteomyelitis of the right leg. Skin ulcers, discharging sinus, necrotic soft tissues (**a**) and bone destruction can be an indication for amputation. Radiograph (**b, c**) and bone scan (**d, e**) of tibial osteomyelitis showing high activity of the bacterial process (courtesy of L. Fényes, Nat. Instit. of Trauma Surg.)

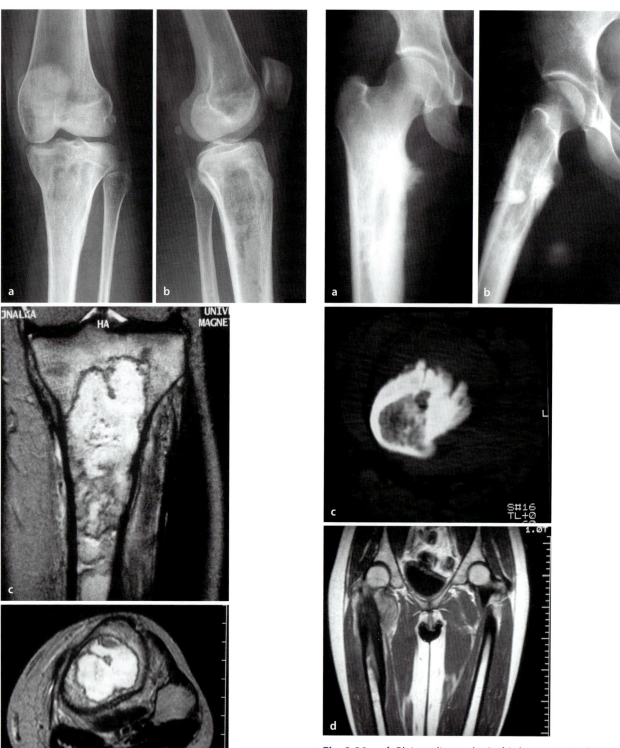

Fig. 2.19 a–d　Plain radiographs (**a**, **b**) and MRI pictures (**c**, **d**) show chronic *Salmonella*-osteomyelitis in the left proximal tibia. *Salmonella spp.* as a causative agent is a very rare condition

Fig. 2.20 a–d　Plain radiographs (**a**, **b**) demonstrate chronic bacterial osteomyelitis of the femur: the diaphysis is enlarged and sclerotic with a central lytic area. There is a prominent periosteal reaction seen in the CT image (**c**), especially at the level of the lesser trochanter. Contrary to the extensive edema in the acute form, MRI picture (**d**) reveals moderate edema in the soft tissues

2.1.4 Special Forms of Bacterial Osteomyelitis

Lower bacterial virulence and higher resistance of young patients may cause special forms of osteomyelitis, which are different from acute hematogenous osteomyelitis in appearance and clinical course. In the second decade of life, two special forms of chronic osteomyelitis may occur. The problem of differentiation between osteomyelitis and primary bone tumors can be difficult. Often the final diagnosis of osteomyelitis is set only after evaluation of histology and bacterial culture.

In *Garré's chronic sclerosing osteomyelitis*, there is a dense sclerotic appearance and often lack of lucency on radiographs. The most common localization is the diaphysis of the tibia. The lesion can involve the entire circumference of the bone and have a fusiform shape. Serial radiographs generally show little or no change within a short period of time. The involved bone is painful, sometimes swollen, fever and lab tests are not characteristic.

Osteomyelitis in the metaphysis of the bones with a sclerotic margin or an oval lytic destruction in the radiograph is called *Brodie's abscess or subacute osteomyelitis*. The most frequent site is the proximal metaphysis of the tibia. Cultures show that *Staphylococcus aureus* may have a role, but normally it can not be proven. The affected joint (mostly the knee) may be painful and swollen (Figs. 2.21–2.24).

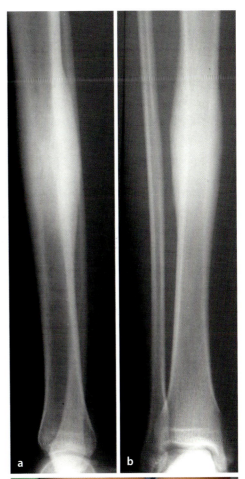

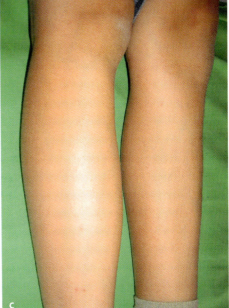

Fig. 2.21 a–c Radiographs of Garré's subacute sclerosing osteomyelitis: fusiform sclerotic change in the diaphysis (**a**, **b**). The photograph shows a characteristic swelling and deformity of the leg (**c**)

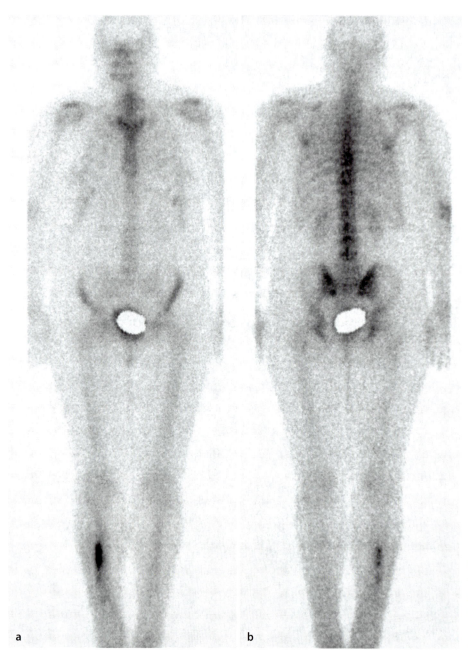

a   b

Fig. 2.22 a, b Garré's subacute sclerosing osteomyelitis on the tibia of a 17 year-old boy: the Technetium bone scan shows osteoblast activity in the diaphysis

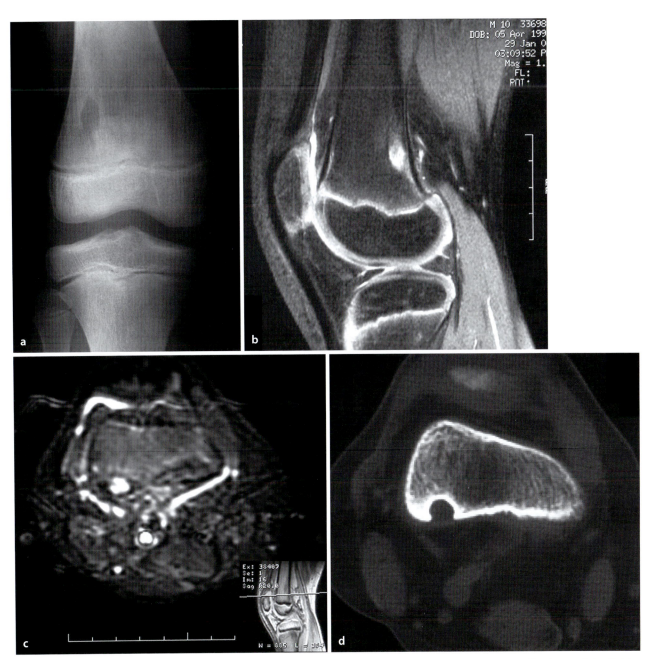

Fig. 2.23 a–d Subacute bacterial osteomyelitis (Brodie's abscess) of the distal–dorsolateral metaphysis of the femur in an adolescent boy. The radiograph shows a lytic lesion with a sclerotic margin (**a**). MR images (**b, c**) reveal the fluid content of the cyst. Note the cortical destruction in the CT scan (**d**)

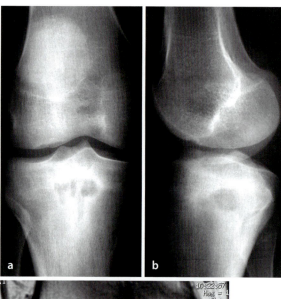

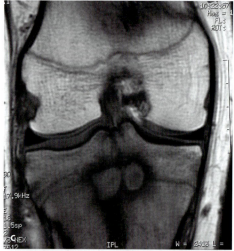

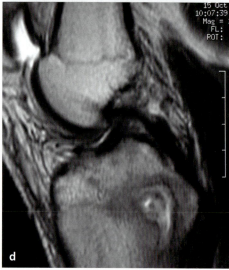

Fig. 2.24 a–d Brodie's abscess in the proximal metaphysis of the tibia in an adolescent. The lesion is seen on the radiographs (**a, b**) sclerotic margin around the cysts. MRI scans (**c, d**) show oval osteomyelitic lesions with perifocal edema

2.1.5 Osteoarticular Skin Syndromes: CRMO and SAPHO

Chronic Recurrent Multifocal Osteomyelitis (CRMO) is a recognized condition that usually affects children and adolescents. It is characterized by insidious onset of local swelling and pain in several metaphyses of affected bones. Clinical, biological and especially radiological abnormalities are suggestive of septic osteomyelitis, and so the diagnosis is delayed. Bone biopsy with culture is certainly necessary to rule out bacterial osteomyelitis and bone tumor. In many cases proper diagnosis can be made only after several years.

A symmetric, recurrent and multifocal pattern is usual. The disease is characterized by a prolonged, fluctuating course with recurrent episodes of pain occurring over several years. CRMO is often multifocal and most often seen in tubular bones, the clavicle, and less frequently the spine and pelvic bones; other locations are rare.

Inconstant association with a cutaneous affection (palmoplantar pustulosis, acne fulminans, psoriasis) or less frequently with an inflammatory chronic bowel disease is described. Disease course is benign and self-limited. The clinical course is characterized by recurrences and remission occurring for 6–10 years.

Synovitis, Acne, Pustulosis, Hyperostosis, and Osteitis (SAPHO) syndrome is an osteoarticular skin syndrome characterized by sterile inflammatory arthro-osteitis of the anterior chest wall. It is associated with various skin conditions, including palmoplantar pustulosis, severe acnes and pustular psoriasis.

SAPHO syndrome mainly affects young and middle-aged adults. Skin bacteria (e.g., *Staphylococcus aureus* and *Corynebacterium acnes*) may have a leading role in the etiology, but the real causative agent is not well known.

Synovitis may be observed in all joints, but the most common sites are the sacroiliac and the sternoclavicular joints. Spondylosis and spondylarthritis are characteristic changes as well. Acne is mostly present on the skin of the face and of the decolté. Palmar and/or plantar pustulosis are very characteristic components of the syndrome. Hyperostotic ribs, clavicles and other flat bones are also characteristic findings, such as osteitis or osteomyelitis of long tubular bones (Figs. 2.25–2.37).

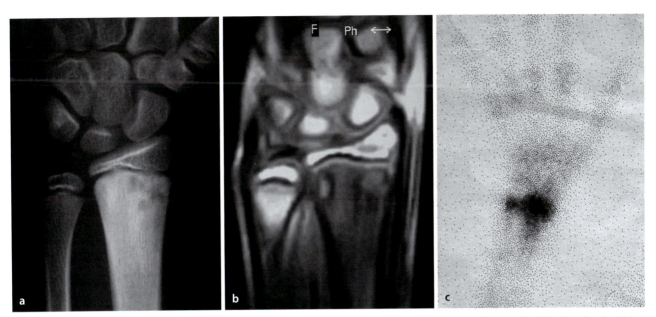

Fig. 2.25 a–c Chronic inflammation in the distal metaphysis of the radius as part of CRMO in a 14-year-old girl. Multicystic lytic foci in sclerotic metaphyseal bone are highly characteristic for CRMO, as presented on the radiograph of the distal radius (**a**). On basis of MR images (**b**), the epiphysis is not involved in this case. A positive bone scan supports the right diagnosis (**c**)

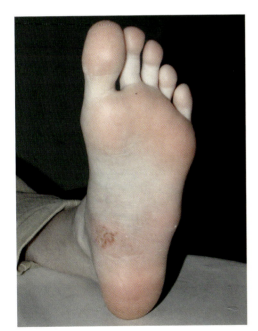

Fig. 2.26 Plantar pustulosis of a 14-year-old CRMO patient. Bacterial cultures show usually no evidence of microorganisms in the pustulae

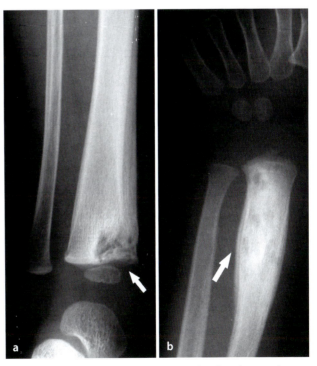

Fig. 2.27 a, b The characteristic multifocal and metaphyseal appearance of CRMO: simultaneous involvement of the right distal tibia (**a**) (*arrow*) and left distal radius (**b**) (*arrow*) in the same patient

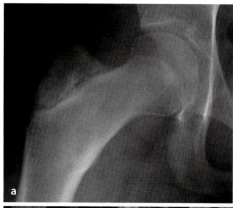

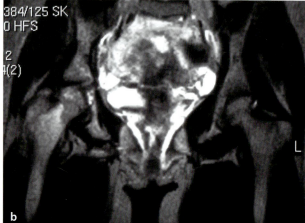

Fig. 2.28 a, b Lytic lesions in the greater trochanter (**a**). Large femur edema is seen on the MR image of the right hip of a CRMO patient (**b**)

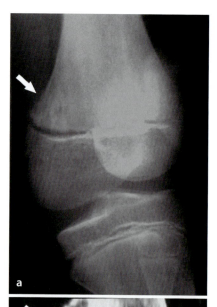

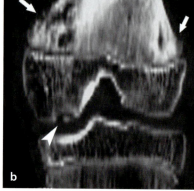

Fig. 2.29 a, b The radiograph (**a**) (*arrow*) and a reconstruction of the CT scan (**b**) (*arrows*) reveal a multicentric destructive process in the meta-epiphysis of the femur of the previous patient

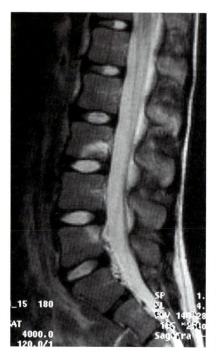

Fig. 2.30 Perifocal edema of L3 vertebral body of a CRMO patient with low back pain (MR image)

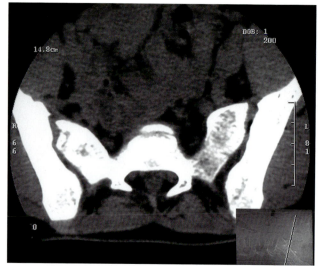

Fig. 2.31 Narrowing of the right sacroiliac joint due to chronic inflammation in CRMO (CT scan)

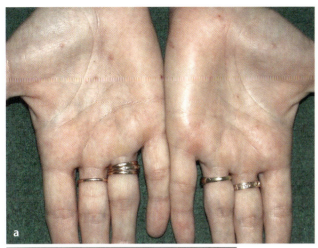

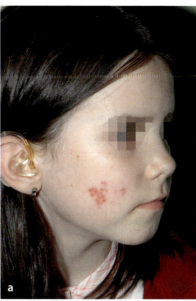

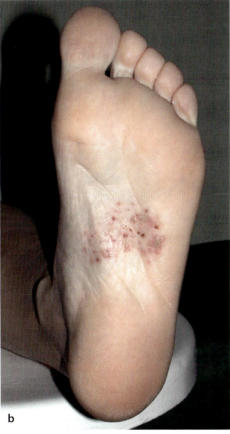

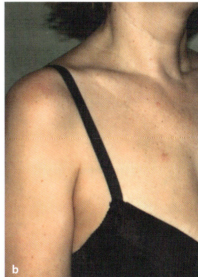

Fig. 2.33 a, b Acne occurring on the skin of the face of a girl (**a**) or on the anterior chest wall of a female SAPHO patient (**b**). Note the protruding sternocostal junction referring to the sterile inflammation process

Fig. 2.32 a, b Palmar (**a**) and plantar (**b**) pustulosis of a patient having SAPHO syndrome: bacterial strains often show the presence of *Staphylococcus aureus*

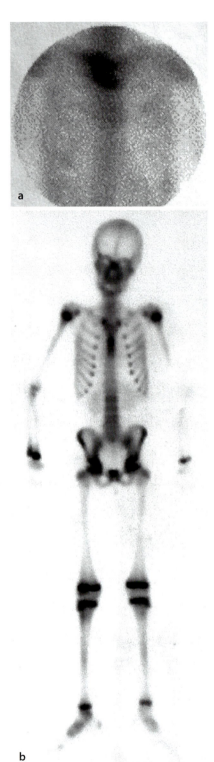

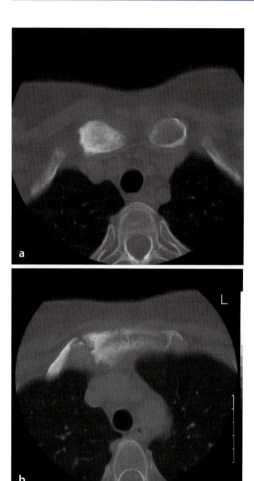

Fig. 2.35 a, b CT scan representing the involvement and destruction of the sternoclavicular joint: note the osteitis of the right proximal clavicle (**a**) and the destruction of the sternal manubrium (**b**)

Fig. 2.34 a, b Bone scan (scintigraphy) findings show hot spots (osteoblast activity) in the affected bones. In the first patient, the sternoclavicular area (**a**) and in the second one, the right distal ulna and sternum are affected (**b**)

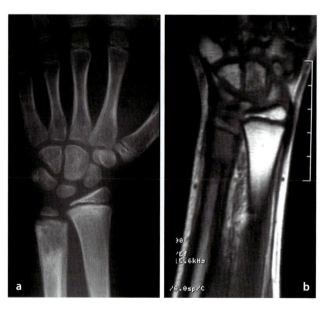

Fig. 2.36 a, b Radiograph (**a**) and MR image (**b**) of the wrist showing an osteomyelitis of the left distal ulna in a SAPHO patient

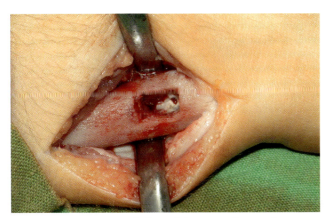

Fig. 2.37 Intraoperative finding of the same ulna: sterile necrotic tissue was found and curetted, with no evidence of bacteria

2.1.6 Postvaccinal Osteomyelitis

Bacillus–Calmette–Guerin (BCG) vaccination often results in local adverse effects; however, serious or long-term complications are rare. Secondary complications after BCG-vaccination are unusual. There is an almost invariably lethal generalized infection affecting the immunodepressed patient. Late dissemination of BCG to bone is characterized by lytic lesions; it is not normally associated with immunologic changes and has a good prognosis. The patients develop pain and swelling in the affected site (calf, arm, thigh, etc.) Sometimes they have no evidence of immunodeficiency. Histopathological examination of biopsy material reveals a chronic granulomatous inflammatory reaction.

Varicella is a common viral infection in childhood, and acute osteomyelitis is one of the rare but serious complications. Osteomyelitis may occur even after vaccination against varicella. It should, however, be considered in any child who develops pain in a limb during or after a varicella infection or immunization. In many cases, *group A beta-hemolytic Streptococcus* is isolated from blood cultures and bone aspirate cultures from the lesion. Serious musculoskeletal complications such as osteomyelitis and necrotizing fasciitis, although uncommon, can be life and limb-threatening (Figs. 2.38–2.40).

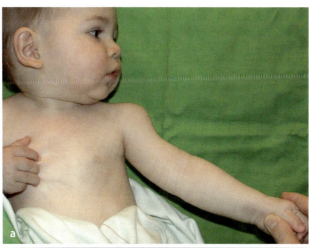
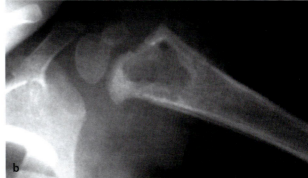
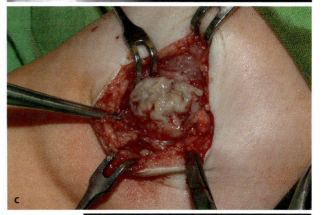
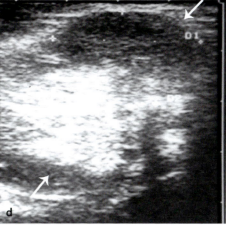

Fig. 2.38 a–d (**a**) A 7-month-old baby with inflammation of the left shoulder following BCG immunization. On the radiograph (**b**), acute osteomyelitis of the proximal metaphysis of the humerus is seen. Ultrasound image (**d**) of the shoulder: cranial to the proximal aspect of the humerus, in the deltoid muscle an echo dense area is detected (*arrow*), more cranially with an echoless zone (*tip of arrow*), which indicates soft tissue collection containing fluid (necrotic-purulent mass) (**c**) due to BCG vaccination

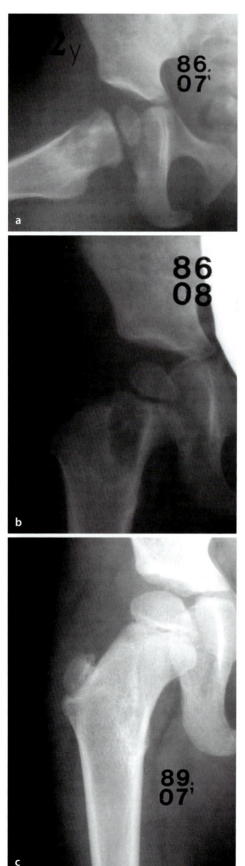

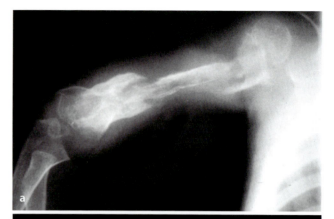

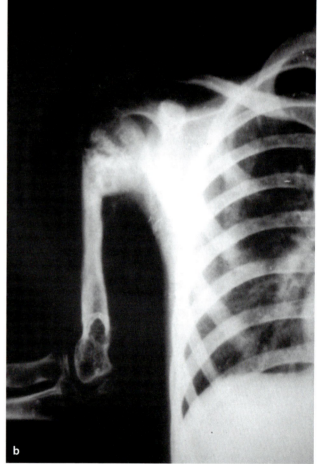

Fig. 2.40 a, b Radiographs of a patient with varicella osteomyelitis of the right humerus: the process with sequester formation destroyed the bone extensively (**a**). The humerus healed with angulation at the surgical neck and the limb could be saved (**b**)

Fig. 2.39 a–c Archive radiographs of a child with femoral BCG-osteomyelitis. Note the metaphyseal osteomyelitis at the age of 2 years (**a, b**), and the outcome following a successful treatment at age 5 (**c**)

2.2 Tuberculous Osteomyelitis and Arthritis

Osteoarticular tuberculosis, although rare, has shown resurgence in recent times, especially in immunocompromised patients. But 10–15% of all tuberculotic manifestations are still involving the bones and joints. The tuberculotic osteomyelitis is caused by *Mycobacterium tuberculosis*, mostly after a primary pulmonary infection and a bacterial spreading on hematogenous way. In the site of infection a caseous necrosis (cheese-like) occurs and causes moderate to severe bone pain and limited articular function with the involvement of the epiphyseal vessels. There are productive forms with tissue granulation and exsudative forms.

Cold abscess is pus formation breaking out of the bone and collected in the soft tissues. The cold abscess may become a sedimentation abscess when flowing down along the soft tissue sheets. When it is breaking through the skin, a discharging sinus is seen.

The general symptoms are pain, subfebrility, fatigue, night sweating, slightly elevated erythrocyte sedimentation rate.

The healing process causes the fusion of the involved bones. In the case of the spine, where tuberculotic spondylitis occurs, the spontaneous fusion of the vertebral bodies results in a *gibbus*. Segmental kyphosis is observed in these cases. In the case of major joints the spontaneous fusion of the involved bones is called an ankylosis, where the joint (e.g. hip, knee) becomes stiff, mostly in flexion position (Figs. 2.41–2.49).

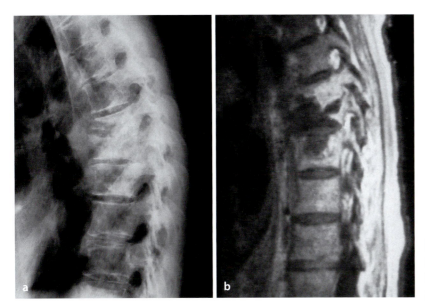

Fig. 2.41 a, b Radiograph (**a**) and MRI (**b**) showing the 7–8–9th thoracic vertebral bodies being destructed by tuberculotic process

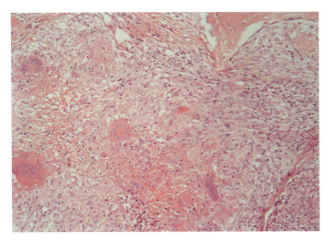

Fig. 2.42 Tuberculous osteomyelitis: the medullar cavity is filled by granulomatous tissue, which consist of Langerhans-type giant cells, chronic inflammatory and epitheloid cells

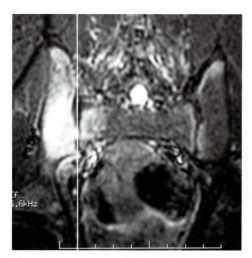

Fig. 2.43 MR image of tuberculotic sacroileitis: note the wide perifocal zone of edema in the iliac bone

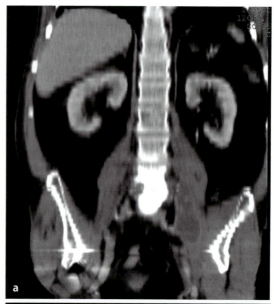

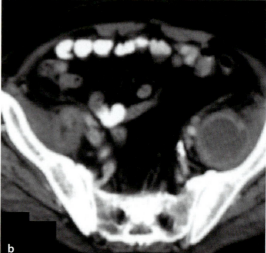

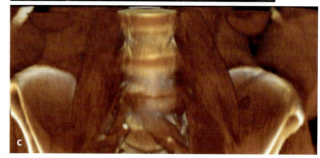

Fig. 2.45 a–c Psoas abscess: pus formation in case of tuberculotic spondylitis. Widening of the left iliopsoas muscle and abscess formation is seen on abdominal reconstruction CT picture (**a**). On conventional CT (**b**) the iliopsoas muscle is thickened, in the caudal part abscess formation is seen. (courtesy of Dr. P. Farkas, OORI, Budapest, Hungary) Widening of the iliopsoas muscle is seen on abdominal 3D color coded CT (**c**) images. (courtesy of Dr. K. Lukács, Szt. Ferenc County Hospital, Miskolc, Hungary)

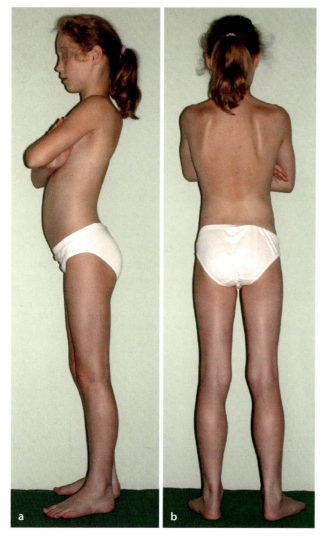

Fig. 2.44 a, b Hyperlordotic (**a**) and antalgic (**b**) posture of the same patient suffering from tuberculous sacroileitis

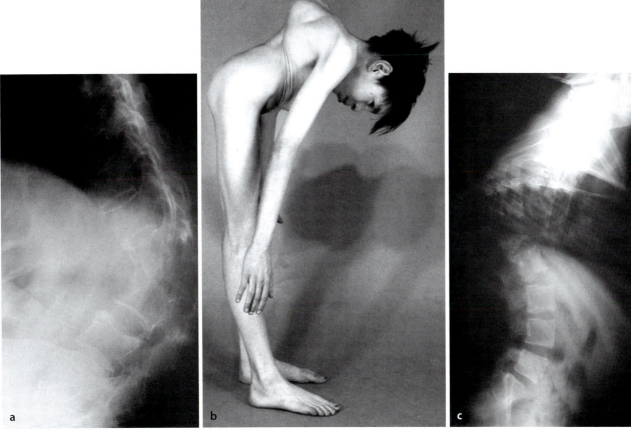

Fig. 2.46 a–c Radiograph showing thoracolumbar spine after healing process of tuberculotic spondylitis. A gibbus is seen with segmental kyphosis of fused vertebral bodies (a). Photograph taken from the patient shows angulated kyphosis caused by tuberculotic vertebral osteomyelitis (archive photograph, b). Lateral view radiograph of the same patient showing extreme hunchback (gibbus) (c)

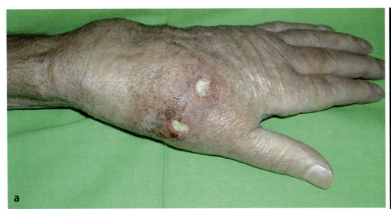

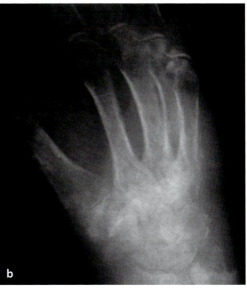

Fig. 2.47 a, b Photograph showing tuberculotic osteomyelitis of the left wrist and hand (a) of an old male patient. The caseous necrotic fluid is braking through the skin, and this condition is called *cutis luposa*. The destruction of the carpal bones and the carpometacarpal joints in the same patient are represented on the radiograph (b)

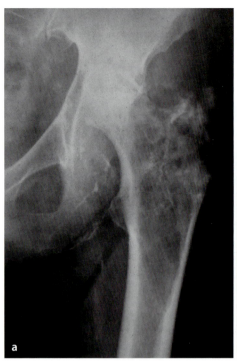
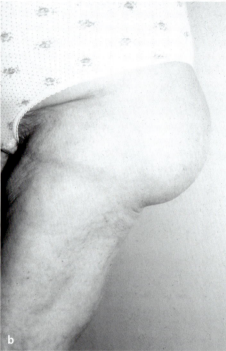

Fig. 2.48 a, b Radiograph presenting so-called *caries trochanterica* (**a**) on the radiograph, where destruction of the greater trochanter and tuberculous coxitis are observed. The skin (archive photograph) above the greater trochanter (**b**) is not affected, yet the fluctuating asymmetric protruding left buttock refers to a huge abscess

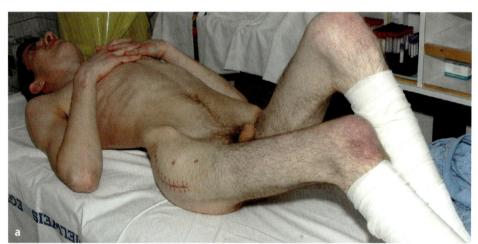

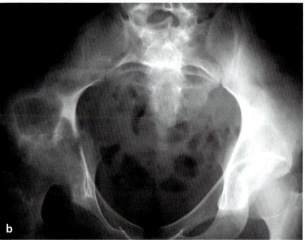

Fig. 2.49 a–d Young cachectic male patient suffering from tuberculotic coxitis in the right hip with enormous pains. Note the flexion contracture in the hip joint (**a**). The radiograph presents the atrophic bone, narrowed joint space of the right hip, with a lytic destruction in the acetabulum – highly characteristic for tuberculotic osteomyelitis (**b**). MRI of the same tuberculotic patient with a tuberculotic osteomyelitis in the right iliac bone (acetabular roof), with edema of the femoral head and fluid formation in the hip joint (**c**). The intraoperative photograph illustrates the tuberculotic oryza (rice corn-like caseous necrotic mass) from the same patient (**d**)

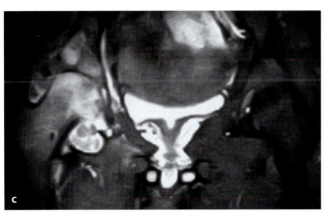
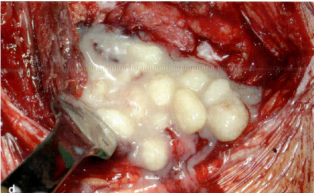

Fig. 2.49 c, d

2.3 Bacterial Arthritis

Septic articular inflammation may occur primarily in the joint, or it is developed secondary due to a septic inflammation in the body elsewhere. The primary bacterial arthritis is most likely in the childhood, and occurs twice as often as osteomyelitis. In 90% of all cases *S. haemolyticus* is responsible for the septic arthritis.

Bacteria may affect the joints on different ways: hematogenous, direct affection in metaphyseal osteomyelitis (e.g. newborn's coxitis), penetrating injury and iatrogenic infection (e.g. intraarticular injection).

In purulent arthritis the joint is swollen, in acute form the skin is red, fever may occur, in chronic form the signs of inflammation are less common. The joint contains pus of yellowish color, a necrotic mass with bacteria and white blood cells. Laboratory tests show elevated C reactive protein levels, high sedimentation rate, high white blood cell counts. The affected joint is painful and the range of motion is significantly decreased.

Punction and bacterial culture are the method of choice to make a certain diagnosis in bacterial arthritis. The quality, cell count and color of the articular fluid (pus) are the characteristics.

The most common sites where a septic arthritis may occur are the knee, the olecranon bursa, the wrist and finger joints, the hip, the glenohumeral joint and the metatarsophalangeal joint (Figs. 2.50, 2.51)

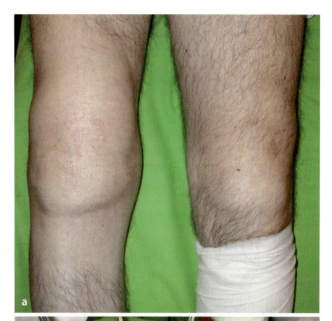
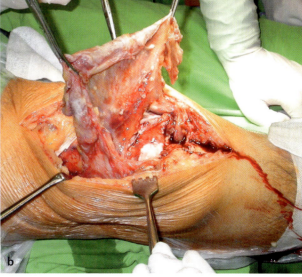

Fig. 2.50 a, b Acute purulent arthritis: the right knee is swollen and the contours are not seen due to enormous articular fluid formation (**a**). During surgical treatment of acute bacterial arthritis, the thickened, red synovial membrane with edematous villi is being removed (**b**)

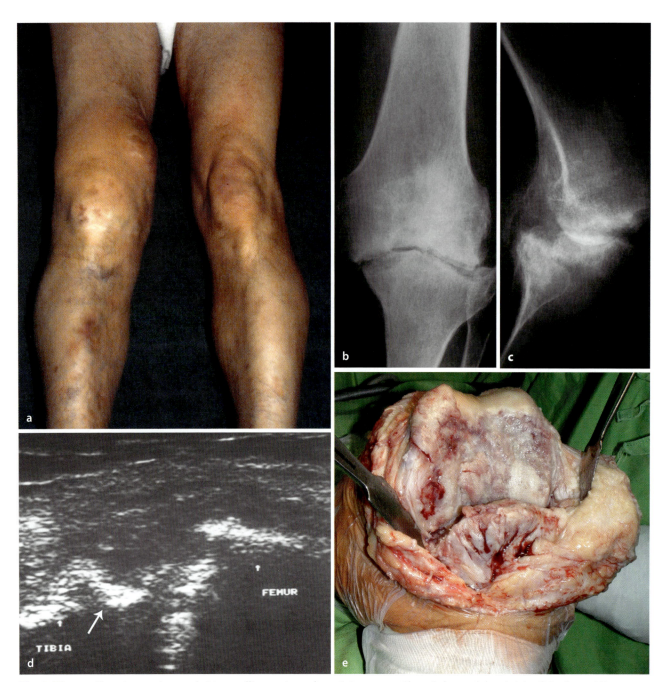

Fig. 2.51 a–e Chronic purulent arthritis: swelling, pain and limited range of motion of the right knee due to bacterial infection and articular destruction (**a**). AP (**b**) and lateral (**c**) view radiographs reveal secondary osteoarthritis of the same patient due to chronic bacterial arthritis: there are secondary osteoarthritic changes, such as subchondral sclerosis, osteophytes, subchondral cyst formation, narrowing of joint space. Chronic bacterial arthritis of the knee: Ultrasonography (**d**) detecting the well visible irregular, rough surface of the medial tibia and femur (*arrow*) The same patient at surgical exposure: the intraoperative picture illustrates serious destruction of cartilage surface of the knee, with osteophytes, edematous soft tissues (**e**)

2.4 Iatrogenic Infections

The range of iatrogenic infections following orthopedic surgical procedures is wide. The less severe condition is a delayed wound healing, seroma formation. More serious complication is the inflammation of the surgical site caused by bacteria (mostly by members of the skin flora) with induration, high fever and pus formation in the deeper soft tissue layers. In total hip and knee arthroplasty, the infection rate is about 0.55–1.27% depending on the design of the surgical theatre, laminar airflow system, antibiotic prophylactic regime, use of antibiotic bone cement, etc.

Bacterial infection around orthopedic implants is one of the most severe complications in orthopedic surgery following arthroplasty. The most important agents are *Staphylococci* (both coagulase-negative and *Staphylococcus aureus*), which are responsible for the infections in about 50% of all cases. The infected implant or other device may become loosened, and the pus produced around the foreign material may come through the skin, causing a draining sinus.

The clinical symptoms of an infected orthopedic implant are pain, limited function of the prosthetic joint, erythema in the involved region, subfebrility, elevated levels of C-reactive protein, erythrocyte sedimentation rate and WBC counts. In case of discharging sinuses fistulography is a useful tool (Figs. 2.52–2.60).

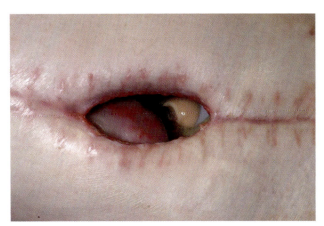

Fig. 2.53 Huge discharging sinus and large skin defect with the total hip implant and green-yellowish pus in the hip joint. If the purulent joint is open, usually no fever is measured (courtesy of Dr. J. Wodtke, Endo-Klinik, Hamburg, Germany)

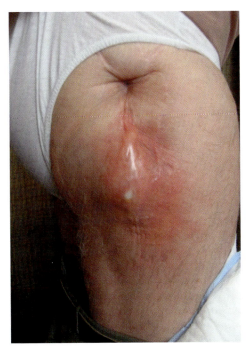

Fig. 2.52 Local signs of inflammation: erythema and induration in the right gluteal region several years following total hip arthroplasty. The pus is about to brake through the skin. The patient had systemic symptoms like fever, too

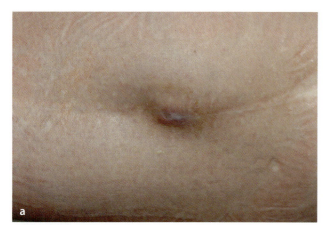

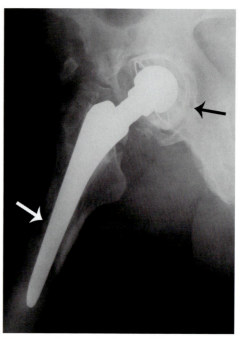

Fig. 2.55 Bacterial infection following total hip replacement. The signs of septic loosening are seen: cortical destruction, para-articular ossification, discreet radiolucent layer between cement and bone surfaces (*black arrow*). The diaphysis at the tip of the prosthesis shaft is blown up and there is a cortical destruction of the femur as sign of septic loosening (*white arrow*)

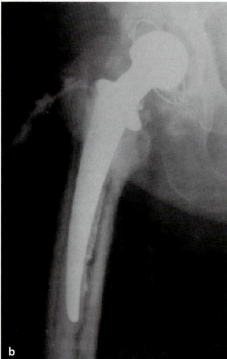

Fig. 2.54 a, b Small discharging sinus following total hip arthroplasty. In this case, fistulography is indicated to see the way of pus running out of the wound (**a**). Fistulography: the radiopaque fluid shows the way of pus through the discharging sinus, which is in direct connection with the infected joint. Note the radiolucency around the entire implant (**b**)

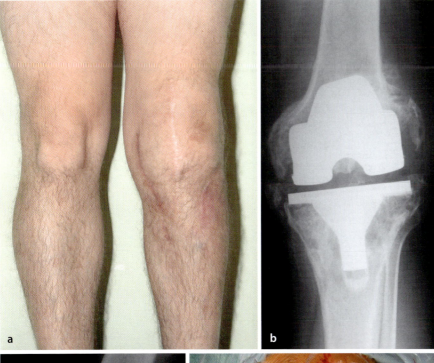

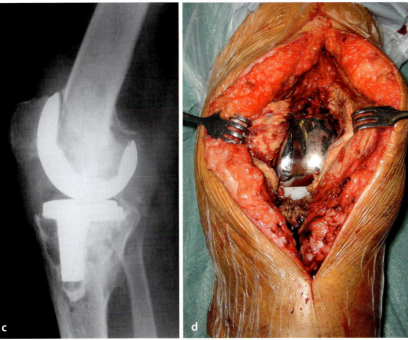

Fig. 2.56 a–d The photograph reveals a chronic infection in the knee following total knee arthroplasty. Several surgical scars are seen; the skin has a red color and the joint is swollen (**a**). The radiographs (**b, c**) show septic loosening of a total knee replacement. In the anteroposterior aspect (**b**) the femoral component is tilted and paraarticular ossification is seen as a sign of septic complication. The lateral view (**c**) represents huge osteolytic changes around the implants. The connection between the implant and the host bone is disturbed by bacterial pseudomembrane. Surgical exposure of the same patient: the implant is covered by slime, produced by coagulase-negative Staphylococci. The soft tissues of the joint are also covered by pyogenic pseudomembrane (**d**)

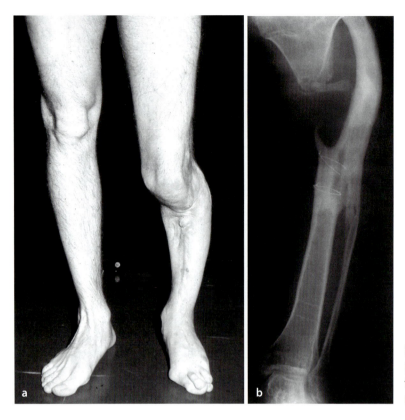

Fig. 2.57 a, b Septic defect tibial non-union (pseudoarticulation) with a severe deformity of the leg and limb length discrepancy (**a**). On the radiograph large bone defect is observed (**b**)

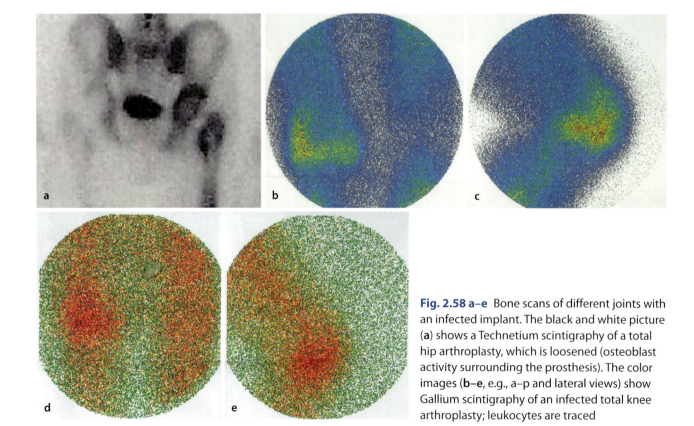

Fig. 2.58 a–e Bone scans of different joints with an infected implant. The black and white picture (**a**) shows a Technetium scintigraphy of a total hip arthroplasty, which is loosened (osteoblast activity surrounding the prosthesis). The color images (**b–e**, e.g., a–p and lateral views) show Gallium scintigraphy of an infected total knee arthroplasty; leukocytes are traced

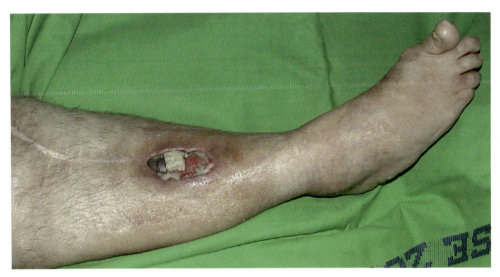

Fig. 2.59 Tumor endopros-thesis was implanted after resection of the proximal tibia. Huge skin defect showing the implant and bone junction. There was a polymicrobal infection, which could only be treated with amputation

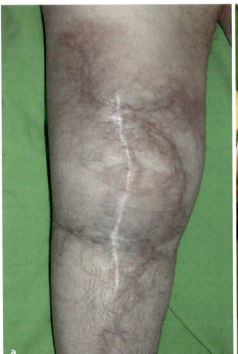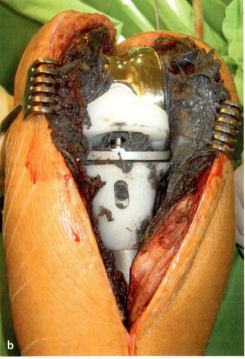

Fig. 2.60 a, b In this case a modular tumor knee endo-prosthesis was infected and metallosis occurred (metal particles in the joint fluid from the implant). The metal particles are transported by phagocytes through the lymphatic vessels; the skin has a grayish color (**a**). After surgical exposure the synovial membrane has a black color, it is full with wear particles (**b**)

Chapter 3
Rheumatoid Arthritis and Related Diseases

Contents

Rheumatoid Arthritis and Related Diseases

I. Böröcz and M. Szendrői

3.1 Rheumatoid Arthritis, Early and Late Stage

Rheumatoid arthritis (RA) is a chronic, progressive polyarticular inflammation of unknown origin, with autoimmune pathomechanism, causes destruction of joints and severe disability, often accompanied by extraarticular changes. Serological signs are the presence of rheuma factor and antifilaggrin positivity.

Incidence of RA is approximately 1% of the adult population, may start in any age, mostly between 35 and 55 years. The female–male proportion is 3:1. Often increased familial occurrence is present; HLA-Dr4 tissue antigen is detectable at 50% of patients. Extrinsic factors are also needed apart from the genetical issues for the development of the disease.

To diagnose RA, criteria of the American Rheuma Association (ARA) are used. The simplified varieties are (1) Morning joint stiffness (minimally 1 h, lasting for more than 6 weeks), (2) arthritis (minimally three areas of joints, lasting for more than 6 weeks), (3) arthritis of hand joints (lasting for more than 6 weeks), (4) symmetrical arthritis lasting for more than 6 weeks, (5) rheumatoid nodule, (6) elevated serum rheumatoid factor, and (7) radiological changes (marginal erosions or striped osteoporosis). RA is considered "confirmed," if at least four criteria are fulfilled.

Progress of the disease is characterized by Steinbrocker's functional and anatomical stages.

Anatomical stages are (1) Early, (2) Moderately severe, (3) Severe and (4) Endstage.

Various stages can be present at the same time on the same patient (Figs. 3.1–3.20).

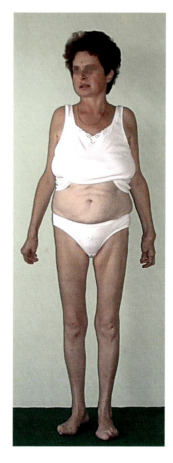

Fig. 3.1 Early stage of RA in a female patient: Typical, symmetrical hand and feet deformities, bilateral mild knee swelling

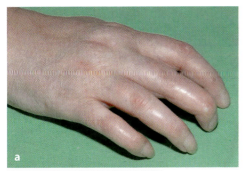

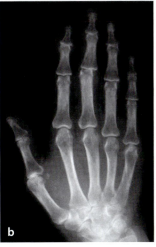

Fig. 3.2 a, b Suspect for early RA, fusiform swelling on the fingers (**a**); radiograph shows striped periarticular atrophy of the phalanxes (**b**)

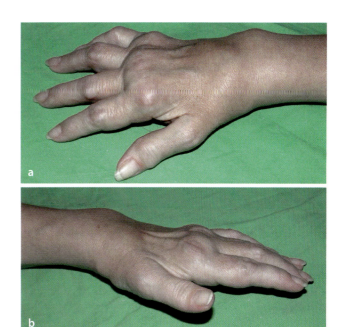

Fig. 3.4 a, b Moderately severe typical RA deformities of the hand. Metacarpophalangeal (*MCP*), proximal interphalangeal (*PIP*) and wrist swelling, synovitis, mild ulnar deviation of fingers (**a**). Atrophy of the intrinsic muscles (**b**)

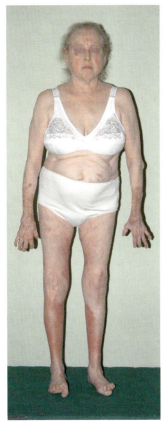

Fig. 3.3 Symptoms of a severe RA case. This female patient has been suffering from RA for 20 years. Note the altered face due to the steroid treatment, the typical hand and foot deformities

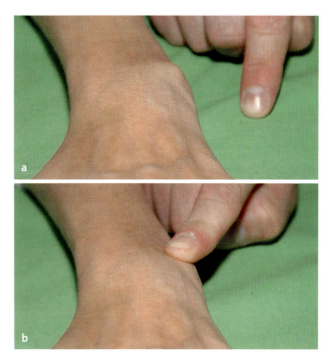

Fig. 3.5 a, b Synovitis of the radioulnar joint, tendon of the extensor carpi ulnaris slides in palmar direction, and the ulnar head dislocates dorsally (**a**). It can be reduced with moderate pressure, but as soon as the pressure is released it returns to the dislocated position: "piano-key" sign (**b**)

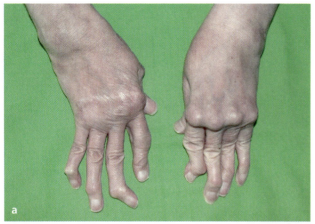

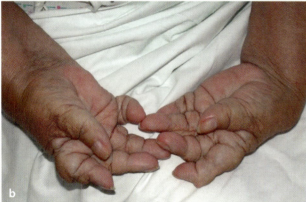

Fig. 3.6 a, b Bilateral severe hand and wrist deformities. Typical swan-neck deformity on the hands: PIP joints in extension, distal interphalangeal (*DIP*) joints in flexion. On the index finger typical buttonhole deformity: PIP joints in flexion, DIP joints in extension. MCP joints are subluxed (**a**). Disorganization of all the joints of the hands results in a mutilans form (**b**)

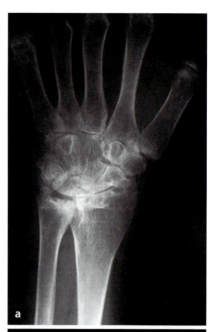

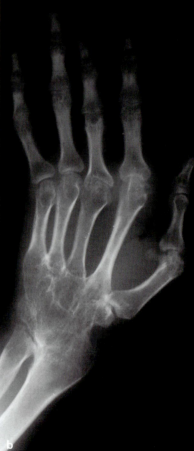

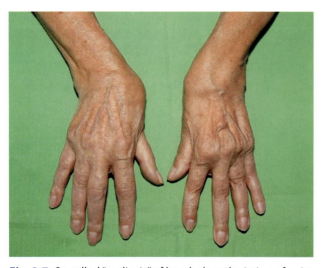

Fig. 3.7 So called "scoliosis" of hand, ulnar deviation of wrist

Fig. 3.8 a, b X-ray appearance of moderately severe and severe wrist changes. Ulnar epiphysis is destroyed, decreased radiocarpal and intercarpal joint spaces (**a**). As end result the wrist is ankylosed, the bones of the carpus are fused creating a single bone (os carpi) (**b**)

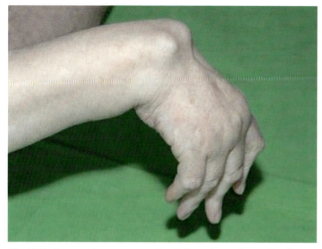

Fig. 3.9 Severe, late stage wrist deformity, palmar displacement, tear of the extensor tendons ("dropped fingers"). The carpus is dislocated palmar below the radius

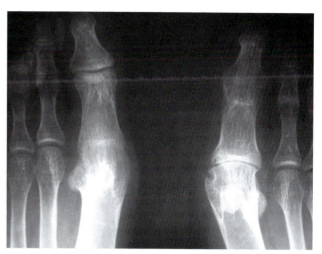

Fig. 3.11 Early diagnostic sign is in RA the marginal, subchondral erosion visible on the distal end of the first metatarsal bone. On the other side spontaneous ankylosis in the MP joint is visible. Various radiological stages can be present at the same time on the same patient

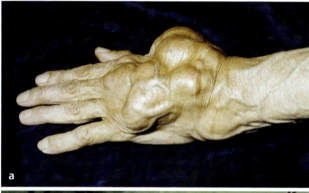

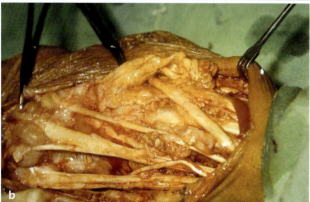

Fig. 3.10 a, b Extensor tenosynovitis (**a**). Intraoperative picture: The hypertrophic synovial tissue is visible penetrating into the tendons (**b**). The hypertrophic synovial tissue and its enzymes damage the ligaments and the tendons running in their sheets. This is the mechanism of development of the joint deformities, subluxations, tendon ruptures

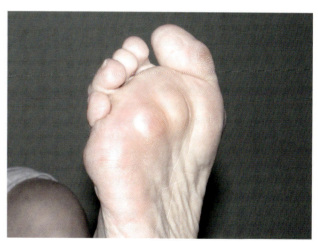

Fig. 3.12 Chronic bursitis, metatarsophalangeal (*MTP*) joint synovitis induced swellings under the dropped metatarsal heads cause severe metatarsalgia

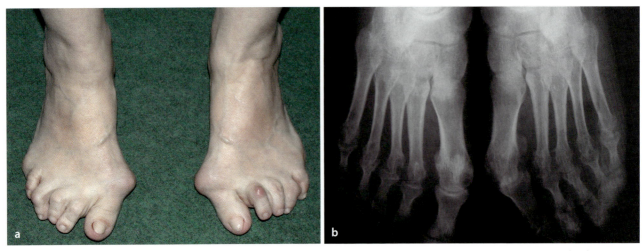

Fig. 3.13 a, b Severe forefoot deformities and flat foot. Hallux valgus and hammer toes, MTP destruction, and flat foot. Lateral deviation of toes (**a**). X-ray confirms fibular deviation of toes, MTP destruction, and erosions (**b**)

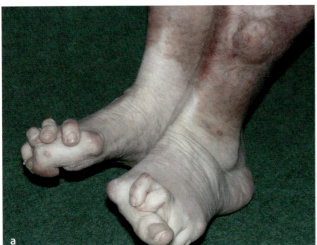
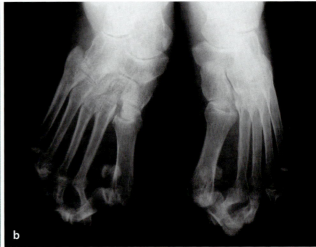

Fig. 3.14 a, b In RA skin hyperpigmentation or pigment loss is characteristic. Atrophy of skin is effected by the disease or steroid treatment. Skin ulcers also occur due to the vasculitis, the scar after the ulcer cured can be seen with severe forefoot deformities and the hind foot in valgus position in the subtalar joint (**a**). X-ray shows severe subluxations and luxations in MTP and PIP joints (**b**)

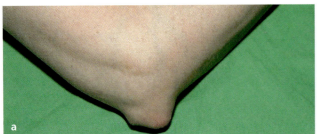
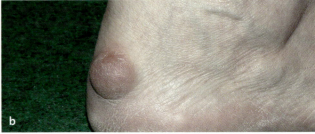

Fig. 3.15 a, b Typical rheumatoid nodules in typical locations: Over the olecranon (**a**) and Achilles tendon (**b**). The nodules appear mainly subcutan at the extensor sides of the limbs on areas subjected to pressure. Their size can extend from the size of rice to walnut. Sometimes they start to drain, get infected, and difficult to cure (fistulous rheumatism)

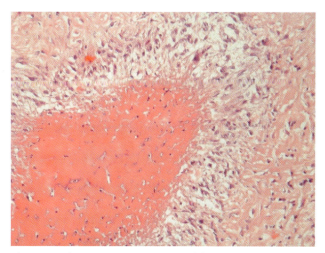

Fig. 3.16 The microscopic picture of rheumatoid nodule is of diagnostic value. Central necrotic area with peripheral histiocytic pallisading

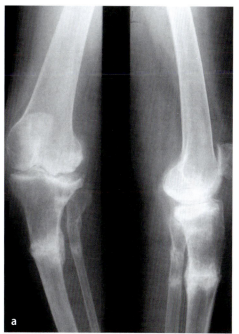

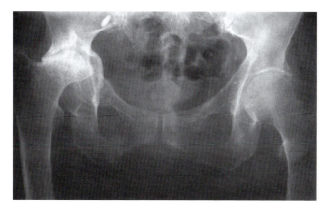

Fig. 3.17 The basic disease, steroid treatment, and inactivity induced osteoporosis result often in secondary hip protrusion, definitely thinner acetabular wall. Femoral head necrosis developed in the right hip, note crush, and deformity of the femoral head, which could be the result of steroid treatment and/or vasculitis

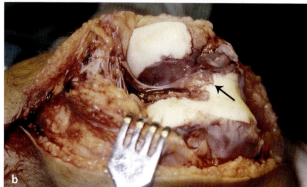

Fig. 3.18 a, b Milkman fracture on tibia and fibula with valgus deformity of the knee (**a**), both are common in RA. Intraoperative picture: Extremely hypertrophic synovium, filling up the intercondylar space, the pannus invades the cartilage surface (*arrow*) (**b**). The proliferative synovial pannus destroys the cartilage partly mechanically, partly by its enzymes. The high intraarticular pressure expands the joint capsule causing pain and joint laxity and leads to muscle atrophy via reflexes

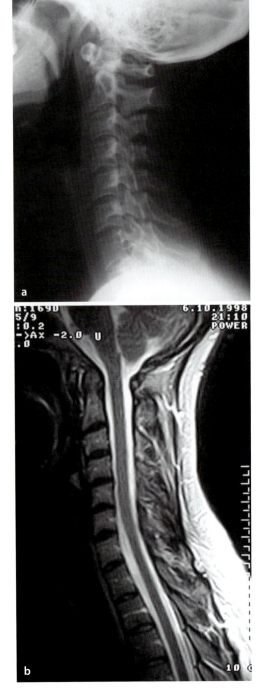

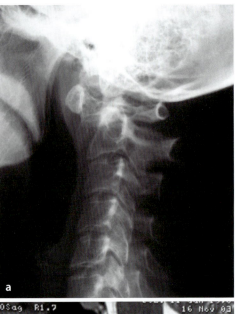

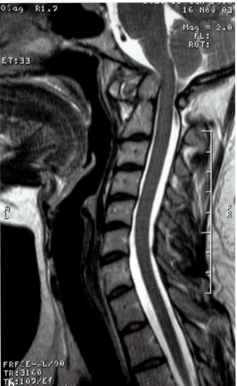

Fig. 3.19 a, b X-ray (**a**) and MR (**b**) in early stage of RA. Incipient atlanto-axial synovitis with moderate subluxation. MR shows normal liquor space around the spinal cord, cordal involvement is not present

Fig. 3.20 a, b X-ray (**a**) and MRI (**b**) in late stage of RA. Severe atlanto-axial synovitis and subluxation, luxation (dorsal and cranial displacement), spinal cord compression. Sudden death of RA patients is often caused by cord compression by the dens. When the distance between the posterior wall of the dens and anterior wall of the posterior arch of the atlas is 14 mm or less, indication of surgery is established regardless of neurological signs. Neurological signs generally are not reversible

3.2 Juvenile Idiopathic Arthritis

Juvenile Idiopathic Arthritis (JIA) is the most common heterogeneous connective tissue disease of childhood, which leads to severe disability and blindness in a number of cases. Diagnosis can be established if according to criteria at least one joint inflammation is present for minimum 3 months and other illnesses causing arthritis (e.g., infection, trauma, hematological disorders, neoplasia, hemophilia, psychogenic rheumatism) are excluded Incidence: 1–2: 10,000 child. This illness may start from age of some month to 16 years, most common between 1–3 and 8–12 years. Girls are more likely to suffer. In the first 6 months JIA can be classified to three well-defined subtypes: (1) systemic 25–30%, (2) polyarticular 30% (more than five joints are involved), and (3) oligoarticular 40–45% (four or less joints are involved) (Figs. 3.21–3.29).

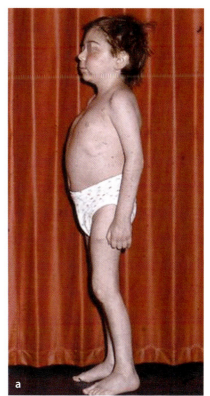

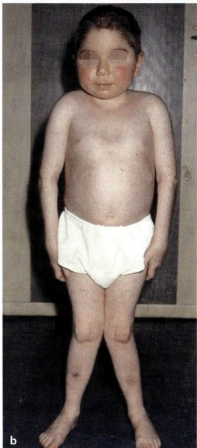

Fig. 3.21 a, b Typical JIA general growth disturbance is present most frequently in systemic and polyarticular types. Note side effects of steroid treatment and the common valgus deformity of the knees (**a, b**)

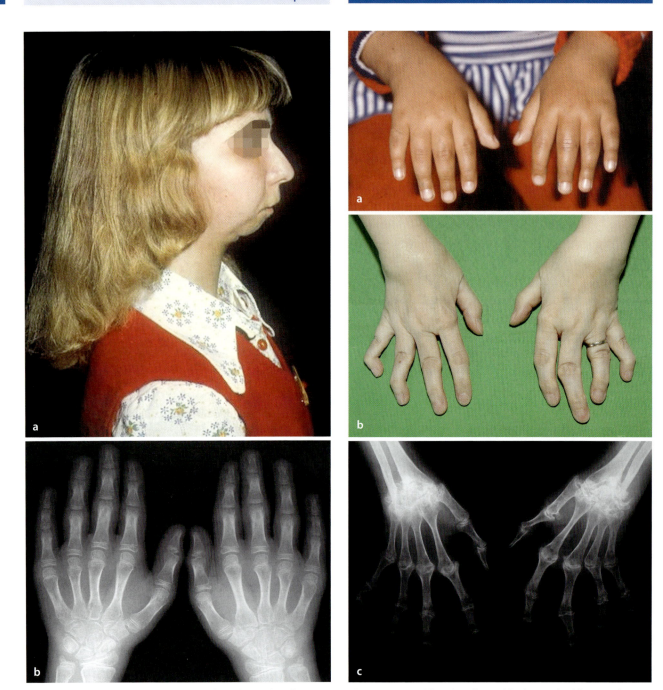

Fig. 3.22 a, b Characteristic growth disorder is also the micrognathia (**a**) and short metacarpals (**b**)

Fig. 3.23 a–c Often hardly visible, but palpable in early stage of JIA swelling of the small joints of the hand (**a**). Later on the disease progresses and a mutilating destruction of the small joints of the hand and wrist develops like in this case of a 22-year-old woman (**b**) and (**c**)

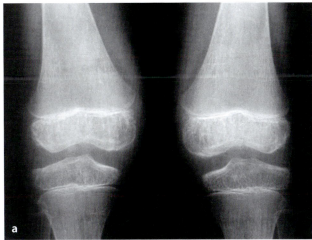

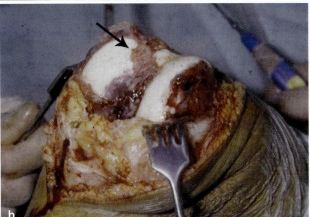

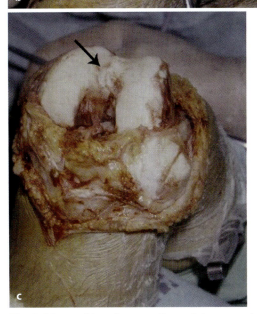

Fig. 3.24 a–c JIA early stage. X-ray: Joint space intact (**a**). Cartilages of the children are thicker and more resistant than the adults. Intraoperative picture of the same patient demonstrates obvious synovial proliferation and pannus formation (**b**, *arrow*). In early stage under the pannus the cartilage could be intact (**c**, *arrow*)

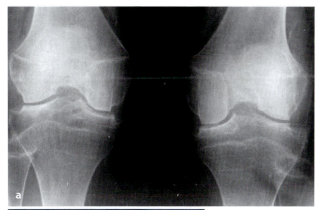

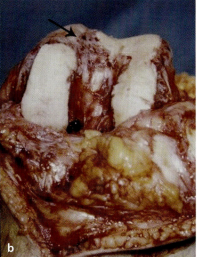

Fig. 3.25 a, b More advanced stage radiograph presents narrow joint space, subchondral erosions (**a**). After removal of extreme proliferation of synovial membrane and pannus, the subchondral bone is visible instead of cartilage (**b**) (*arrow*)

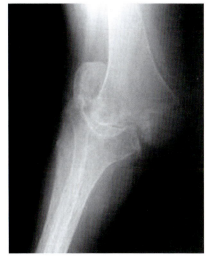

Fig. 3.26 Late stage, severe knee joint deformity, subluxation, extreme valgus deformity

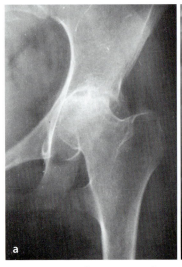
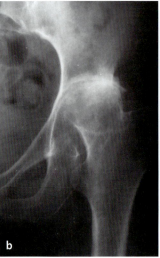
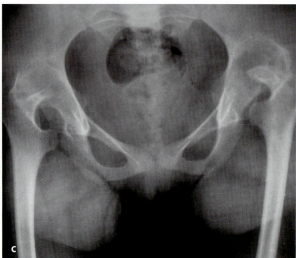

Fig. 3.27 a–c Characteristic features are the short femoral neck and relatively large greater and lesser trochanter (the synovitis caused earlier closure of the growing plate of the femoral neck of a 14-year-old female patient) (**a**). Other typical changes are the valgus neck and central cranial migration (**b**). The extreme small sizes due to the growing disturbance and bilateral serious destruction and proximal migration of the femoral heads are characteristic for serious cases. This patient was 17-year-old only (**c**)

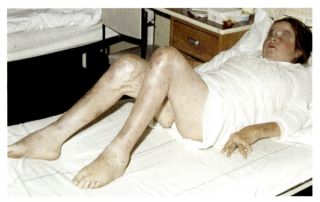

Fig. 3.28 Hip and knee ankylosis with severe flexion deformity, hand deformity, and skin signs of steroid treatment; striates are present in a 21-years-old female JIA patient

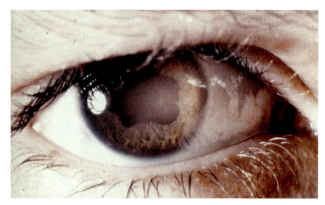

Fig. 3.29 Slit-lamp picture of iridocyclitis, which frequently accompanies JIA, difficult to detect, and often ends up in blindness

3.3 Ankylosing Spondylitis

Ankylosing spondylitis (AS) (Marie-Strümpell disease, Bechterew's disease, pelvospondylitis ossificans) is an inflammatory disease of unknown etiology characterized by ascending and progressive inflammation of spinal joints and adjacent structures, with bony fusion of the spine in the end stage. In one third of cases, hips and shoulders may become involved, and less frequently, inflammatory lesions of extraarticular organs such as eye and heart may occur. AS is characterized by a close association with the HLA-B27 antigen, which is found in more than 90% of the patients. Male/Female frequency: 3–5/1, age at onset range from adolescence to age 35 years, peak around 28 years. Incidence of AS is approximately 6.6/100,000 population. Modified New York criteria for the diagnosis of AS: (1) Low-back pain of more than 3 months' duration/improved by exercise and not relieved by rest, (2) Limitation of movement of lumbar spine in sagittal and frontal planes, (3) Chest expansion decreased relative to normal values for age and sex, and (4) Bilateral sacroileitis, grade 2–4, or unilateral sacroileitis, grade 3–4 (Figs. 3.30–3.38).

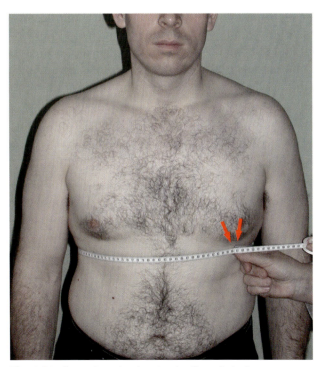

Fig. 3.30 Apart from back pain, the first clinical symptom in the AS, limited chest expansion, less than 1 in. at forced inhale

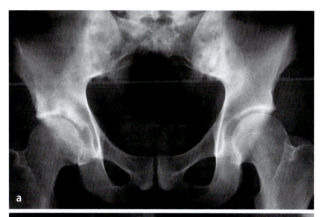

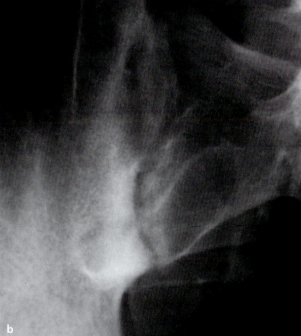

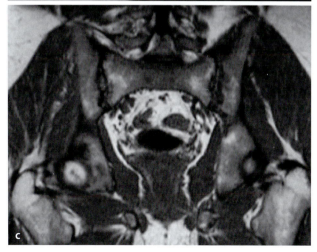

Fig. 3.31 a–c Radiograph of the pelvis reveals bilateral grade 2–3 sacroileitis (**a**). Radiograph focused to the right sacroiliac joint (**b**) and MRI (**c**): Grade 2 moderate sacroileitis with sclerosis and erosions

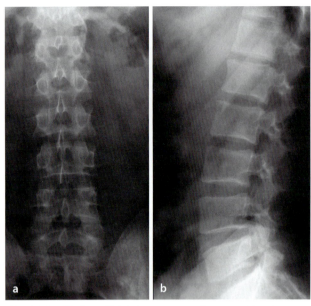

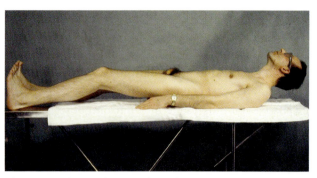

Fig. 3.33 Advanced stage of AS: The entire spine is stiff and ankylosed. The patient can not turn his head or rest it on the flat examining table

Fig. 3.32 a, b Sacroileitis but apparently normal lumbar vertebral column

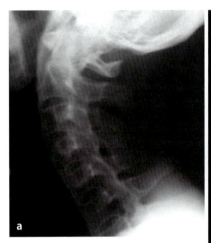

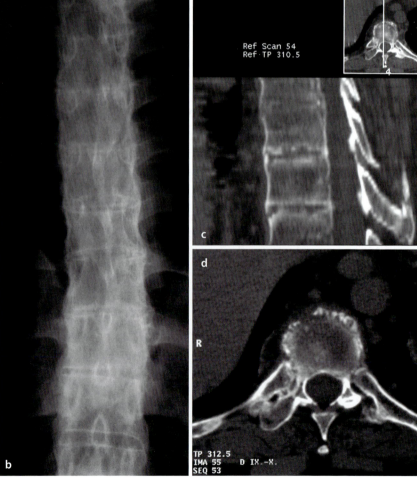

Fig. 3.34 a–d Bony fusion of the cervical spine (**a**). Typical "bamboo" appearance of the thoracic vertebral column (**b**). Reconstruction CT picture reveals erosions of the end-plates of the vertebral bodies and marginal syndesmophytes (**c**). CT scan of a thoracic vertebra with bony fusion of the costovertebral joint (**d**)

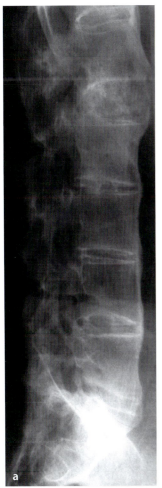

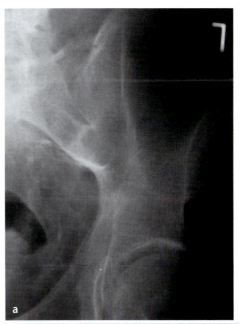

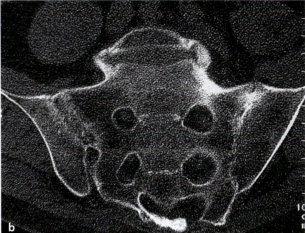

Fig. 3.36 a, b Ankylosis of the left sacroiliac joint (**a**). CT scan of the partly ankylosed sacroiliac joints (**b**)

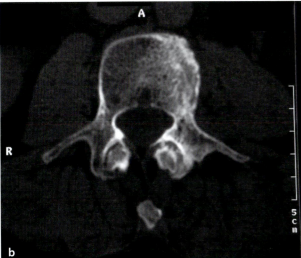

Fig. 3.35 a, b Lateral radiograph of the lumbar spine in AS. Typical marginal syndesmophytes (**a**). CT scan of the lumbar spine: Bony union of the lumbar facet joints (**b**)

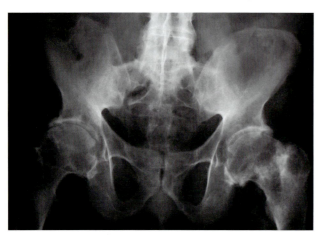

Fig. 3.37 Radiograph of pelvis affected by AS: Ankylosis of sacroiliac joints, bony ankylosis of the apophyseal joints, and ossification of the interspinous ligaments, so-called "trolley-track" sign; in about one-third of the AS cases sever bilateral osteoarthritis of the hips occur, which can progress to a spontaneous ankylosis of the hips

3.4 Psoriatic Arthritis

Psoriatic arthritis is one form of seronegative spondylarthritis (SNSA) involving combinations of a number of organs. Psoriatic changes of skin and nails appear along with polyarthritis. The skin changes usually precede the joint manifestations, but can happen vice-versa ("arthritis psoriatica sine psoriasis"). Polyarthritis is erosive, destructive, and involves most commonly the DIP joints. Often occurs with sacroileitis and/or spondylitis.

Incidence of psoriasis vulgaris is 0.5–2%; out of this population 5–10% suffer joint involvement. Familial accumulation is characteristic. The disease appears between 30 and 50 years of age, women get it earlier, but the gender proportion is equal. HLAB27 antigen is positive only on cases of spinal spread.

Diagnosis of psoriatic arthritis is established in presence of skin or nail psoriasis and seronegative arthritis. Destructive arthritis of distal joints may be manifest in so-called sausage fingers. Enthesopathia is common, presenting usually on the plantar surface of the heel and at the attachment of Achilles tendon (Figs. 3.39–3.42).

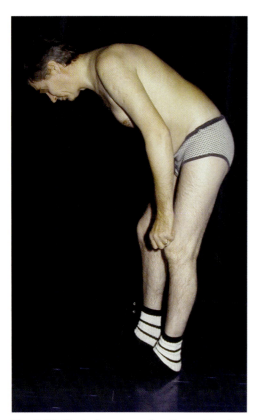

Fig. 3.38 Typical posture of patient with advanced AS: Cervical fixation in flexion, pronounced dorsal kyphosis, involution of the chest, and compensatory flexion of the knees. At insufficient physiotherapy management, the patient neck and trunk is fixed in a fully bent position, so that he can not see ahead

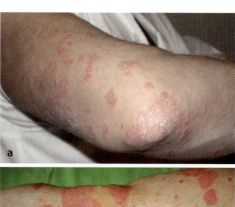

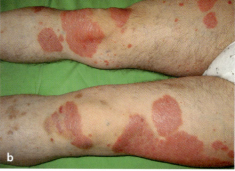

Fig. 3.39 a, b Typical psoriatic skin lesions in the characteristic locations. Well-defined erythematosus papulae and plaques covered with silver–gray lamellae. Most commonly involves the hairy area of the skull and the extensor surfaces of the limbs

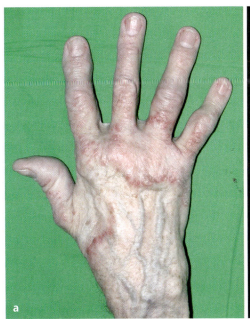

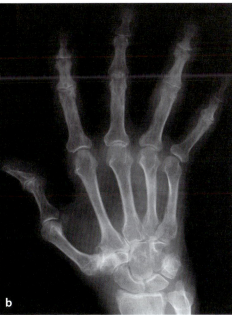

Fig. 3.40 a, b Hand and nail psoriasis (**a**) and typical DIP joint changes (**b**). Nail changes are present in 30% in cases of psoriasis vulgaris, this proportion in psoriatic arthritis exceeds 80%

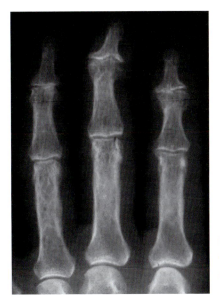

Fig. 3.41 Distal interphalangeal joint involvement and periostitis

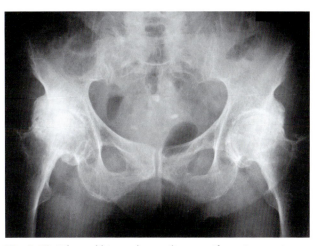

Fig. 3.42 Bilateral hip and sacroiliac manifestation, periosteal reaction at sciatic bone, "beard feature," enthesopathia are characteristic for psoriatic arthritis

Chapter 4

Neurogenic Osteoarthropathy (Charcot's Joint)

Contents

Neurogenic Osteoarthropathy (Charcot's Joint)

A. Deli and M. Szendrői

Neurogenic osteoarthropathy can be defined as the bone and joint changes that occur secondary to loss of sensation and accompany a variety of disorders. Charcot first described the relationship between loss of sensation and arthropathy in 1868.

The pathophysiology of the disease is that the loss of proprioception and deep sensation result in recurrent trauma, and ultimately lead to progressive destruction. Another theory postulates that neurally mediated vascular reflex results in hyperemia, which can cause osteoclast bone resorption.

Charcot's joint is associated with some degenerative diseases of the spinal cord and other peripheral neuropathies, including syringomyelia, tabes dorsalis, diabetes mellitus, transverse myelitis, traumatic paralysis, spinal dysraphism, and alcohol abuse (late stage with peripheral neuropathy).

4.1 Syringomyelia

Syringomyelia is a generic term referring to a disorder in which a cyst or tubular cavity forms within the spinal cord. This syrinx expands and elongates over time, destroying the center of the spinal cord. This damage results in pain, weakness, and stiffness in the neck, back, shoulders, arms or legs, and other symptoms (e.g., headaches and loss of the ability to feel extremes of hot or cold, especially in the hands) (Figs. 4.1–4.7)

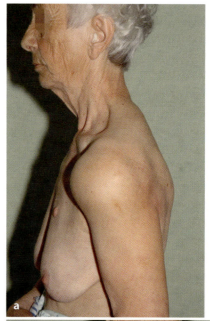

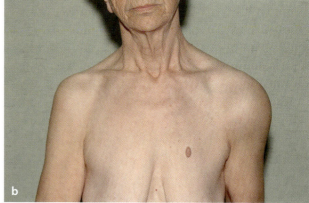

Fig. 4.1 a, b Photographs of a patient with syringomyelia. Note the significantly enlarged left shoulder joint and upper part of the arm. In syringomyelia, neuropathic changes are common in the shoulder joint, followed by the elbow and wrist. Symptoms are due to spinal cord damage; decreased sensation of touch and pain, weakness, and loss of muscle tissue

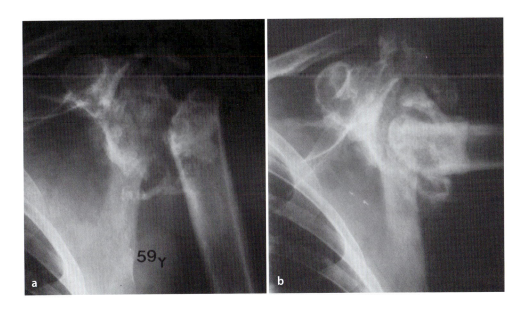

Fig. 4.2 a, b Neuropathic arthropathy of shoulder in a patient with syringomyelia demonstrated on radiographs. Note the extensive destruction of the bones adjacent to the shoulder, and extensive calcification in the soft tissues, which are pathognomic for a neuropathic joint

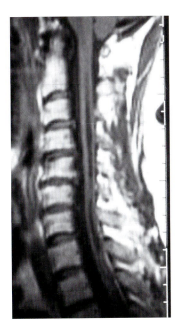

Fig. 4.3 The MRI finding – the syrinx formation in the cervical cord – confirms the correct diagnosis of syringomyelia

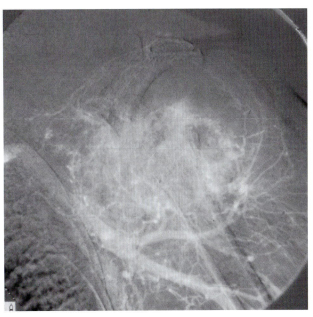

Fig. 4.4 Digital subtractive angiography demonstrates hypervascularization in the parenchymal phase around the glenohumeral joint

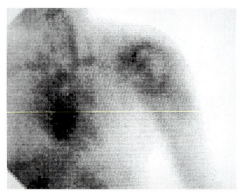

Fig. 4.5 Bone scintigraphy: increased isotope uptake above periarticular ossification

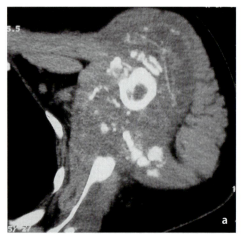

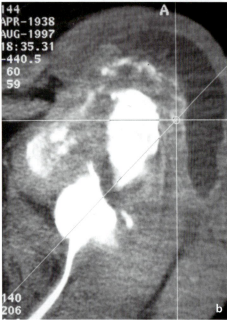

4.6 a, b CT scan shows destroyed humeral head and disorganized gleno-humeral joint, ossification in the soft tissues (**a**). Subdeltoid bursa is also visualized, filled with fluid (**b**)

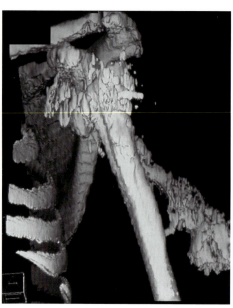

Fig. 4.7 3D CT visualizes better the destruction of the shoulder joint and the extensive soft tissue ossification

4.2 Arthropathy in Tabes: Syphilitic Myelopathy

Tabes dorsalis is the slowly progressive degeneration of the spinal cord that occurs in the tertiary phase of syphilis, a decade or more after originally contracting the infection. Among the serious features of tabes dorsalis are lancinating lightning-like pain, ataxia, deterioration of the optical nerves leading to blindness, urinary incontinence, loss of sense of position, and degeneration of the joints (Charcot's joint).

Neuropathic arthropathy is seen in 10–20% of patients with tabes dorsalis (Figs. 4.8–4.10).

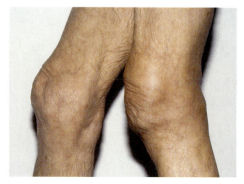

Fig. 4.8 The joints of the lower extremity (hip and knee) are commonly affected in patients with tabes dorsalis

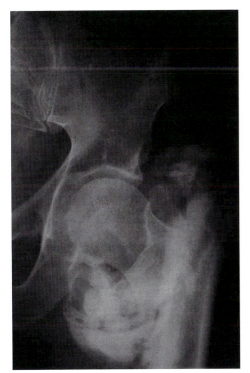

Fig. 4.9 Disorganization of the hip joints with soft tissue ossification in a patient with tabes dorsalis (courtesy of Dr. H.W. Wouters, Utrecht, Holland)

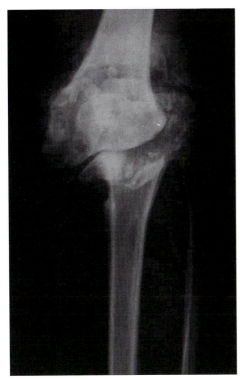

Fig. 4.10 Extensive destruction and subluxation of the knee joint, and massive periarticular ossification (courtesy of Dr. H.W. Wouters, Utrecht, Holland)

4.3 Alcoholic Arthropathy

Neuropathic arthropathy due to chronic alcohol abuse commonly involves the metatarsophalangeal, interphalangeal joints with dislocation of the midtarsal bones (Lisfranc joint). Besides impaired sensitivity, severe arthropathy can develop without major pain and with considerable swelling, causing significant destruction (Figs. 4.11–4.15).

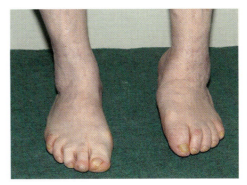

Fig. 4.11 Swollen and deformed ankle and left foot of an alcoholic patient

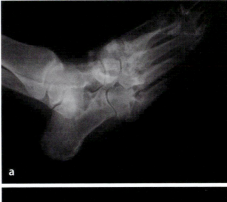

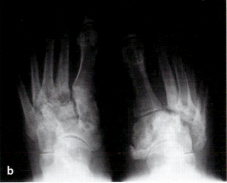

Fig. 4.12 a, b Lateral view of the foot shows extensive destruction of the tarsal bones (Lisfranc joint) (**a**).The a–p radiograph reveals the affected tarsal bones of both mid-foot. Note the dislocation of the metatarsal bones in the Lisfranc joint with widening of the first intermetatarsal space of the right foot (**b**)

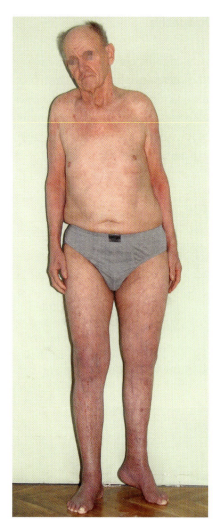

Fig. 4.13 Patient with a history of chronic alcohol abuse. Note the shortened left lower extremity, the skin pigmentation, and color due to the circulatory abnormality, polyneuropathy. The distal involvement of the limbs may be associated with severe destruction of the large joints

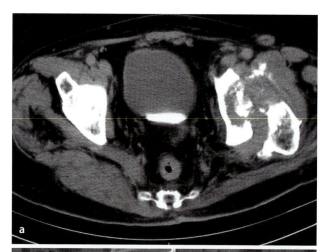

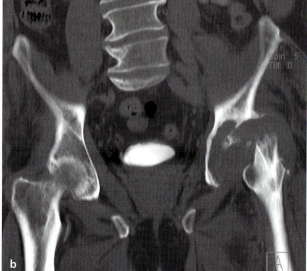

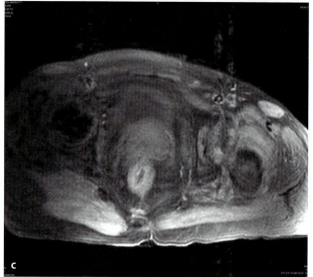

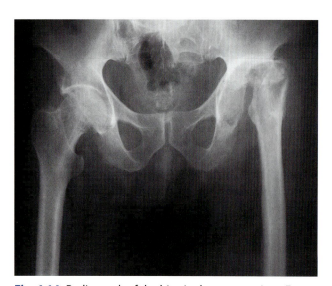

Fig. 4.14 Radiograph of the hips in the same patient. Extensively destructed left hip joint with disappearance of the femoral head

Fig. 4.15 a–c CT (**a**), reconstruction CT (**b**) pictures reveal the disorganization of the femoral head and calcification in extensive connective tissue formation, which is best assessed by MRI (**c**)

4.4 Reflex Sympathetic Dystrophy

4.4.1 Algodystrophy, Sudeck syndrome

Algodystrophy is a colorful combination of clinical signs and symptoms, including pain, tenderness, hyperesthesia, vasomotor changes, and swelling of the distal part of the limb involved.

The etiology is often trauma, occasionally other diseases neurological, rheumatologic conditions, metabolic diseases, drugs and alcohol abuse, direct tissue damage (due to burning, frost, irradiation) are the causative factors. The inappropriate immobilization after minor injuries and the personality of the patient (psychological changes) are also contributive factors.

Disturbance of circulation (precapillary sphincter spasm, opening of arteriovenous shunts, capillary stasis) develops following neurogen stimulus; then metabolic changes (acidosis, activation of osteoclasts, consecutive osteoporosis) progress.

Algodystrophy often involves the foot as well as the hand. In case of upper limb involvement, it may result in restricted range of motion of the ipsilateral shoulder (hand–shoulder syndrome).

Clinical stages: Acute, dystrophic, and atrophic stage (Figs. 4.16–4.20).

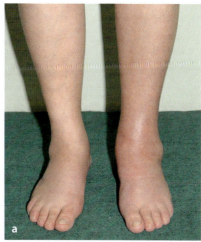

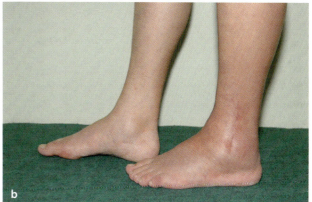

Fig. 4.17a, b This patient was operated for a left ankle fracture (*note the scar formation*). The RSD appeared during immobilization in the plaster

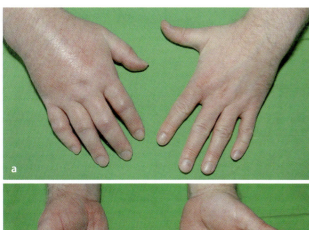

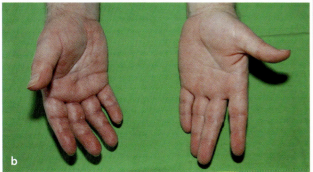

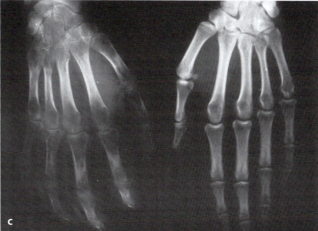

Fig. 4.16 a–c Photograph presents a patient with acute stage of the RSD. Right hand is swollen; there is an evidence of vasodilatation, causing warmth, redness of the skin, marked joint stiffness (**a**, **b**). At the beginning of the acute stage, there are no characteristic alterations on the radiograph. Two months later, a characteristic patchy osteoporosis developed in the bones of the hand of previous patient (**c**)

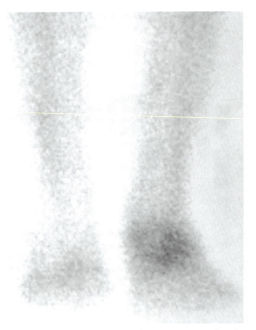

Fig. 4.18 The bone scan shows increased radioisotope uptake of the tarsal bones in the acute stage

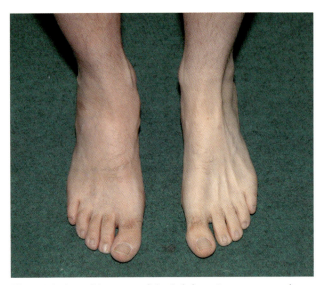

Fig. 4.19 Atrophic stage of the left foot. Symptoms and signs: Pain extends proximally on the limb involved. Note the atrophy of the skin, subcutaneous tissue and general soft tissue, flexion contracture of the joint

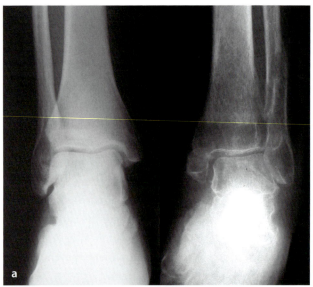

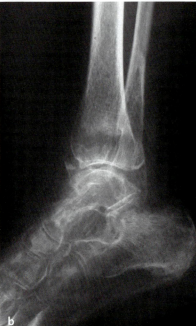

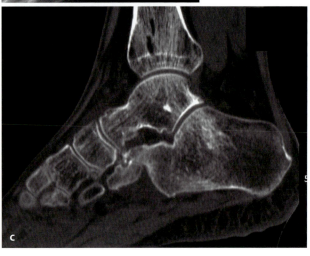

Fig. 4.20 a–c Radiographs of the same patient: Note the diffuse osteoporotic changes of the bones on the left compared to the opposite side (**a**), diffuse and patchy loss of bone density (**b**) in the tarsal bones. Reconstruction CT picture reveals osteoporosis, lytic areas, and thickened scarce bony trabeculae (**c**)

Chapter 5

Stress Fractures (Fatigue Fractures, Marsh-Fractures)

Stress Fractures (Fatigue Fractures, Marsh-Fractures)

M. Szendrői

In consequence of cyclic long-continued or oft-repeated stress like prolonged walking, dancing, or running, infraction or complete fracture can develop on certain sites of the skeleton. There is no specific single causative injury in the history, like in trauma-related fractures. It occurs mostly in two groups of young adults: in those who are not accustomed to sudden physical activity (fresh recruits in the army, etc.) or professional sportsmen with overestimated training programs. Ninety five percent of stress fracture occur in the bones of the lower extremity, most often in the tibia (30–35%, e.g., middistance runners), fibula (20–25%, e.g., ballet dancing, walking, aerobics), in the metatarsal bones (20%, e.g., marching, walking, tennis), femur (10–15%, e.g., ballet, athletics), or pelvis (4–8%, e.g., athletics), but it can affect many other sites, too. Leading symptom is the tenderness above the fracture and pain, which increases at physical activity and decreases at rest (Figs. 5.1–5.6).

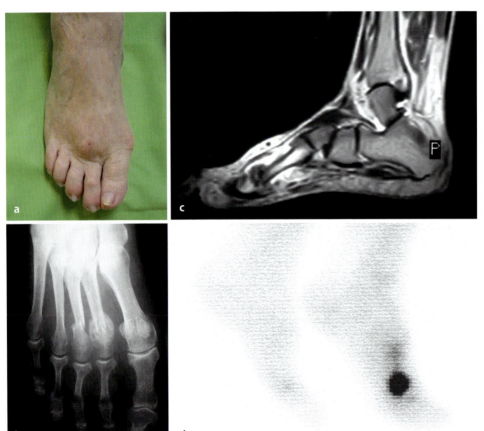

Fig. 5.1 a–d Swelling above the second and third metatarsal heads (**a**). New subcapital stress fracture in the third metatarsal bone and old one in the second, which is already surrounded and fixed by extensive callus formation (**b**). MR picture reveals the edema in the surrounding soft tissue (**c**). Bone scan shows a "hot spot" above the callus (**d**)

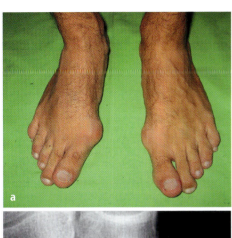

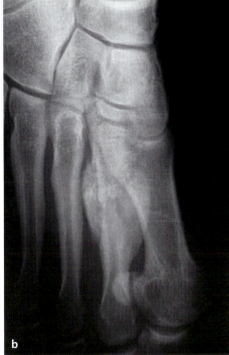

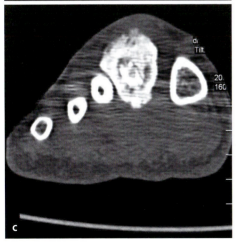

Fig. 5.2 a–c Swollen forefoot of a young athlete (**a**). Massive callus formation mimicking tumor around the diaphysis of the second metatarsus (**b**). CT pictures reveal the fractured bone within the callus (**c**)

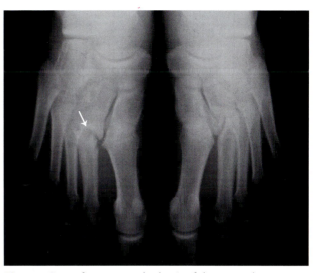

Fig. 5.3 Stress fracture on the basis of the second metatarsal bone (*arrow*)

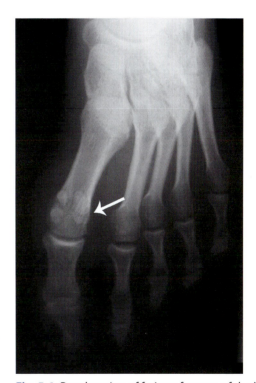

Fig. 5.4 Rare location of fatigue fracture of the lateral sesamoid bone in a ballet dancer (*arrow*). The medial sesamoid bone is of bipartite type

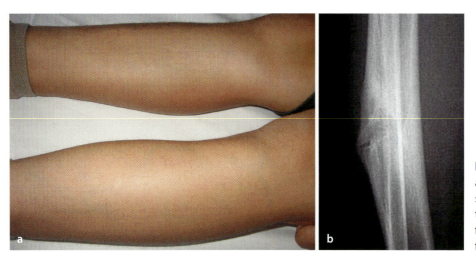

Fig. 5.5 a, b Local tenderness and swelling above the midshaft of the left tibia (**a**). Note the faint hairline crack of the infraction and beginning of callus formation on the radiograph (**b**)

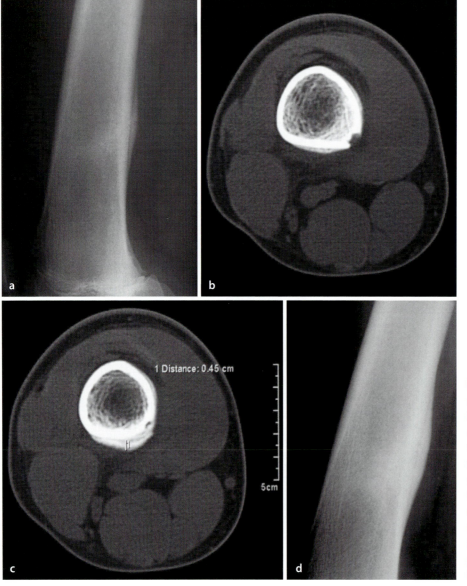

Fig. 5.6 a–d Early stage of stress fracture in the femur: the infraction is not recognizable on the radiograph only, but the transverse dense line and the fine periosteal reaction (**a**). CT slides present the atypical fracture line that mimics osteoid osteoma, but in this latter case there is no callus formation (**b, c**). Three months later, the process healed by solid callus formation (**d**)

Chapter 6

Hemophilia

Hemophilia

L. Bartha

Hemophilia is an inherited bleeding disorder affecting certain proteins of the blood-clotting cascade. The severity of hemophilia is determined by the level of clotting activity of factor VIII or factor IX in the blood. Low activity of these factors may result in excessive bleeding. Bleeding is mostly internal, affecting joints, muscles, and other soft tissues, and can happen spontaneously without an external cause or as a result of injury. Spontaneous bleeding is more likely as the severity of the disorder increases.

Hemophilia A, often referred to as classical hemophilia, is the most common type of hemophilia affecting approximately one person in 5,000–10,000 births. Hemophilia A is due to a deficiency of factor VIII.

Hemophilia B, often called Christmas Disease, named after the first person diagnosed with the condition, is caused by a deficiency in factor IX and affects one in 30,000 males.

Mild hemophilia: Blood clotting activity is between *5 and 25%* compared to normal. Someone with mild hemophilia will usually have few problems and will only need treatment for their condition after tooth extraction, surgery, or an injury. Spontaneous bleeding is rare.

Moderate hemophilia: Blood clotting levels are between *2 and 5%*. Spontaneous bleeding in moderate hemophilia is more likely but still infrequent.

Severe hemophilia: Less than 1% of clotting factor activity is classified as *severe hemophilia*. Bleeding occurs excessively, after trauma and injury, into joints, muscles, and soft tissues.

Von Willebrand's (vW) disease is a blood-clotting disorder, which is usually inherited, and affects less than 1% of the population. Unlike hemophilia, vW can affect both males and females and has symptoms similar to hemophilia (Figs. 6.1–6.11).

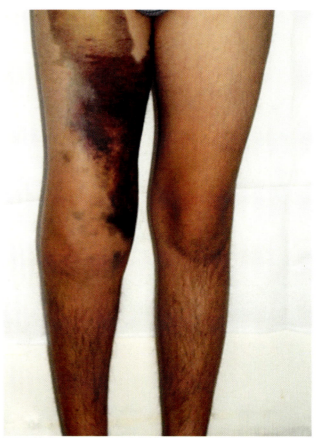

Fig. 6.1 Acute and spontaneous bleeding into the soft tissues of the right lower extremity and knee joint in a patient with severe hemophilia. Bleeding into muscles and soft tissues. The most common joints affected by bleeding are the knees, ankles, elbows, shoulders, and hips

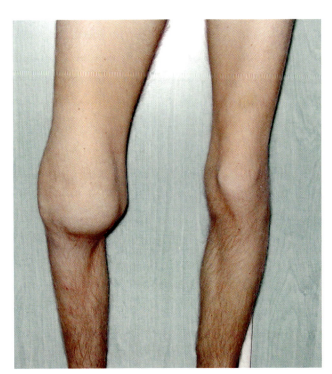

Fig. 6.2 Hemophilic arthropathy in the right knee. A diffuse hematoma first develops in the synovium, which eventually extends into the joint cavity. A joint that displays a tendency towards recurrent bleeding is termed a "target joint." The most common joints affected by bleeding are the knees, ankles, elbows, shoulders, and hips

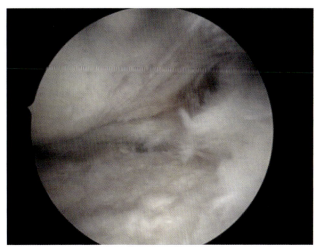

Fig. 6.4 Second stage of hemophilic arthropathy: Arthroscopic view of the cartilage damage of the hemophilic knee joint. In response to the ongoing complex inflammatory response, the cartilage breaks down and becomes rough. These changes eventually result in an arthritic and destroyed joint

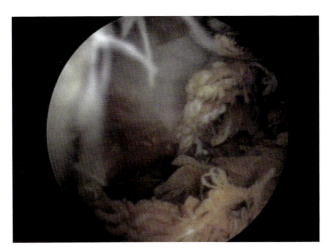

Fig. 6.3 Arthroscopic picture: first stage of hemophilic arthropathy. Hypertrophic hemophilic synovial tissue provoked by the previous bleedings

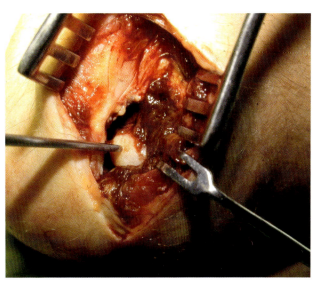

Fig. 6.5 Open view of hypertrophic synovium of the hemophilic elbow joint. The characteristic "mahogany brown" synovium secondary to hemosiderin deposition in a hemophilic elbow joint affecting already the cartilage

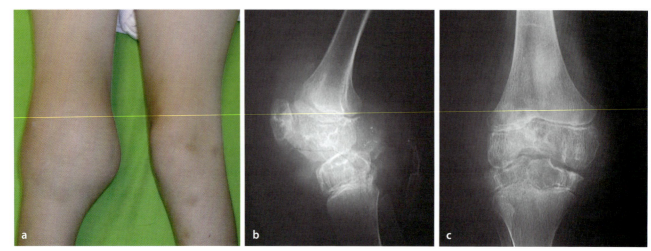

Fig. 6.6 a–c A typical manifestation of hemophilia is articular bleeding (hemarthrosis). When hemarthroses become frequent and/or intense, the synovium may not be able to reabsorb the blood. To compensate for such reabsorptive deficiency, the synovium will become hypertrophic, resulting in what is called chronic hemophilic synovitis (**a**). Thus, it is very important not only to avoid acute hemarthrosis, but also to manage it as efficiently as possible, with the aim of avoiding the development of synovitis. *Secondary osteoarthritis* due to hemophilia may develop already in childhood (**b, c**). Note the narrowing of the joint spaces, indirect sign of cartilage destruction, bony erosions, juxta-articular cyst formations, and the presence of open physis

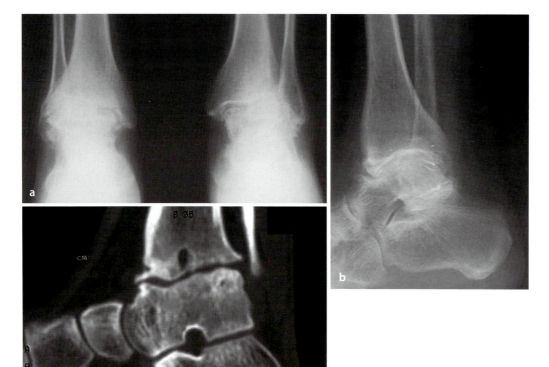

Fig. 6.7 a–c Hemophilic arthritis affecting both the ankles and causing serious destruction of talar and subtalar joints as presented on a–p (**a**) and lateral views (**b**). The juxta-articular cysts, destroyed articular surfaces, and diffuse osteoporosis in a young hemophilic patient are best evaluated on the reconstructive CT pictures (**c**)

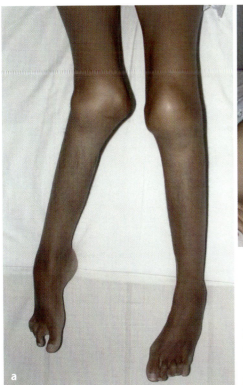

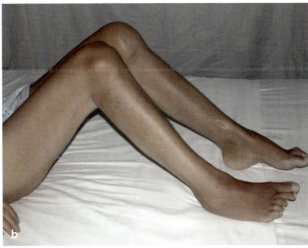

Fig. 6.8 a, b Late stage of hemophilic arthritis in adult patients: axial deformities, secondary contractures of the knees, (**a**) hips and equinus of the ankles (**b**) are frequently seen. These contractures compromise an efficient joint replacement

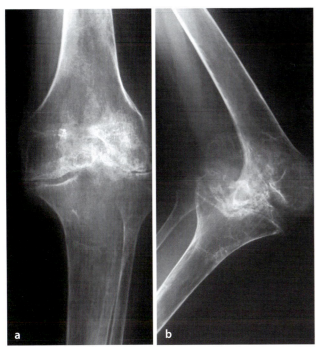

Fig. 6.9 a, b Radiological signs of knee arthritis of the same adult "A" – hemophilic patient. If a joint bleeding is not adequately treated, it tends to recur. The inflamed, swollen synovium bleeds more easily than the normal synovium and causes further swelling and inflammation. This vicious cycle must be broken to prevent the development of arthritis

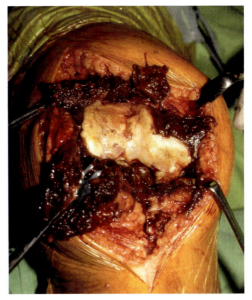

Fig. 6.10 Destroyed cartilage surfaces of the knee joint of a young hemophilic male Synovium shows marked vascular hyperplasia, hemosiderin deposits. Hemosiderin-stained pannus begins to creep over the joint surfaces. Degenerative changes are similar to those seen in osteoarthritis: thinning and erosion of articular cartilage are caused by altered configuration and mechanics of the joint; progressive fibrosis of synovium may contribute to joint contracture and restriction of joint motion

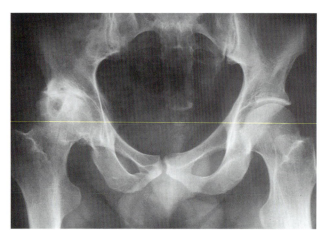

Fig. 6.11 The radiograph of a hemophilic hip joint of an adult patient reveals a common osteoarthritis of the hip. Hemophilia causes less characteristic changes in the hip than in other joints

Chapter 7

Metabolic and Endocrine Diseases

Contents

Chapter 7

Metabolic and Endocrine Diseases

P. Somogyi, A. Deli, and M. Szendrői

7.1 Gout

The gout (arthritis urica) is inflammation of joints caused by the deposit of mononatrium-urate-monohydrate (MNU) crystals in the tissues. The manifestation of the illness is also due to environmental as well as genetic, sexual, and ethnic factors.

Its prevalence is 5–28‰ in males and 1–6‰ in females.

There are two kinds of gout: Primary gout is caused by hyperuricaemia, which is the consequence of hereditary disorder of metabolism. Secondary gout is associated with hyperuricaemia, triggered by other causes, e.g., increased disintegration of the cells because of myeloproliferative disease or decreased excretion of urate because of the malfunction of the kidney.

The presence of MNU crystals in the tophus specimen or in the synovial fluid leads to a safe diagnosis (Figs. 7.1–7.13).

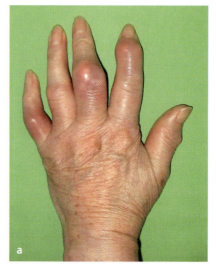

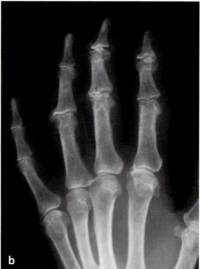

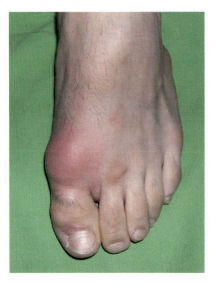

Fig. 7.1 Acute gout spasm: the inflammation is usually monoarticular, e.g., metatarsophalangeal joint (podagra), less frequently present on feet, ankles, and knees. In early stage of the gouty arthropathy, no alteration in the bones can be seen radiograph

Fig. 7.2 a, b Exacerbation of a chronic gout process in the hand: the fingers are deformed, the joints of the phalanges are swollen, with tight, hot, and dark-red skin, frequently accompanied by some general symptoms (fever, higher sedimentation rate, increased number of white blood cells) (**a**). The radiograph of the same patient presents the characteristics of chronic gouty arthropathy, narrowed joint spaces, and typical punched-out periarticular lytic lesions (**b**)

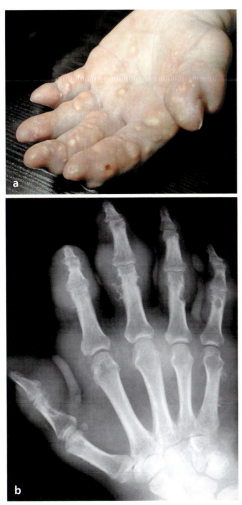

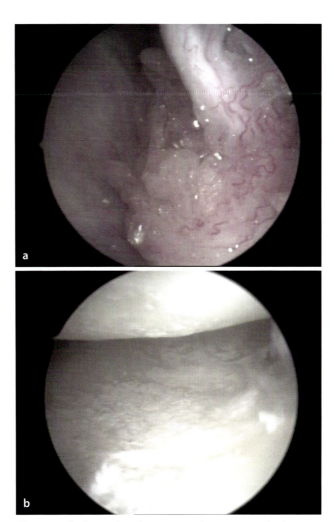

Fig. 7.3 a, b Late stage of gout: numerous subcutaneous tophi are present in the palmar region (**a**). These tophaceus gouty deposits are also visible in the radiograph around the small joints of the hand (**b**) (courtesy of Gy. Poór, Inst. For Rheumat. Budapest,Hungary)

Fig. 7.5 a, b Deposits of urate crystals may occur in the synovium (**a**) and in the cartilage of the knee joint (**b**) as visualized by arthroscopy

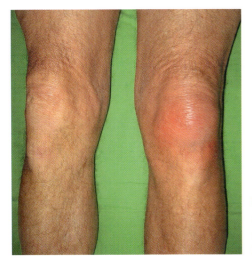

Fig. 7.4
Acute gout spasm of the left knee

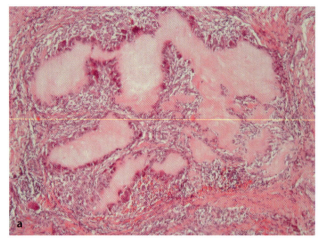

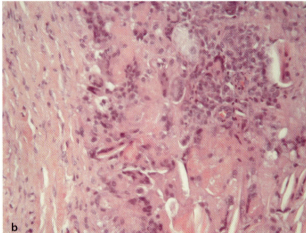

Fig. 7.6 a, b Tophus formation is characteristic of gout: eosinophile-stained amorphous central area represents the urate crystals, which dissolved in processing through water-based solutions (**a**). Higher magnification illustrates the histiocytic and giant cell reaction to urate deposits (slit-like space) in tophus (**b**)

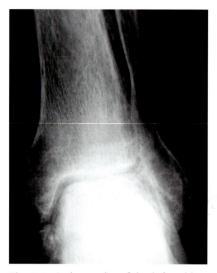

Fig. 7.8 Arthropathy of the left ankle joint in a patient suffering from gout for a long time. Note the narrowed joint space and the deposits around the joint, visible on the radiograph

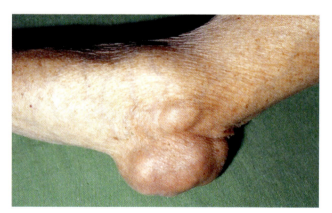

Fig. 7.9 Bursitis olecrani due to the massive tophaceus deposit of urate crystals

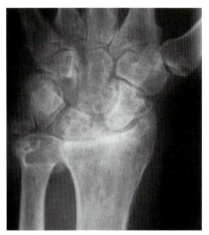

Fig. 7.7 Radiograph reveals a secondary osteoarthritis of the wrist joint because of gout

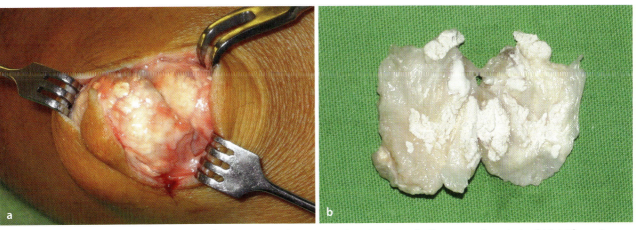

Fig. 7.10 a, b The intraoperative picture demonstrates the encapsulated yellow chalky mass of gouty tophi (**a**). The cut surface of a gouty tophus (**b**)

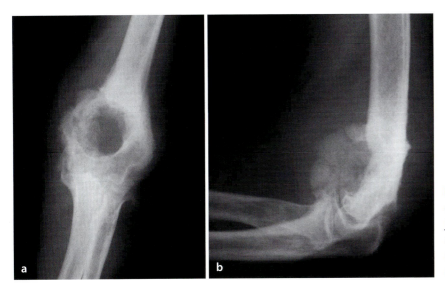

Fig. 7.11 a, b Late stage of gout with extensive destruction of the elbow joint and tophaceus gouty deposits around it are demonstrated on the anterior–posterior(**a**) and lateral (**b**) radiographs

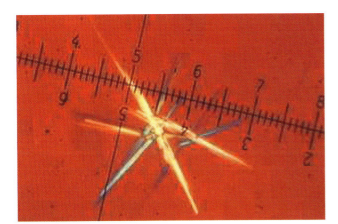

Fig. 7.12 Sodium urate crystal image on polarization microscope: characteristic negative double refraction (courtesy of Dr. G. Ferencz, Institute of Rheumatology, Budapest)

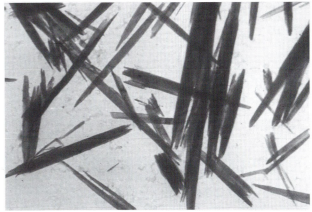

Fig. 7.13 The electron microscope image of sodium urate crystals (magnification: ×6,600). (courtesy of Dr. G. Ferencz, Institute of Rheumatology, Budapest)

7.2 Postmenopausal and Senile Osteoporosis

Osteoporosis is a silent, progressive disease characterized by decreased bone density and increased bone fragility, with a consequent susceptibility to fracture. Women are at the greatest risk. One third of Caucasian women over the age of 50 have osteoporosis. After menopause, a woman's risk of suffering an osteoporotic spine or femur fracture is 30% or three times that of a man's. Risk factors for osteoporosis are low trauma fracture since age 40, maternal history of osteoporotic fracture, age ≥65, thin body build (body weight <57 kg), prolonged amenorrhea, early menopause, chronic corticosteroid use (>6 months), disease predisposing to osteoporosis.

Symptoms of osteoporosis: Back pain with little or no exertion, acute and severe pain or chronic lower-grade back pain, pain localized to specific vertebra, pain may radiate anteriorly, pain associated with limited back mobility, pain relieved by bed rest; worsened when upright, coughing, sneezing (Figs. 7.14–7.27).

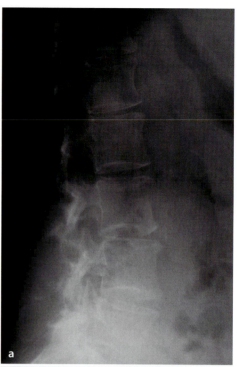

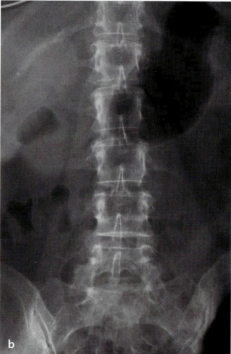

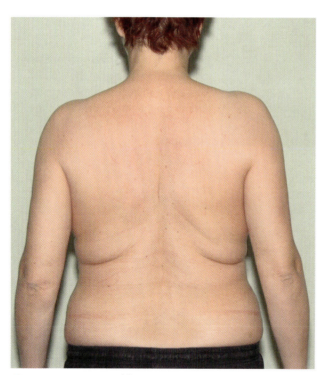

Fig. 7.14 A 55-year-old osteoporotic patient without vertebral fractures

Fig. 7.15 a, b Lateral lumbar spine radiograph: generalized osteopenia is present, the cortices are thinned, and the vertebral bodies have exaggerated vertical striations because of loss of secondary trabeculae and reinforcement of sharply defined primary trabeculae (**a**). Anteroposterior lumbar spine radiograph demonstrates intact vertebrae (**b**)

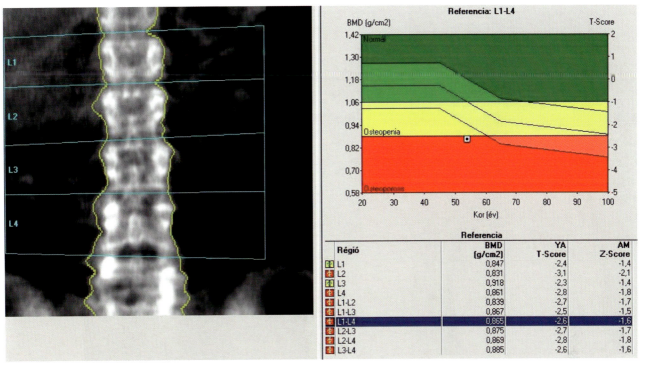

Región	BMD (g/cm2)	YA T-Score	AM Z-Score
L1	0,847	-2,4	-1,4
L2	0,831	-3,1	-2,1
L3	0,918	-2,3	-1,4
L4	0,861	-2,8	-1,8
L1-L2	0,839	-2,7	-1,7
L1-L3	0,867	-2,5	-1,5
L1-L4	0,865	-2,6	-1,6
L2-L3	0,875	-2,7	-1,7
L2-L4	0,869	-2,8	-1,8
L3-L4	0,885	-2,6	-1,6

Fig. 7.16 Lumbar dual-energy X-ray absorptiometry (DEXA) demonstrates low bone density. The fracture risk in this patient is 6–8 times higher than that in healthy people. Fractures are round the corner

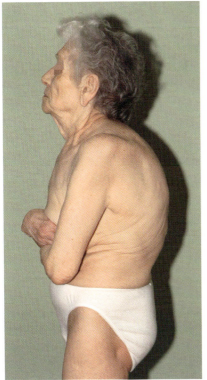

Fig. 7.17 This photograph demonstrates the typical posture of a senile osteoporotic patient. Multiple vertebral fractures over time because of osteoporosis, occurrence of chronic back pain, loss of height, and kyphosis. Continued vertebral fractures can result in the ribcage tilting downward toward the hips, leading to a forward curvature of the upper spine, called kyphosis. This resulting deformity is also known as the dowager's hump

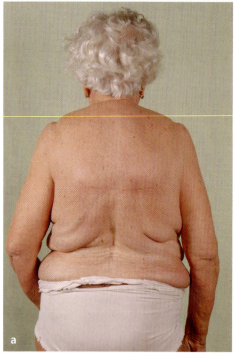

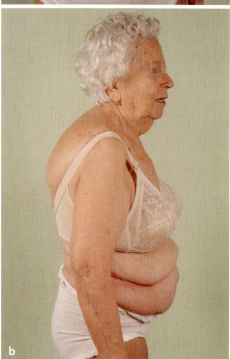

Fig. 7.18 a, b As this shift in posture continues, there is a compensatory anterior shift of the lower spine, called lordosis, resulting in protrusion of the abdomen. These characteristic changes in physical appearance can lead to a presumptive clinical diagnosis of osteoporosis

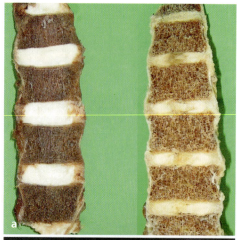

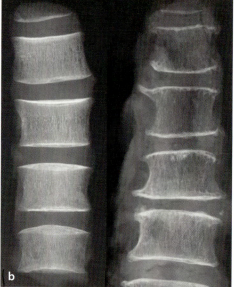

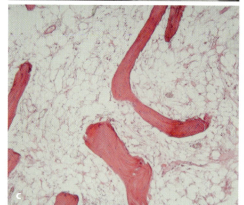

Fig. 7.19 a–c Normal and porotic bony architecture of lumbar vertebral bodies on gross specimen (**a**), and on their radiographs (**b**). Histological appearance of osteoporosis. Note the thinning of the trabecular bones. Little osteoblast activity is present on their surfaces (**c**)

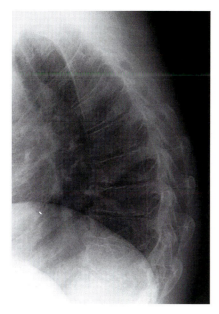

Fig. 7.20 Lateral spine radiograph demonstrates early wedge fractures with moderate kyphosis

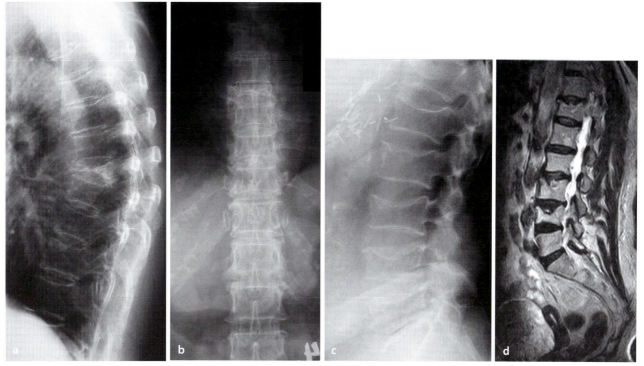

Fig. 7.21 a–d Lateral and anteroposterior spine radiographs: Involution osteoporosis. Note the overall reduction in the bone density and moderate kyphosis of the dorsal spine and a typical wedge fracture (**a**, **b**). Osteoporosis is often called a "silent disease" because bone loss occurs without symptoms. People may not know that they have osteoporosis until their bones become so weak that a sudden strain, bump, or fall causes a fracture or a vertebra to collapse. Lateral spine radiograph: Involution osteoporosis with typical biconcave vertebral fractures (**c**). Chronic benign compression fractures. Sagittal MRI scan shows preservation of normal bone marrow in multiple collapsed vertebrae. (**d**)

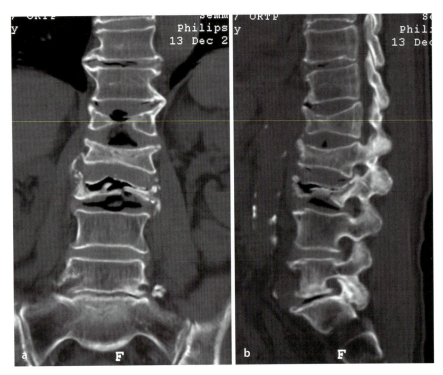

Fig. 7.22 a, b MRI can be used to differentiate between acute and chronic fractures of the vertebrae and occult stress fractures of the proximal femur. These osteoporotic fractures demonstrate characteristic changes in the bone marrow that distinguish them from other uninvolved parts of the skeleton and the adjacent vertebrae. In this case, reconstructive CT pictures show L 1, 2, and 3 fractures with biconcave deformities

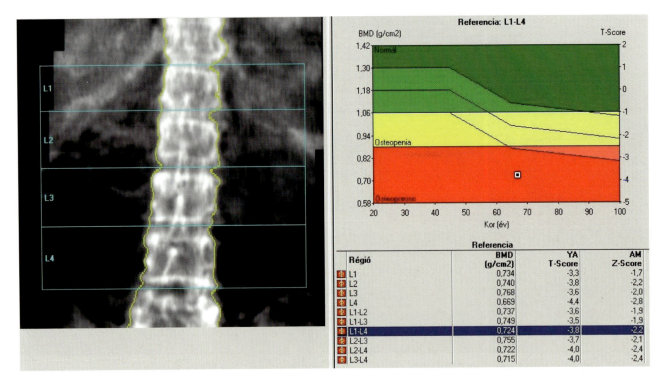

Fig. 7.23 Dual-energy X-ray absorptiometry (DXA) image of the lumbar spine. Measurements of areal bone mineral density (BMD) are generated in L1–L4 of the lumbar spine and average values calculated (total). T-scores and Z-scores are also provided in the printout. T-score is used to estimate the risk of one developing a fracture. Z-score reflects the amount of one's bone compared with other people in the same age group and of the same size and gender

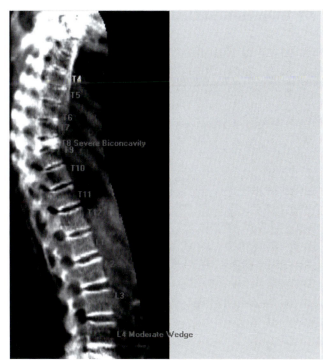

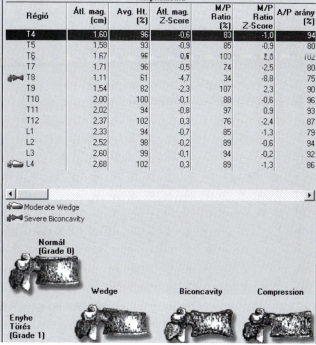

Morphometria						
Régió	Átl. mag. (cm)	Avg. Ht. (%)	Átl. mag. Z-Score	M/P Ratio (%)	M/P Ratio Z-Score	A/P arány (%)
T4	1,60	96	-0,6	83	-1,0	94
T5	1,58	93	-0,9	85	-0,9	80
T6	1,67	96	0,5	100	2,0	102
T7	1,71	96	-0,5	74	-2,5	80
T8	1,11	61	-4,7	34	-8,8	75
T9	1,54	82	-2,3	107	2,3	90
T10	2,00	100	-0,1	88	-0,6	96
T11	2,02	94	-0,8	97	0,9	93
T12	2,37	102	0,3	76	-2,4	87
L1	2,33	94	-0,7	85	-1,3	79
L2	2,52	98	-0,2	89	-0,6	94
L3	2,60	99	-0,1	94	-0,2	92
L4	2,68	102	0,3	89	-1,3	86

Moderate Wedge
Severe Biconcavity

Normál (Grade 0)

Wedge   Biconcavity   Compression

Enyhe Törés (Grade 1)

Fig. 7.24 Dual-energy vertebral assessment provides a dual-energy image of the anteroposterior and lateral spine, allowing clinicians to visually assess the presence of vertebral fractures. An existing vertebral fracture has been shown to double the risk of subsequent fractures. Vertebral fractures are most common in patients over age 70. This patient has a severe vertebral fracture (Th8) and a moderate fracture (L4)

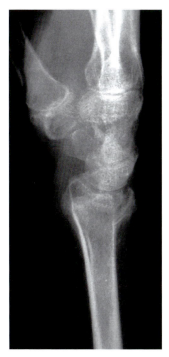

Fig. 7.25 Osteoporotic patients experience most often wrist fractures as a result of a fall on the outstretched hand. The peak incidence of Colles's fractures in postmenopausal women is between ages 60 and 70. The rate is stable thereafter, and this may be because older individuals are more likely to fall on the hip rather than on the hand

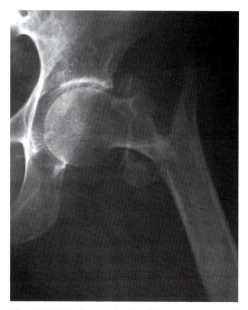

Fig. 7.26 Radiograph of a dislocated, unstable pertrochanteric fracture. The second most common site for osteoporotic fractures is the trochanteric region of the femur

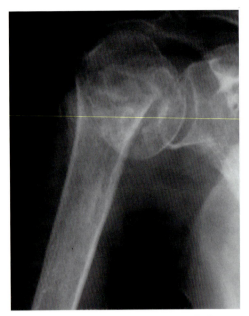

Fig. 7.27 Anteroposterior radiograph demonstrating a proximal humerus fracture (surgical neck) in an elderly woman. Proximal humerus fractures usually result from a fall onto an outstretched hand and are more common in people of middle age or older as the humerus can be weakened by osteoporosis

7.3 Glucocorticoid Induced Osteoporosis

Long-term glucocorticoid therapy is used for a number of conditions, including respiratory diseases (e.g., asthma, chronic obstructive pulmonary disease), autoimmune diseases (e.g., rheumatoid arthritis, systemic lupus erthythematosus), and gastrointestinal diseases (e.g., Crohn's disease and ulcerative colitis), and for immunosuppression in solid organ transplant recipients. Although glucocorticoid therapy is the most frequent cause of drug-induced osteoporosis, recent surveys have reported that despite the availability of effective therapeutic options for glucocorticoid-induced osteoporosis prevention and treatment, less than one-half of patients receiving significant doses of glucocorticoids were investigated for osteoporosis, and less than one-quarter were treated (Figs. 7.28–7.31).

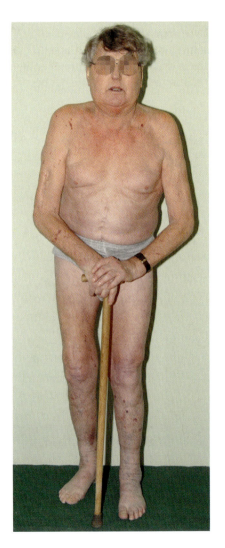

Fig. 7.28 This photograph illustrates the typical phenotype of a patient who was treated with steroids for years because of autoimmune disease. Patients may have increased adipose tissue in the face (moon face), upper back at the base of neck (buffalo hump), and above the clavicles (supraclavicular fat pads). Muscle weakness tends to be more evident in those patients with more severe disease

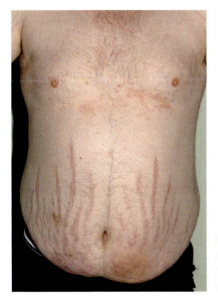

Fig. 7.29 The corticosteroids change the skin. Striation may be present and are typically purple. Striae are due to the combination of rapid weight gain and impaired collagen synthesis (commonly observed on the thighs, proximal arms, abdomen, and breasts)

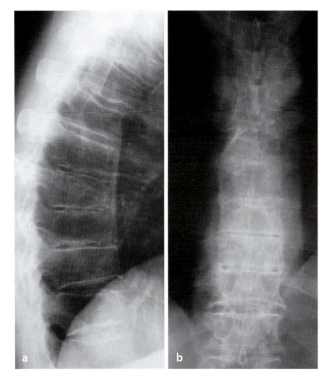

Fig. 7.30 a, b Lateral and anteroposterior views of the dorsal spine demonstrating osteoporosis and some fractured vertebral bodies

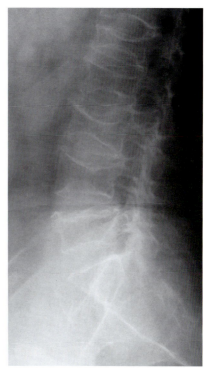

Fig. 7.31 Lateral view radiograph of the lumbar spine demonstrates osteoporosis and biconcave vertebral bodies

7.4 Osteomalacia, Osteoporomalacia

Osteomalacia is a disease in which insufficient mineralization leads to a softening of the bones. Usually, this is caused by a deficiency of vitamin D, which reduces bone formation by altering calcium and phosphorus metabolism. Osteomalacia can occur because of reduced exposure to sunlight, insufficient intake of vitamin D-enriched foods, or improper digestion and absorption of food with vitamin D. It can also be related to tumor (oncogenic osteomalacia) or to renal tubular disorders (Fanconi's syndrome). This disease causes the bending and misshaping of bones, such as bow-legging of the lower limbs, and is called rickets when it occurs in children. Symptoms in adults are often delayed until the disorder has advanced. These include easy fatigability, malaise, diffuse bone pain, and spasms. Very often the osteomalacia and the osteoporosis are together (Figs. 7.32–7.41).

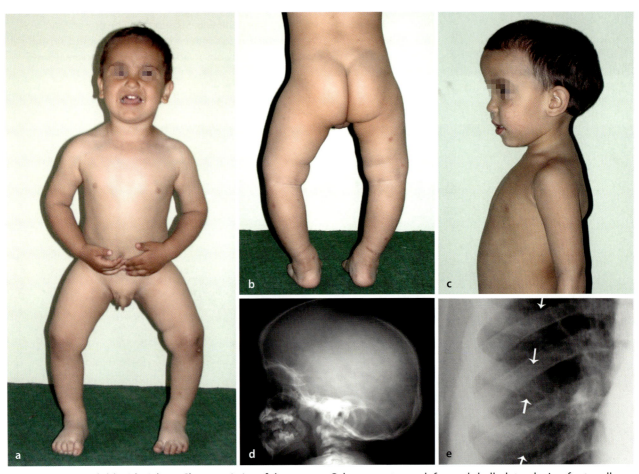

Fig. 7.32 a–e A child with rickets. Characteristics of the disease are bowing of legs under weight (**a**, **b**), spinal deformity, proximal muscle weakness, and bone pain. The height is low, the skull is cubical, "caput quadratum" (**c**, **d**). Other symptoms: deformed skulls, late-closing fontanelles, rib–breastbone joint enlargement (**e**), delayed sitting, delayed crawling, delayed walking, and knobby enlargements on the ends of bones

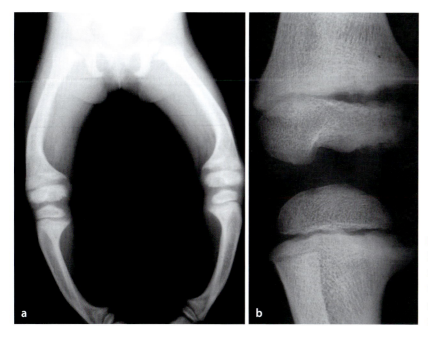

Fig. 7.33 a, b AP radiograph of the knee in rickets demonstrates diffuse osteopenia and an "O" curvature – varus deformation (**a**). The growth plates are widened and protrude into the soft and weakened metaphyseal region (**b**)

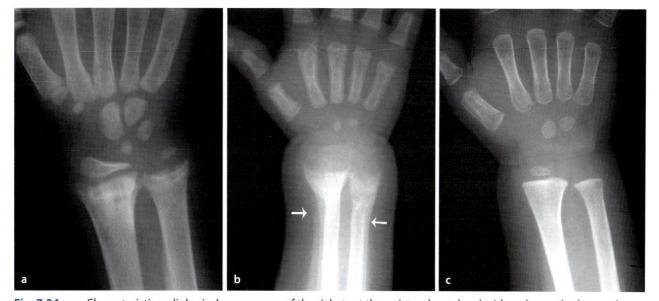

Fig. 7.34 a–c Characteristic radiological appearance of the rickets at the wrist: enlarged and widened growth plate and metaphysis. A boy at age 2 with rickets demonstrates cupping and fraying (*arrows*) of the metaphyseal region of wrist before (**b**) and at 1 year after adequate substitution vitamin-D treatment (**c**)

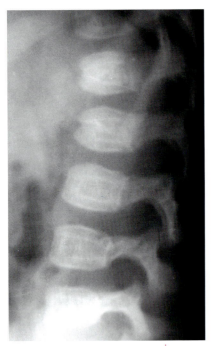

Fig. 7.35 Lateral radiograph of thoracal vertebral bodies. After a longer period of Vitamin-D treatment, the contours of the former vertebral bodies can be observed in the newly formed vertebral bodies. (It is also called "bone in bone")

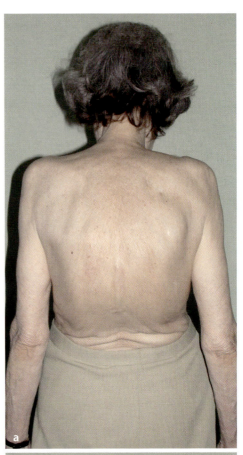

a

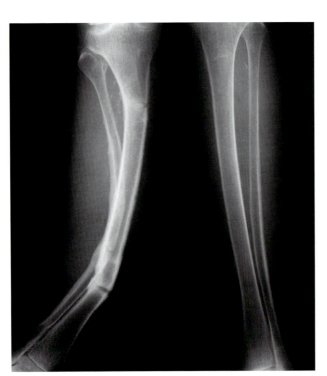

Fig. 7.37 Anteroposterior radiograph of the leg shows generalized osteopenia (it is present in approximately two-thirds of the cases). Bowing and infractions are characteristic for advanced osteomalacia

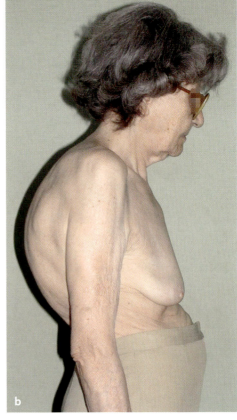

b

Fig. 7.36 a, b Posterior (**a**) and lateral (**b**) clinical view of a 78-year-old female patient with osteoporomalacia. Loss of height and kyphosis, as well as the bulging abdomen, are characteristic

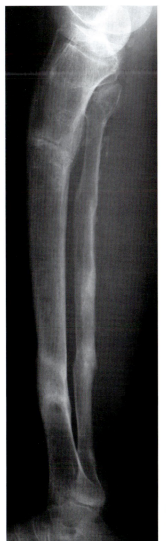

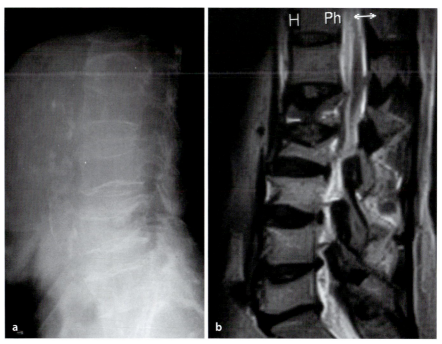

Fig. 7.40 a, b The radiograph of lumbar vertebral column in patient with osteomalacia demonstrates fractures and biconcave vertebral bodies. The trabeculae in the vertebral bodies appear indistinct or blurred and there is evidence of bone softening with bowing of the endplates, as presented on lateral radiograph (**a**) and MR picture (**b**)

Fig. 7.38 Lateral radiograph of the leg in an old women with chronic renal failure reveals osteopenia, anterior bowing of the distal tibia, and lucent areas perpendicular to the long axis of the bone (Looser zones, Milkman's fractures)

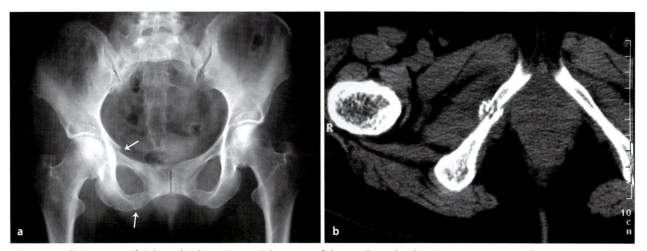

Fig. 7.39 a, b Fracture of right pubic bone (*arrows*) because of the weakened pelvic ring in a patient with osteoporomalacia presented on anteroposterior radiograph (**a**) and CT (**b**)

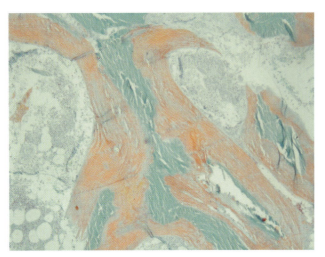

Fig. 7.41 Osteomalacia: this trichrome stain demonstrates well the increased amount of nonmineralized osteoid (*orange*) covering the normal mineralized trabeculae (*green*)

7.5 Hyperparathyroidism

Hyperparathyroidism is overactivity of the parathyroid glands resulting in excess production of parathyroid hormone (PTH). Increased PTH consequently leads to increased serum calcium, increased bone resorption, allowing flow of calcium from bone to blood, reduces renal clearance of calcium, and increases intestinal calcium absorption.

Primary hyperparathyroidism results from dysfunction in the parathyroid glands themselves, with oversecretion of PTH. The most common cause is a benign parathyroid adenoma that loses its sensitivity to circulating calcium levels. The other causes are hyperplasia and rarely carcinoma. Secondary hyperparathyroidism is due to resistance to the actions of PTH, usually because of chronic renal failure or malabsorption.. The bony involvements are also named as brown tumors. The majority of patients with hyperparathyroidism are asymptomatic. Manifestations of hyperparathyroidism usually involve the kidney (stones) and the skeletal system (bone pain due to fibrous tissue replacement, termed osteitis fibrosa cystica) (Figs. 7.42–7.50).

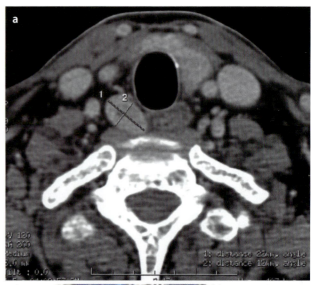

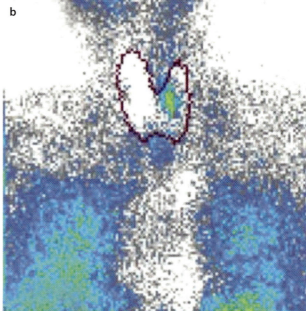

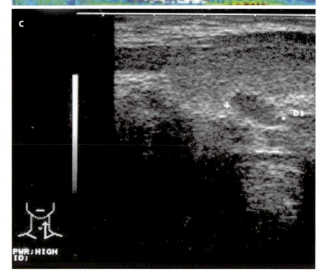

Fig. 7.42 a–c Large parathyroid adenoma presented by CT (**a**), isotope (^{99m}Tc-MIBI–^{99m}Tc-pertechnetate enhanced isotope uptake in the left parathyroid gland) (**b**), and by ultrasound (**c**) examinations (courtesy of Dr. Györke and Dr. J. Horányi, Semmelweis University, Budapest)

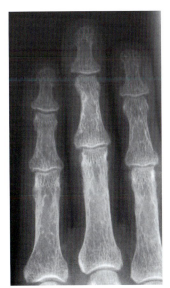

Fig. 7.43 Primary hyperparathyroidism with subtle subperiostal bone resorption and local osteopenia of the phalanges

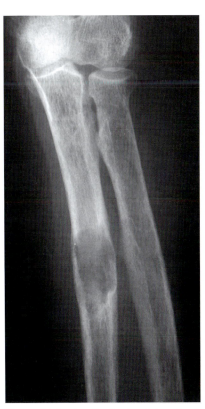

Fig. 7.45 In the diaphysis of the ulna is a cystic-lytic lesion, the so-called brown tumor of hyperparathyroidism thinning the cortical bone. There is a diffuse osteopenia and subperiostal resorption of the long tubular bones

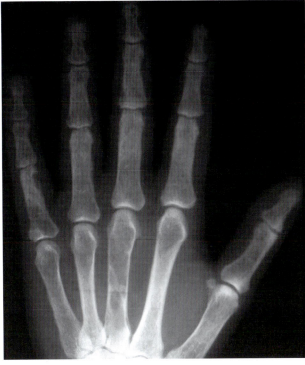

Fig. 7.44 Metacarpals and phalanges show different sized cyst-like bone resorption

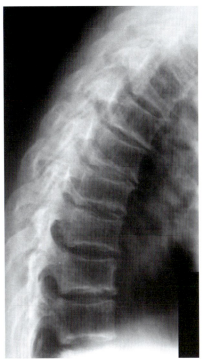

Fig. 7.46 Lateral spine radiograph demonstrates diffuse osteopenia, trabecular bone loss. The vertebral bodies have a striated appearance due to loss of trabeculae

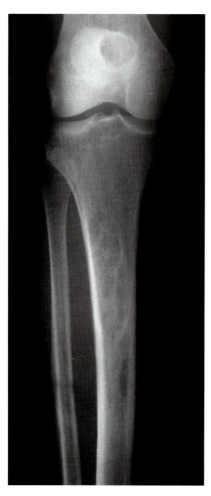

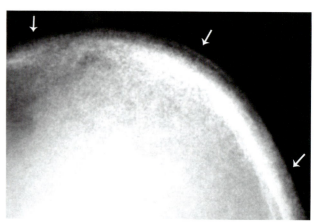

Fig. 7.49 Bone resorptions in the skull – dominantly in the external cortical region (*arrows*)

Fig. 7.47 Different sized cystic-lytic lesions of the tibia and patella. The well-defined lytic appearance of these lesions is characteristic of brown tumors

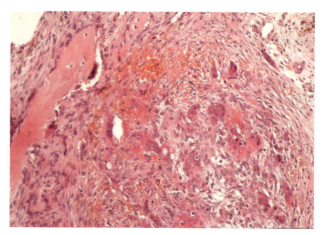

Fig. 7.50 This photomicrograph illustrates the characteristic histological feature of a brown tumor in hyperparathyroidism. Note the relative clustering of the osteoclast-type giant cells in fibrous tissue and reactive bone formation

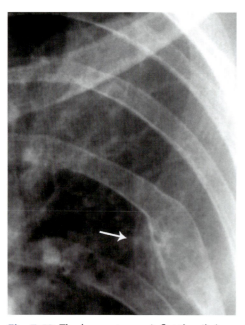

Fig. 7.48 The brown tumor inflat the rib (*arrow*)

7.6 Paget's Disease: Osteitis Deformans

This is a disease of unknown etiology, which is characterized by the disturbance of bone remodeling, pathologically active osteoclast cell activity, and accordingly increased osteoblast function, which results in producing robust, however, often fragile bone tissue.

Paget's disease involves 2–8% of the population aged over 60. Male to female ratio is 2:1.

Bone changes in Paget's disease are characterized by the development of "woven" bone and lamellar pattern of collagen. In the active phase with high turnover, the abnormal osteoclast activity creates lytic cavities, and the consequent increased bone production by active osteoblasts produces abnormal growth of the bone cortex. The deformed bone is fragile.

The most often involved bones are pelvis, spinal column, skull, femur, and tibia, but it may be present in any bone (Figs. 7.51–7.58).

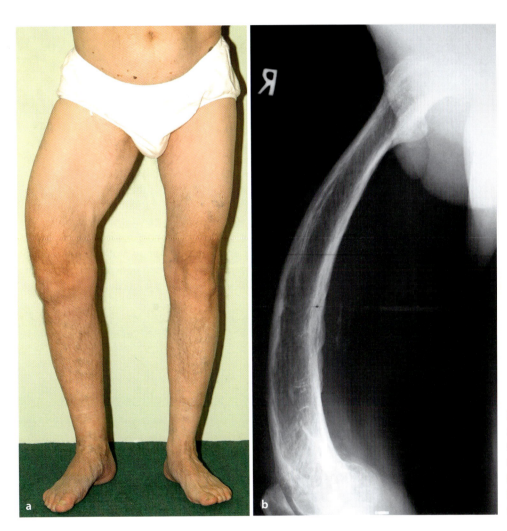

Fig. 7.51 a, b Patient with monostotic Paget's disease affecting the right femur (a). Radiograph of the right femur of the same patient. Note the laterally and anteriorly bowed long bone (b)

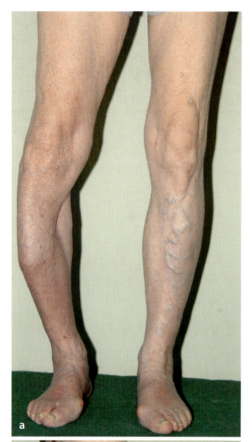

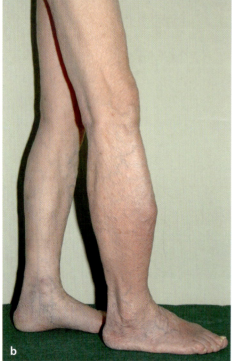

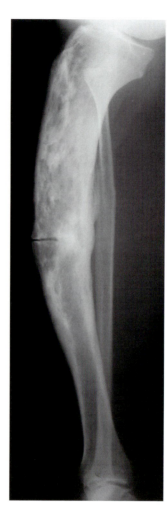

Fig. 7.53 Radiograph taken from the right tibia of the same patient. The Paget's disease involves the whole proximal and mid-part of the bone. The cortex is thickened, the medullary canal is filled by rough, coarse, irregular, trabecular bone. Note the infraction at the punctum maximum of the bowing

Fig. 7.52 a, b photograph of a patient with progressed Paget's disease localized to the tibia (monostotic form). The anterior bowing of the enlargened tibia ("sabre tibia") is highly characteristic

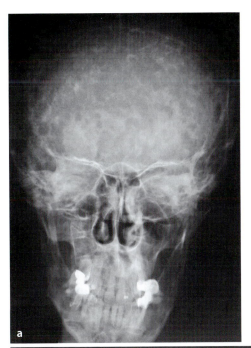

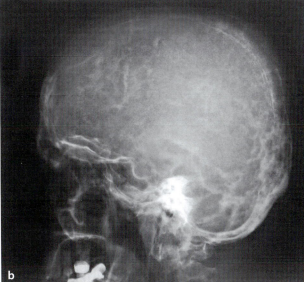

Fig. 7.54 a, b The skull shows typical changes in the acute phase known as osteoporosis circumscripta

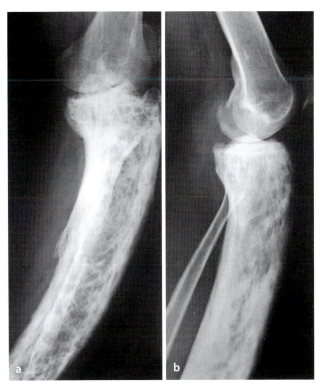

Fig. 7.55 a, b Early osteoarthritis of the knee in a patient with Paget's disease

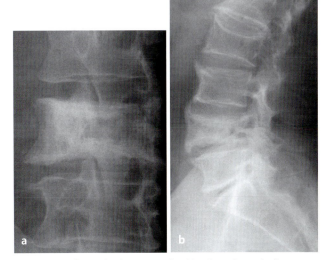

Fig. 7.56 a, b Radiodens vertebral body in Paget's disease (**a**) and "picture frame" appearance of vertebral bodies with Paget's disease (**b**). Note the compression fracture of L4 vertebral body

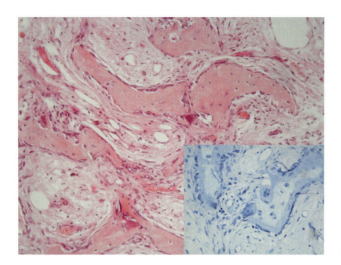

Fig. 7.57 This photomicrograph illustrates the irregular and thickened bony trabeculae in a Paget's disease. The medullar cavity is filled by loose connective tissue, rich in vessels. *Insert*: higher magnification of the pagetoid bone reveals active large osteoclasts aggravating tunnels into the trabeculae, which are lined by active osteoblasts (toluidin blue stain)

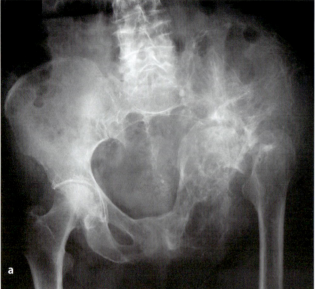

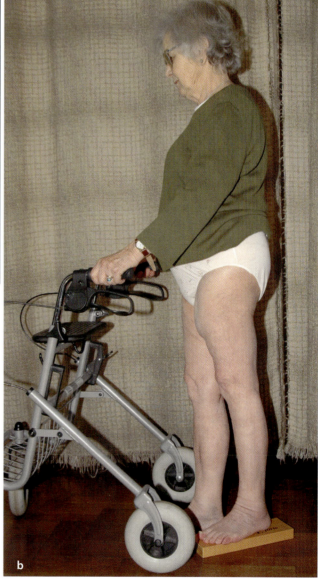

Fig. 7.58 a, b Florid lytic phase of the disease affecting the innominate bone and vertebra. Note the marked osteopenia, the extensive destruction of the left pelvic bone, and proximal femur that mimics metastatic carcinoma (**a**). The patient has 4-cm absolute shortening of the left extremity and required support for walking (**b**)

Chapter 8

Bone Tumors

Contents

Bone Tumors

F. Sim, R. Esther, and D.E. Wenger

Primary neoplasm of the skeleton is relatively uncommon. Bone tumors account for 0.2–0.5% of all malignant tumors. These tumors are quite different from the other tumors of the body. Most of them are highly malignant and affect children frequently. The pathway of metastasis formation is different from that of carcinoma, the primary filter is the lung followed by other parts of the skeleton. Regional lymph nodes are rarely affected. Bone neoplasms change or destroy the structure of the bone, and accordingly they show up as characteristic lesions in the radiographs. As clinical features such as pain, swelling and discomfort are nonspecific, a long period of time may elapse until the correct diagnosis is achieved. As consequence, most of the bone sarcomas are recognized in an extracompartmental advanced stage.

8.1 Primary Bone Tumors

8.1.1 Osteoid Osteoma

Osteoid osteomas are uniquely painful benign lesions that most commonly occur during adolescence. Males are affected more commonly than females. Most lesions occur in the meta- or diaphysis of the long bones (proximal femur and tibia) although, as with osteoblastoma, spinal lesions can lead to painful scoliosis. Ten per cent has an intraarticular location. At least 2/3 of patients will have the classic clinical symptoms of intense, throbbing, night pain that is largely relieved by nonsteroidal anti-inflammatory medicines. Patients have minimal findings on clinical examination, although some will have swelling, muscle atrophy, or spasm (Figs. 8.1–8.12).

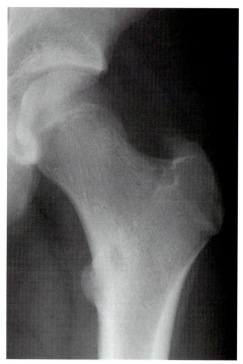

Fig. 8.1 Plain radiograph of an osteoid osteoma in the proximal femur. There is a well-circumscribed radiolucent lesion with surrounding sclerosis. The area of lucency is by definition less than 1.5 cm

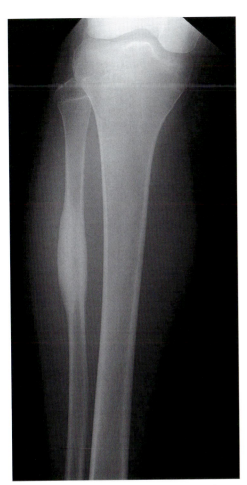

Fig. 8.2 AP radiograph showing osteoid osteoma of the fibula. Note the benign-appearing cortical reaction and enlargement of bone

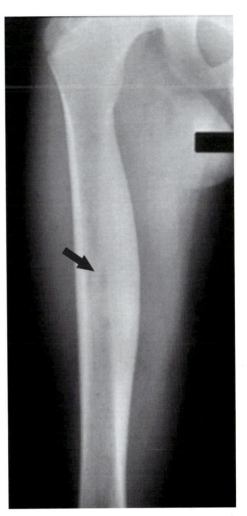

Fig. 8.3 Diaphyseal osteoid osteoma in the femur. Note the cortical thickening and benign periosteal new bone. The lesion also demonstrates intramedulary sclerosis (*arrow*), another hallmark of the lesion

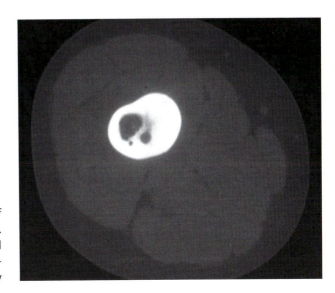

Fig. 8.4 Following plain films, CT is the imaging modality of choice for the detection and diagnosis of osteoid osteomas. CT is very sensitive for detecting the intra-or juxtacortical nidus. This lesion is associated with marked cortical thickening. Note the adjacent incidental nutrient artery

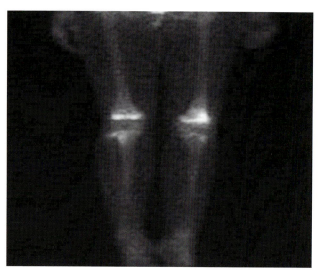

Fig. 8.5 Bone scans are very sensitive for detecting osteoid osteomas. This distal femoral lesion displays characteristic flows of intense tracer activity

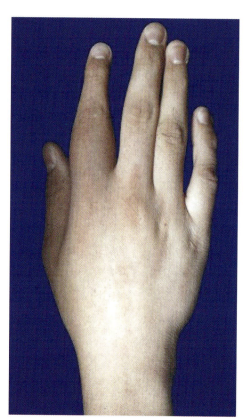

Fig. 8.7 Swelling in proximal phalanx of index finger secondary to osteoid osteoma

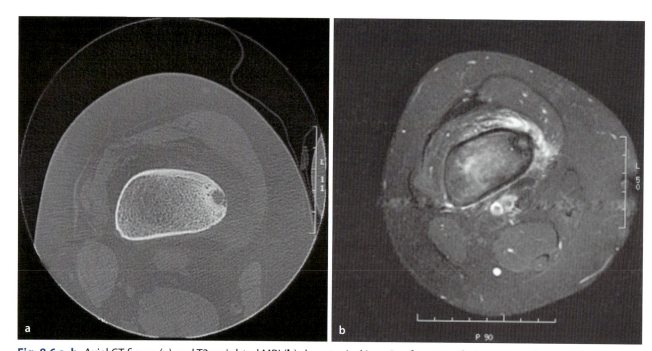

Fig. 8.6 a, b Axial CT figure (**a**) and T2 weighted MRI (**b**) show typical imaging features of a juxtacortical osteoid osteoma of the distal femur. The CT shows typical surrounding medullary sclerosis. The MRI shows significant associated edema and adjacent periostitis

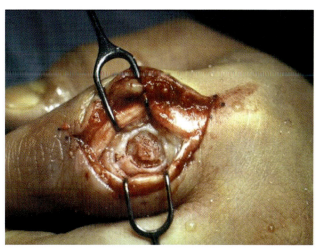

Fig. 8.8 Surgical photograph of nidus

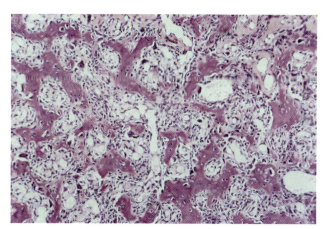

Fig. 8.10 Thin, irregular osteoid trabeculae are evident on microscopic evaluation. There is loose fibrovascular connective tissue between the trabeculae

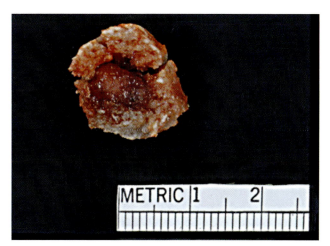

Fig. 8.9 Gross pathologic image. The nidus is typically "cherry-red" on gross examination

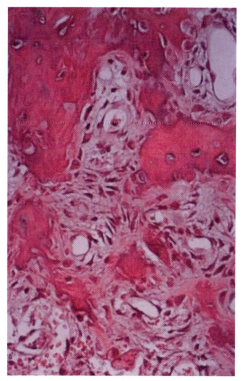

Fig. 8.11 Higher power examination shows osteoid with uniform osteoblasts without nuclear atypia

8.1.2 Osteoblastoma

Osteoblastoma is a rare benign bone tumor. Patients often complain of intermittent episodes of pain. The clinical course is usually slow and indolent, but osteoblastomas can progress rapidly, mimicking a malignant process. The usual age of onset is adolescence to early adulthood, but the clinical presentation is variable. Males are affected more commonly than females. Patients have minimal physical findings, although some have muscle atrophy or muscle spasm. Spinal osteoblastomas occur in the posterior elements; muscle spasm in this area can lead to a painful scoliosis.

Osteoblastomas typically have loose fibrovascular connective tissues intermixed with irregular osteoid. Radiographic correlation is essential (Figs. 8.12–8.19).

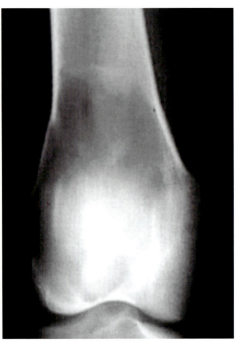

Fig. 8.13 AP radiograph of the distal femur shows a purely lytic osteoblastoma in the epiphysis and metaphysis with mild osseous expansion but no evidence of sclerosis or mineral production

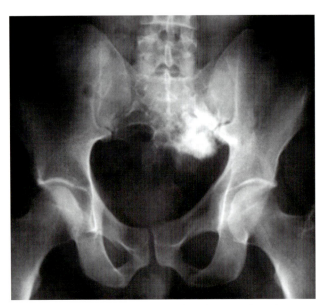

Fig. 8.12 AP radiograph of the pelvis shows a densely sclerotic osteoblastoma in the left sacrum. Due to the extent of sclerosis, this lesion was initially mistaken for an osteosarcoma

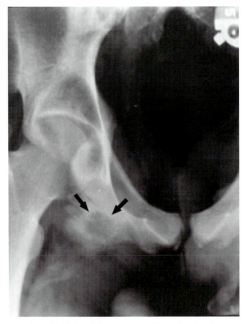

Fig. 8.14 Osteoblastoma of the right inferior pubic ramus (*arrows*). There is a central lucent area surrounded by abundant reactive bone. This exuberant mineralization could also be mistaken for malignancy

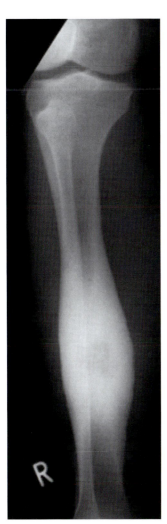

Fig. 8.15 Marked bony enlargement and sclerosis with central lucency classical for osteoblastoma

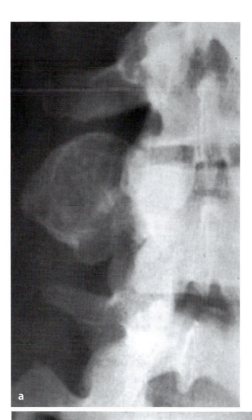

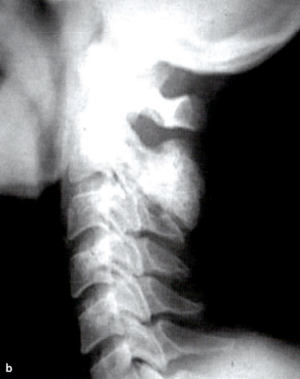

Fig. 8.16 a, b AP radiographs of the lumbar spine (**a**) and lateral radiographs of the cervical spine (**b**) both illustrate osteoblastomas in their typical locations in the posterior elements of the spine. Osteoblastoma in the spine are typically expansile, but may be primarily lytic (**a**) or sclerotic (**b**)

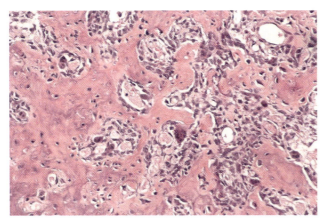

Fig. 8.17 Photomicrograph of osteoblastoma. The low-power figure demonstrates a permeative growth pattern, with mature cortical bone on the left surrounded by osteoblastoma

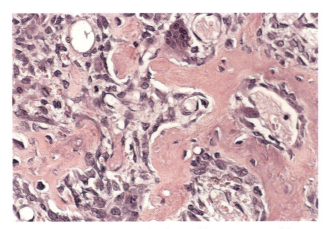

Fig. 8.18 Photomicrograph of osteoblastoma. Osteoblastomas typically have loose, fibrovascular connective tissue intermixed with irregular osteoid. Mitotic figures may be present

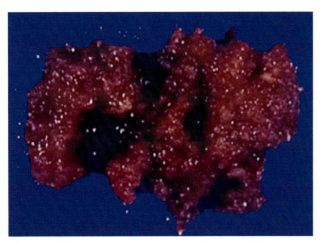

Fig. 8.19 Gross appearance of curetted osteoblastoma

8.1.3 Enchondroma

Enchondromas are relatively common benign intramedullary cartilaginous lesions that often are detected incidentally. The peak age is the second decade. Half of enchondromas occur in the short tubular bones of the hands and feet followed by proximal humerus and proximal and distal femur. Some enchondromas are painful and appear more aggressive radiographically but still display the bland, benign histology typical of asymptomatic lesions (Figs. 8.20–8.24).

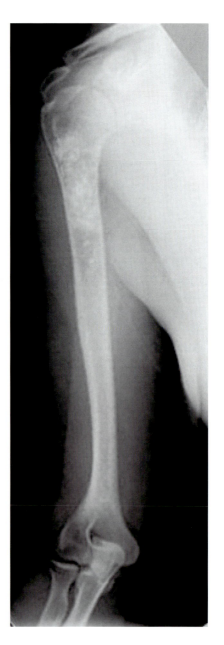

Fig. 8.20 AP radiograph showing proximal humeral enchondroma. Note the lesion's central location, characteristic calcification, and lack of periosteal reaction. The lesion was detected on a chest radiograph obtained during a medical work-up. There is no evidence of cortical destruction or periosteal reaction

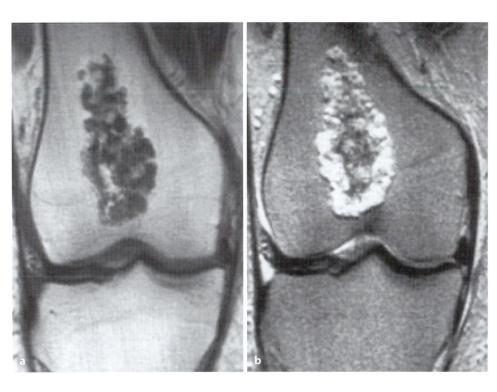

Fig. 8.21 a, b T1–T2 weighted images (**a**, **b**) of a distal femoral enchondroma. The lesions typically have a lobulated morphology with low signal on T1 with areas of high and low signal on T2 images

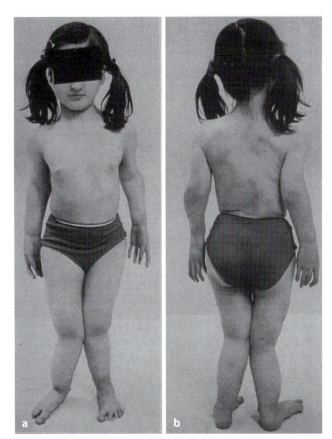

Fig. 8.22 a, b Short stature and osseous deformity secondary to Ollier's disease

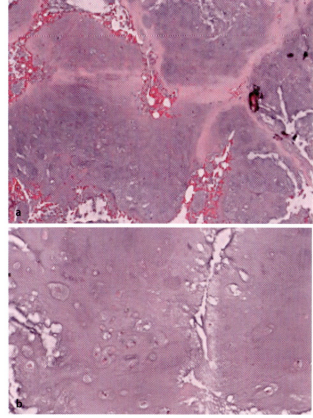

Fig. 8.23 a, b Low-power images demonstrate the lobular growth pattern and hypocellular nature of enchondromas. The nuclei are uniform

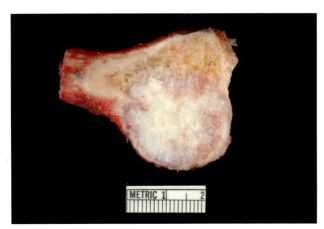

Fig. 8.24 Gross image of an enchondroma of the proximal fibula. Note the bone's cortical integrity and the mature-appearing cartilaginous tissue

8.1.4 Periosteal Chondroma

Periosteal chondromas are benign intracortical cartilaginous lesions. Most patients are asymptomatic. Lesions that become especially large may cause local mechanical symptoms or bursitis. Depending on the size of the lesion and the patient's body habitus, lesions may be palpated on physical examination. The majority of the patients present within the second through the fourth decades of life (Figs. 8.25–8.29).

Fig. 8.26 Periosteal chondroma of the distal femur. Again note the chronic benign appearing concave scalloped defect medially with a partially visualized peripheral shell laterally

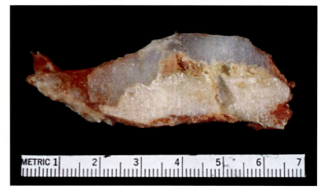

Fig. 8.27 Periosteal chondroma gross specimen. The lesion resembles hyaline cartilage

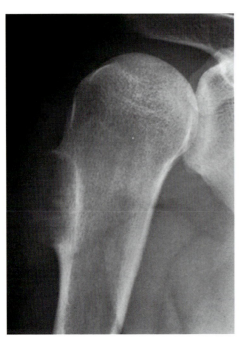

Fig. 8.25 Periosteal chondroma of the proximal humerus. The lesion is arising in the cortex of the proximal humeral metadiaphysis laterally. These lesions frequently result in a concave, scalloped deformity of the cortex with a sclerotic rim along the medullary side. Some lesions have an identifiable shell of bone along the soft tissue margin. They may or may not have identifiable calcified matrix mineralization

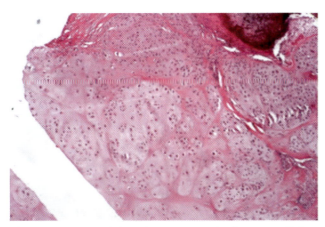

Fig. 8.28 Periosteal chondromas are typically more cellular than their intramedullary counterparts

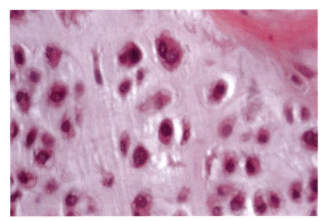

Fig. 8.29 They often display a lobular growth pattern, as shown in this example

8.1.5 Osteochondroma

Osteochondromas are benign cartilage capped bony projections arising from the external surface of the bone that are often asymptomatic. They may become painful due to compression of overlying structures or due to overlying bursa formation. Sudden pain may be due to a fracture through the stalk. Most patients present in the first three decades. Patients with multiple osteochondromatosis or with lesions close to physes frequently have developmental deformity. There is a small (less than 1%) risk of transformation to a low-grade chondrosarcoma. Lesions that continue to grow after skeletal maturity and that have cartilage caps greater than 1–2 cm should be examined carefully for malignant degeneration.

Histologically, osteochondromas resemble physes (enchondral ossification) (Figs. 8.30–8.38).

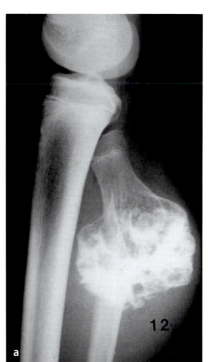

Fig. 8.30 a–c Large osteochondroma of the proximal fibula is shown on radiograph (**a**), 3D CT (**b**) and on CT (**c**). Lesions in this area can cause a peroneal neuropathy. There is a prominent concave deformity of the adjacent tibial cortex reflecting chronic extrinsic deformation secondary to mass effect from the osteochondroma

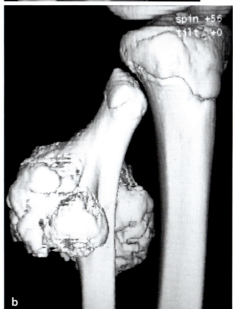

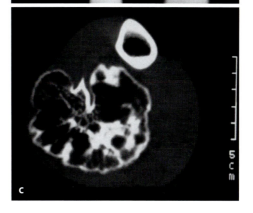

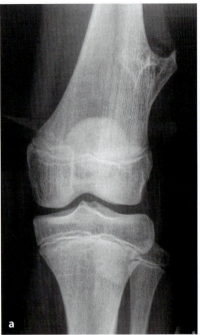 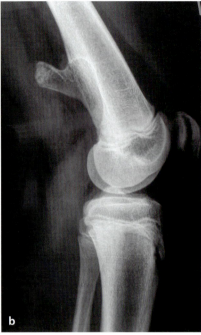

Fig. 8.31 a, b Pedunculated osteochondroma of the distal femur. Lesions typically grow away from the joint. The cancellous portion of the osteochondroma communicates with the intramedullary portion of the involved bone. This lesion demonstrates cortical and medullary continuity between the lesion and parent bone that is a radiographic hallmark of osteochondroma

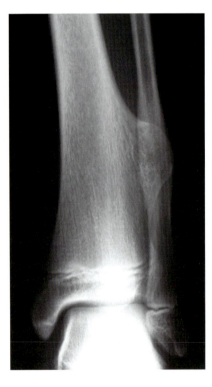

Fig. 8.32 Sessile osteochondroma of the distal tibia. Note the angular deformity of the tibial plafond. Lesions in this area can cause growth abnormalities and angular deformity

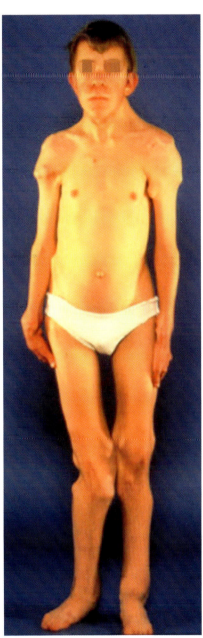

Fig. 8.33 Multifocal osteochondromatosis with associated bony deformities. This represents an autosomal dominant inheritance

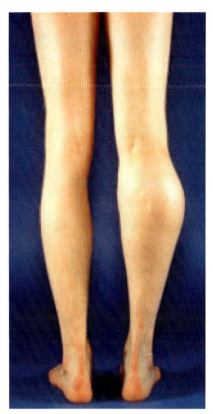

Fig. 8.34 Patient presented with symptoms related to compression of the tibial nerve

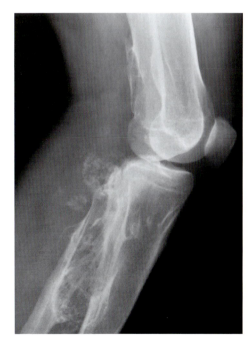

Fig. 8.35 Knee radiograph of a patient with multiple osteochondroma. There are multiple lesions in the distal femur and proximal tibia with associated developmental deformity

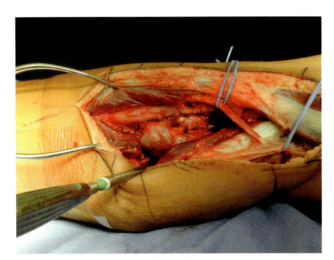

Fig. 8.36 Intraoperative photo of an osteochondroma. Note the continuity with the underlying cortex and cap of mature-appearing cartilage

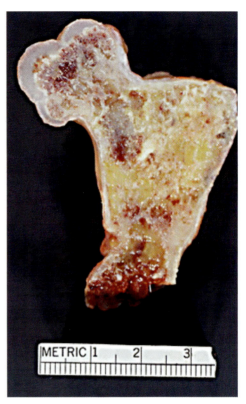

Fig. 8.38 Gross photo of an osteochondroma. Note again the cartilage cap and the continuity between the marrow space of the osteochondroma and that of the involved bone

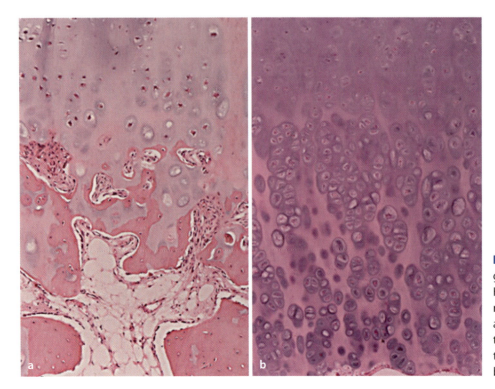

Fig. 8.37 a, b Photomicrographs of osteochondroma. Histologically these lesions resemble growth plates with a cartilaginous cap maturing through enchondral ossification to normal-appearing bony trabeculae

8.1.6 Chondroblastoma

Chondroblastoma is a benign cartilage-producing tumor usually occurring in patients in adolescence or early adulthood. Pain is the most common clinical finding any may be present for many years before diagnosis. These lesions occur in primary or secondary ossification centers and are two times more common in males than in females. Although usually localized to the epiphysis or apophysis, these lesions occasionally cross an open growth plate. Tenderness is the most common finding on physical examination; patients may also present with regional muscle atrophy and an antalgic gait (Figs. 8.39–8.44).

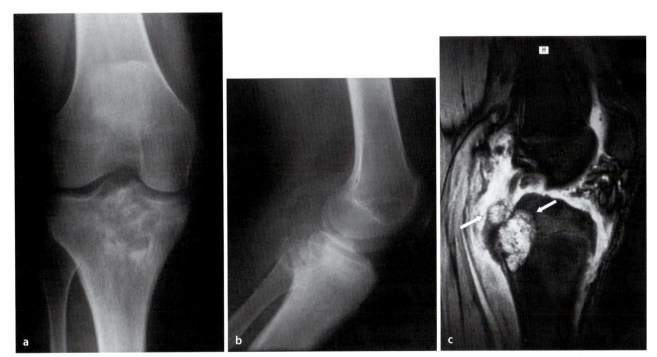

Fig. 8.39 a–c Chondroblastoma in a 16-year-old who underwent knee arthroscopy prior to referral (**a**: ap radiograph). The lateral radiograph (**b**) and the MR picture in sagittal plane show a lytic lesion in the proximal tibial epiphysis posteriorly. Matrix calcifications are present in approximately one-quarter of chondroblastomas

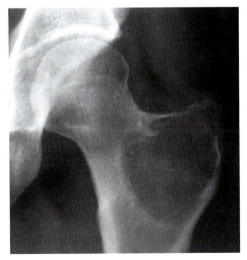

Fig. 8.40 Radiograph demonstrating a chondroblastoma of the greater trochanter of the proximal femur. Here the lesion is in a secondary ossification center, the greater trochanter. The lesion shows typical imaging features of a lytic lesion with well-defined margins and subtle sclerotic rim

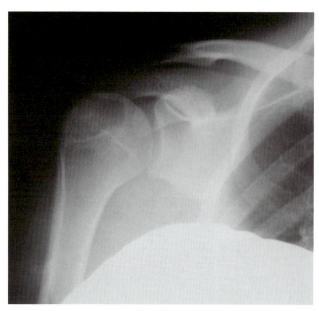

Fig. 8.41 14-year-old female with a proximal humerus chondroblastoma. As in this lesion, chondroblastomas are often eccentric

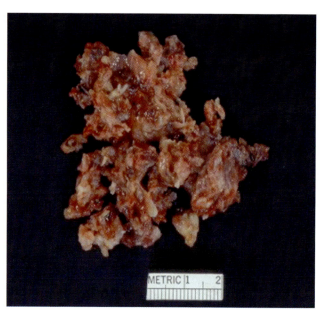

Fig. 8.43 Grossly, chondroblastoma is usually grey or pink, with occasional areas of calcification in the tissue

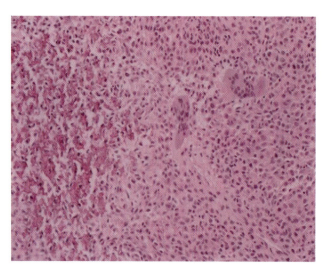

Fig. 8.42 Low magnification histology shows a uniform background of mononuclear cells with occasional giant cells

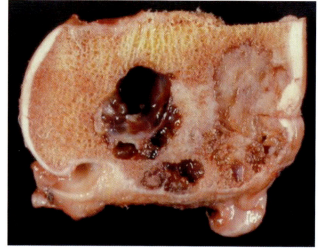

Fig. 8.44 This gross specimen shows an area of chondroid-appearing tissue as well as more cystic regions. Chondroblastomas can have components of secondary aneurysmal bone cyst

8.1.7 Chondromyxoid Fibroma

Chondromyxoid fibromas are rare benign cartilaginous tumors. They more commonly occur in males and most patients present in the first 3 decades. Pain and local swelling are the most common patient complaints. Physical exam may reveal tenderness but many lesions have minimal findings on examination (Figs. 8.45–8.51).

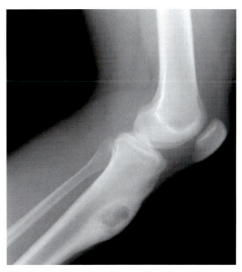

Fig. 8.46 Lateral radiographs of a patient with a chondomyxoid fibroma of the proximal tibia. These lesions, as in this case, frequently present as an intracortical tumor. This lytic intracortical lesion is associated with osseous expansion and chronic benign cortical thickening

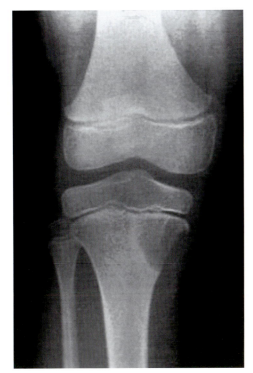

Fig. 8.45 The majority of chondromyxoid fibromas are eccentric, metaphyseal lesions with sharp, well-demarcated borders as presented in this proximal tibia. Matrix calcification may be seen in a minority of lesions

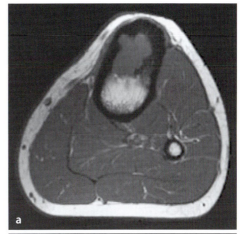

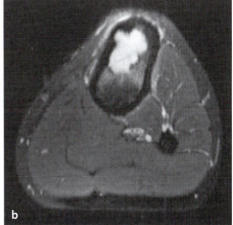

Fig. 8.47 a, b. Axial T1 (**a**) and Axial T2 weighted image with fat saturation (**b**) of the lesion. The MR pictures confirm the intracortical location of the lesion. It has nonspecific signal characteristics with low signal intensity on T1 and high signal intensity on T2

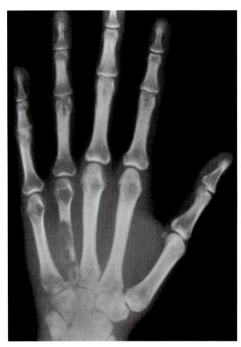

Fig. 8.48 Chondromyxoid fibroma of the metacarpal. Lesions occur most commonly in the tibia, followed by small bones of the hands and feet, femur, and humerus

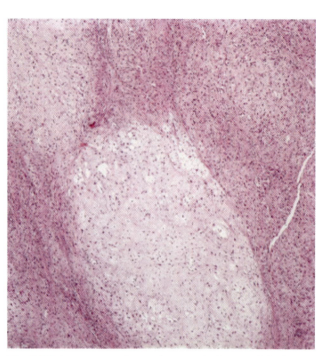

Fig. 8.50 Low power photomicrograph showing lobular growth pattern

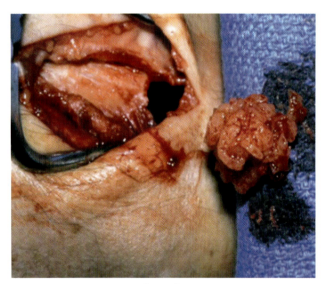

Fig. 8.49 Intraoperative photo showing gross appearance of chondromyxoid fibroma. The tissue often resembles hyaline cartilage

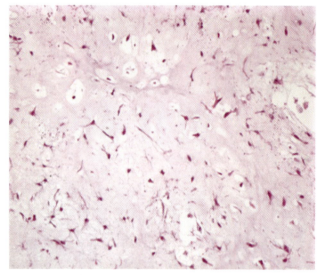

Fig. 8.51 Higher power photomicrograph showing myxoid/chondroid stroma and lobules of spindle shaped or stellate cells with abundant myxoid or chondroid intercellular material

8.1.8 Giant Cell Tumor of Bone

Giant cell tumor is a benign aggressive bone lesion that occurs in the epiphysis or apophysis (secondary ossification center). Giant cell tumors usually occur in patients between the age of 20 and 40. Clinical presentation includes pain, swelling, limitation of joint motion, regional muscle atrophy, and occasionally (5%) pathologic fracture. Spine lesions usually occur in the anterior column and may present with radicular or compressive symptoms. Approximately 2% of the patients develop lung metastases, which usually run a benign course. Malignancy in giant cell tumor occurs in 5–15%, at the site of a previous giant cell tumor (usually associated with radiation) or rarely de novo associated with benign giant cell tumor (Figs. 8.52–8.56).

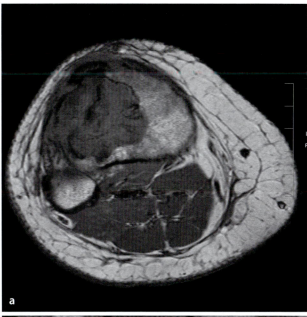

a

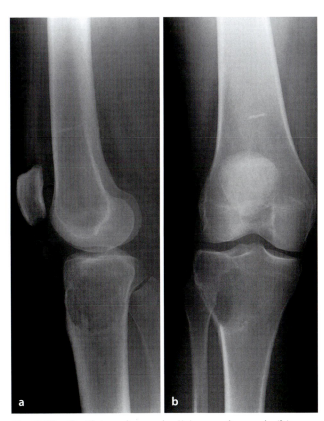

a

b

Fig. 8.52 a, b Plain radiographs ((**a**): ap radiograph, (**b**): lateral view radiograph) showing giant cell tumor of the proximal tibia. Note the epiphyseal location, absence of matrix mineralization, and lack of sclerosis surrounding the lesion

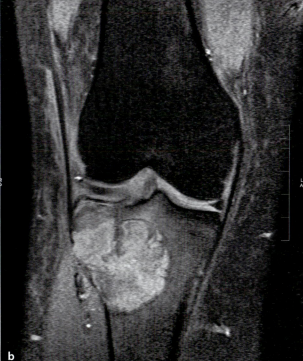

b

Fig. 8.53 a–e MRI of lesion seen in plain radiographs above. Giant cell tumors have low to intermediate signal on T1(**a**) or proton density (**b**) sequences, high signal on STIR

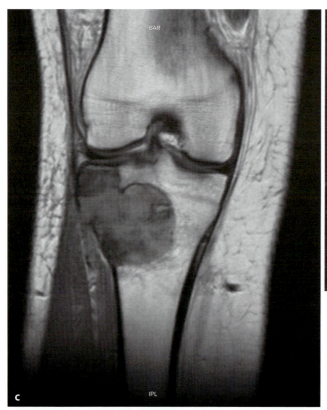

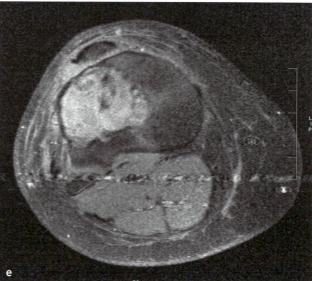

(**c**) or T2 sequences (**d**), and enhance with administration of gadolinium (**e**)

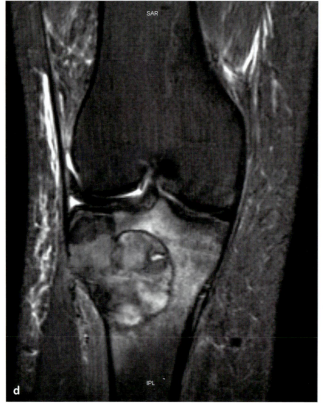

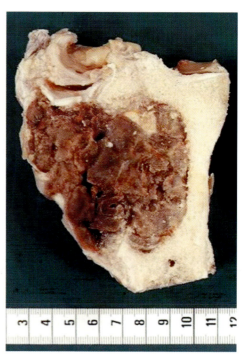

Fig. 8.54 Cross section of surgical specimen

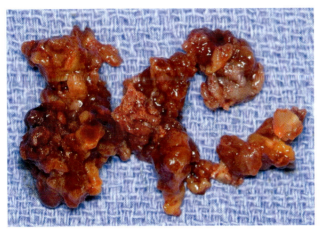

Fig. 8.55 Grossly, lesions are composed of friable, brownish–red material

8.1.9 Massive Osteolysis (Gorham's Disease)

Gorham's disease is an idiopathic process involving massive, progressive osteolytic changes. Many patients report antecedent trauma. Clinical symptoms vary depending on the anatomic site, with many patients reporting pain, swelling, and mechanical symptoms. Lesions of the vertebral column may cause neurologic findings.

Radiographically, findings include extensive osteolytic changes of the involved bone. Local soft tissues may also be involved. Over time, sclerotic bone may accompany healing.

Pathology: Gross specimens have a sponge-like consistency. Microscopic examination shows varying amounts of vascular changes without reactive bone formation (Figs. 8.57–8.63).

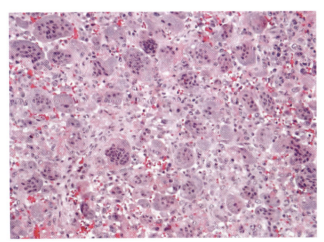

Fig. 8.56 Microscopically, lesions have giant cells interspersed against a background of mononuclear cells with round or oval nuclei. The cells composing the giant cells should be similar in appearance to the background cells. Mitotic figures may be present

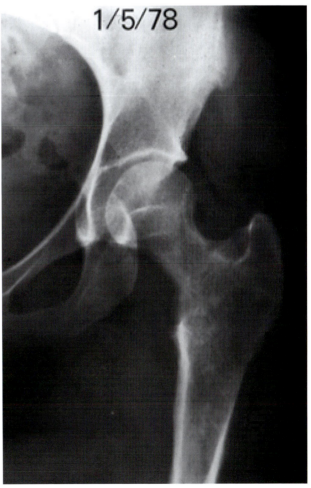

Fig. 8.57 Lytic destruction in the proximal femur with concentric narrowing of the femoral neck

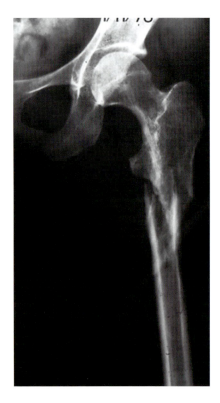

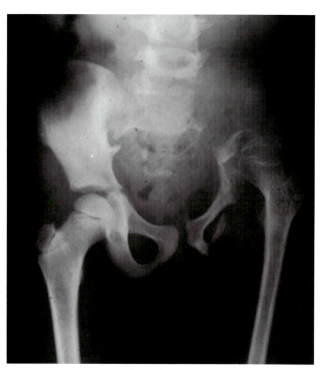

Fig. 8.58 Following pathological fracture

Fig. 8.60 Massive osteolysis showing complete resorption of left hemipelvis

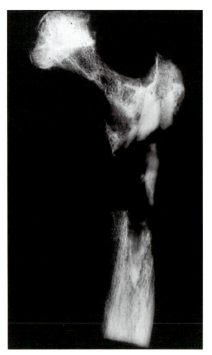

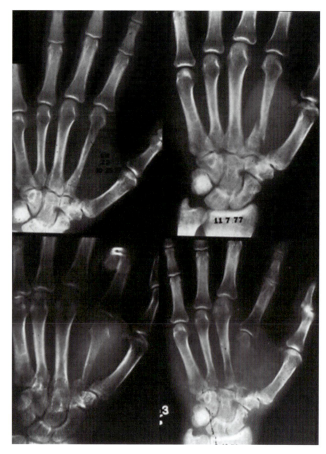

Fig. 8.59 Following surgical resection

Fig. 8.61 Progressive erosion and absorption in left hand and wrist

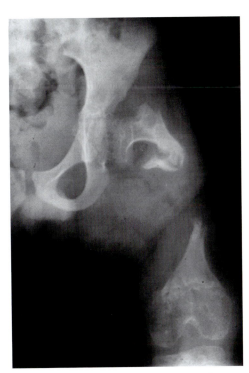

Fig. 8.62 AP left femur showing complete resorption of diaphysis

8.1.10 Intraosseous Lipoma

Intrasseous lipomas are rare lesions. Most lesions are symptomless and detected incidentally. As the lesions are entirely contained within the bone, no masses are appreciated on physical examination. Occasionally, regional tenderness or joint irritability may be present.

Radiographically, lesions have a benign appearance with a narrow zone of transition between the more radiolucent lesion and the surrounding bone. A sclerotic rim is often present. MR imaging of intraosseous lipomas is diagnostic, showing that the lesion is comprised entirely of fat.

Histology shows mature adipocytes and no atypia. The lesion appears grossly and microscopically like normal fat Fig. 8.64.

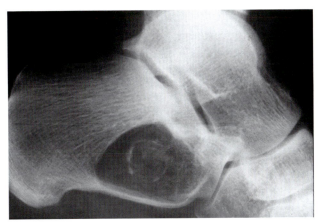

Fig. 8.64 Intraosseous lipoma demonstrated on a lateral radiograph of the calcaneus. The lesion is benign-appearing and has a secondary degenerative calcification pattern seen in these lesions. The calcaneus is a common location for intrasseous lipoma

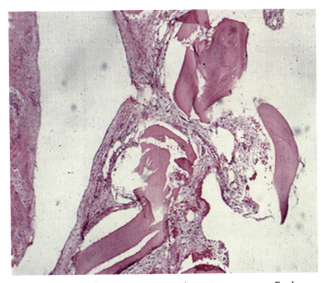

Fig. 8.63 Note the cavernous angiomatous spaces. Endothelial cells show no cytological atypia

8.1.11 Osteosarcoma

Osteosarcoma is a malignant bone-forming tumor that most often occurs in the first three decades of life. Osteosarcoma developing as a secondary process may occur in older individuals (60s and above). Patients almost always present with local pain. The pain is usually a classic tumor pain, often occurring at night or rest and without apparent provocation. Local swelling and tenderness is often present. Patients will usually develop an associated soft-tissue mass that can be appreciated on physical examination. Most patients present with a relatively short time course, usually from weeks to 6 months in the case of high grade tumors.

8.1.11.1 Classic Osteosarcoma

Osteosarcomas typically present radiographically as aggressive malignant destructive lesions with a wide zone of transition and malignant periosteal new bone formation. Although they may be purely lytic, they usually show a mixed lytic or sclerotic or purely sclerotic pattern of bone destruction. The lesions frequently reveal variable quantities of osteoid production that manifest as hazy cloud-like, amorphous regions of increased density in the bone and/or adjacent soft tissues. Osteosarcomas are typically metaphyseal or metadiaphyseal and show intense activity on bone scan.

CT and MRI is an invaluable adjunct in the imaging work up of osteosarcoma. The lesions present as destructive lesions with nonspecific signal characteristics. They frequently have cortical destruction with an associated soft tissue mass. MRI is the most accurate imaging tool for determining intraosseous and extraosseous extent of the tumor. It is important to image the entire bone involved with osteosarcoma to evaluate for skip metastasis.

8.1.11.2 Parosteal Osteosarcoma

Parosteal osteosarcoma presents as a heavily mineralized mass on the surface of the bone with no cortical or medullary continuity between the masses and the parent bone. Parosteal osteosarcomas are usually metaphyseal in origin with the most common site being the posterior aspect of the distal femoral metaphysis. CT and MRI nicely demonstrate the relationship between the lesion and the parent bone with little or no medullary invasion. Parosteal osteosarcomas grow slowly and as grade 1 tumors rarely result in distant metastases.

8.1.11.3 Periosteal Osteosarcoma

Periosteal osteosarcomas are grade 2 surface tumors usually affecting the diaphysis of long bones. There will be no involvement of underlying marrow in the early stage. They usually present with a partially mineralized mass on the surface of the bone with ill-defined margins. The mass is denser near the cortex with an unmineralized soft tissue component on the surface of the lesion.

8.1.11.4 High Grade Surface Osteosarcoma

Lesions are incompletely mineralized and occur on the surface of long bones. There is frequently abundant periosteal reaction with cortical thickening and irregularity. The high grade surface osteosarcomas are difficult to differentiate from periosteal and conventional eccentric central osteosarcomas.

8.1.11.5 Classic Osteosarcoma Pathology

Lesions will be somewhat variable but consistently show malignant cells producing bony matrix (osteoid). Cells are pleomorphic and mitotic figures are often present.

8.1.11.6 Parosteal Osteosarcoma Pathology

Lesions appear low-grade. There will be trabeculae of osteoid and a fibrovascular stroma. The lesions are well-circumscribed and there will be little cytologic atypia.

8.1.11.7 Periosteal Osteosarcoma Pathology

The tumor has a blue appearance on gross examination. Microscopically there will be chondroid matrix intersperced with osteoid. There will be mild cytologic atypia. There will be more spindle cells toward the lesion's periphery.

8.1.11.8 High Grade Surface Osteosarcoma Pathology

Lesions are variable. There will be significant atypia and mitotic activity. There may be areas that appear more chondroid than some regions of osteoid formation (Figs. 8.65–8.79).

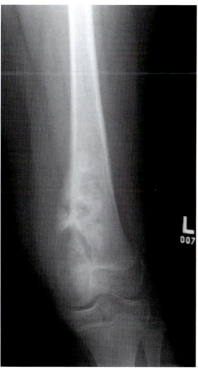

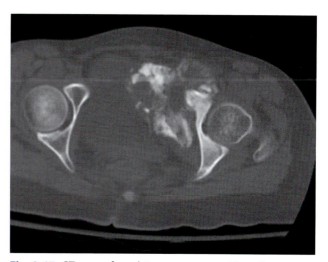

Fig. 8.67 CT scan of a pelvic osteosarcoma There is a destructive lesion in the pubic bone with a large soft tissue mass that contains abundant mineral production. The mineral has an amorphous pattern typical of osteosarcoma

Fig. 8.65 Conventional osteosarcoma (high-grade, osteoblastic) of the distal femur. Note the mixed radiodense and radiolucent areas, broad zone of transition, periosteal reaction, and extraosseous extension

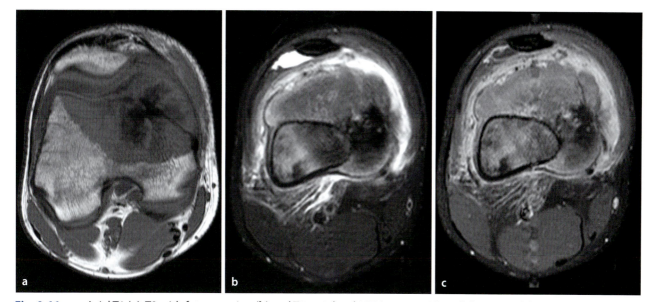

Fig. 8.66 a–c Axial T1 (**a**), T2 with fat saturation (**b**) and T1 weighted MRI images with gadolinium and fat saturation (**c**) show typical findings of an osteosarcoma. There is a large heterogeneous destructive mass in the bone with a large associated soft tissue mass

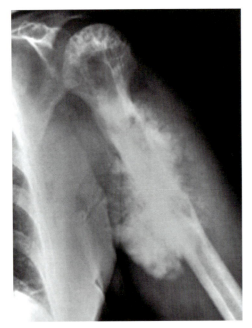

Fig. 8.68 Secondary osteosarcoma originating in a patient with Paget's disease of the humerus

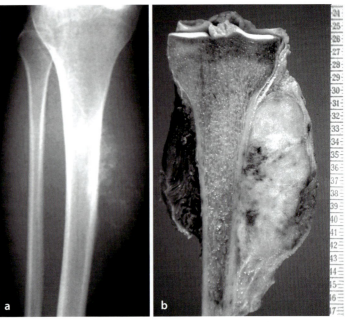

Fig. 8.70 a, b Radiograh (**a**) and cross specimen (**b**) of a periosteal osteosarcoma of the tibial diaphysis. The lesion shows slight cortical irregularity, malignant periosteal new bone formation and a large mineralized soft tissue mass

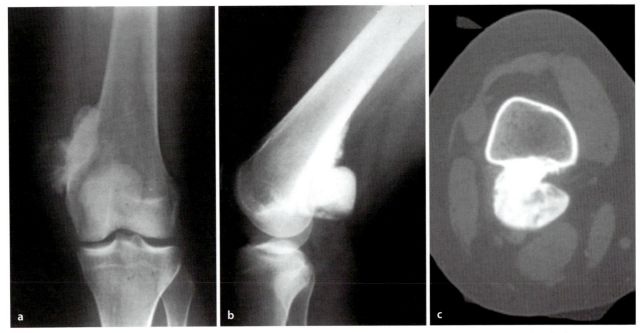

Fig. 8.69 a–c AP radiograph of a bone forming lesion classical for parosteal osteosarcoma (**a**). Lateral radiograph demonstrating parosteal osteosarcoma (**b**) originating from the posterior aspect of the distal femur. CT scan (**c**) of a distal femoral parosteal osteosarcoma. There is a heavily mineralized lesion intimately associated with the cortex on the posterior aspect of the distal femur. Note the absence of marrow involvement in addition to lack of cortical and medullary continuity between the lesion and adjacent bone

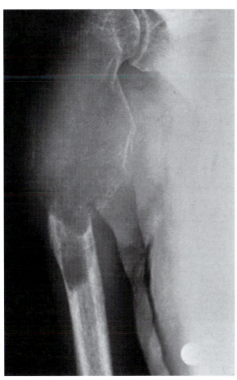

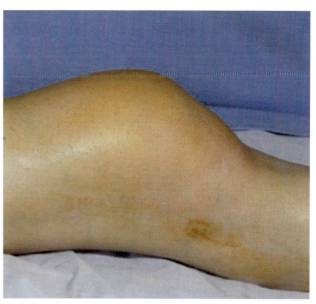

Fig. 8.73 Clinical photo of a 19-year-old patient with osteosarcoma of the distal femur and large soft tissue mass

Fig. 8.71 Teleangectactic osteosarcoma with lytic expansile destruction

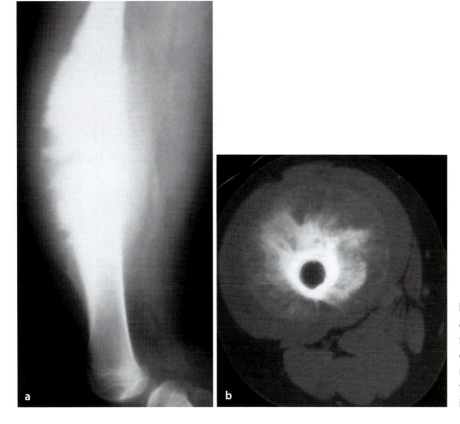

Fig. 8.72 a, b Lateral radiograph (**a**) and axial CT (**b**) show a high grade surface osteosarcoma of the femoral diaphysis. The lesion forms a heavily mineralized circumferential mass that encircles the bone, but does not involve the medullary canal

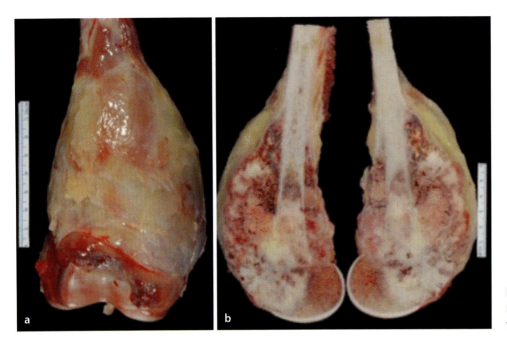

Fig. 8.74 a, b Gross specimen of a distal femoral osteosarcoma

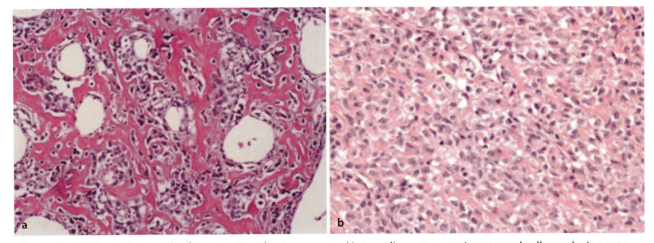

Fig. 8.75 a, b Photomicrograph of a conventional osteosarcoma. Note malignant appearing stromal cells producing osteoid. Low (**a**) and high (**b**) powered photomicrographs of conventional high-grade osteosarcoma

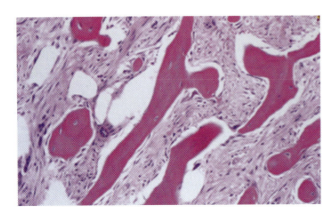

Fig. 8.76 Parosteal osteosarcoma. Note the parallel trabeculae and relatively hypocellular fibrovascular stroma

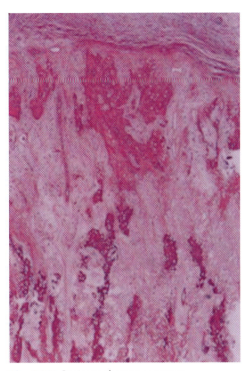

Fig. 8.77 Periosteal osteosarcoma

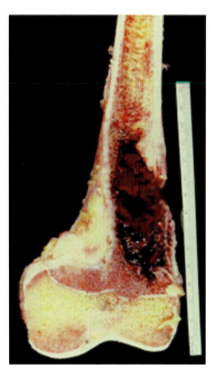

Fig. 8.79 Resection specimen of telangiectatic osteosarcoma. Note blood-filled areas of destruction

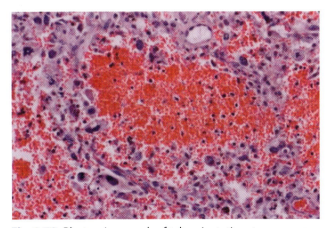

Fig. 8.78 Photomicrograph of telangiectatic osteosarcoma. Note malignant spindle cells and osteoid and associated blood-filled spaces

8.1.12 Chondrosarcoma

Chondrosarcoma is a malignant cartilage-forming tumor. Patients usually present with local or regional pain, although spinal lesions may have a significant component of referred pain. Local tenderness and a mass may be present. In patients with dedifferentiated tumors, a sudden change in pain or increase in the size of a mass may be present. Secondary chondrosarcomas can arise from osteochondroma, enchondroma, etc., and these tumors are usually grade 1 malignant tumors similar to those 60% of primary conventional chondrosarcomas. There is a close relationship between histological grading and survival of the patients. Primary chondrosarcoma is a tumor of adulthood.

8.1.12.1 Conventional

Most lesions are partially mineralized. There may be areas of chondroid calcification as well as areas of lysis and cortical destruction. Periosteal reaction and new bone may be present. Soft tissue extension may be appreciated on CT or MRI.

Grossly, the lesion will appear cartilaginous, although areas of myxoid change or liquefaction may be present. Microscopically, the lesion will appear cartilaginous with varying amounts of cytologic atypia (Figs. 8.80–8.84).

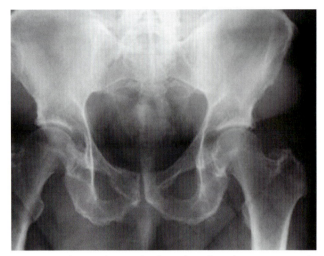

Fig. 8.80 Plain radiograph of a pelvic chondrosarcoma and associated pathologic fracture of the right superior pubic ramus

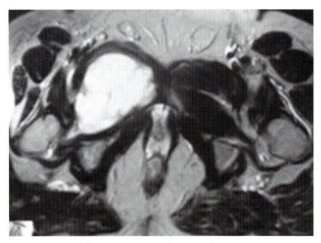

Fig. 8.81 MRI demonstrating a large soft tissue mass

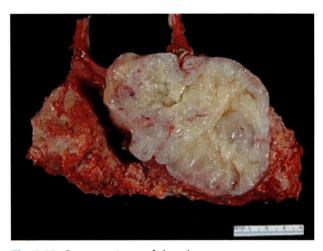

Fig. 8.82 Gross specimen of chondrosarcoma

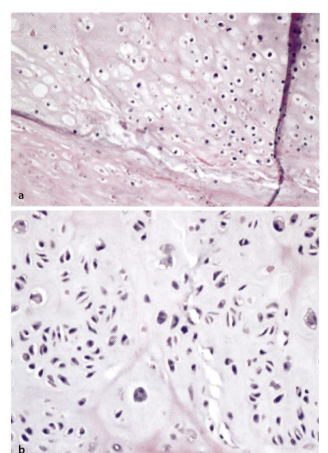

Fig. 8.83 a, b Low (**a**) and high (**b**) power photomicrographs of pelvic chondrosarcoma

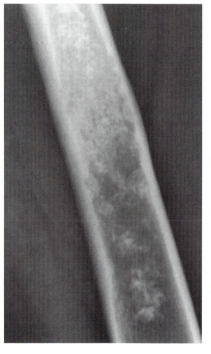

Fig. 8.84 Chondrosarcoma of the femoral diaphysis. Note the chondroid-type calcifications throughout the lesion as well as the significant lucency and endosteal erosion in the center of the radiograph

8.1.12.2 Mesenchymal Chondrosarcoma

Lesions will appear nonspecific and aggressive on radiographs. There is usually some component of calcification in the lesion. There will be a broad zone of transition and cortical destruction.

There will be more mature cartilage-appearing areas interspersed with groups of hypercellular round or spindle cells. There will be little cytologic atypia (Figs. 8.85–8.89).

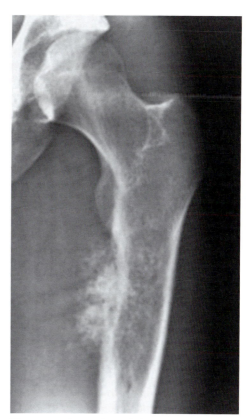

Fig. 8.87 Mesenchymal chondrosarcoma arising from the proximal one-third of the femur

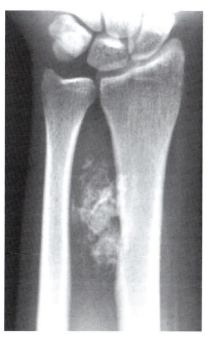

Fig. 8.85 Mesenchymal chondrosarcoma of the distal one-third of the radius

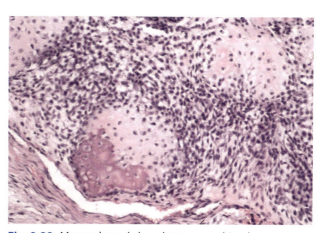

Fig. 8.88 Mesenchymal chondrosarcoma, histology

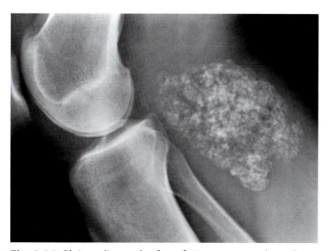

Fig. 8.86 Plain radiograph of a soft tissue mesenchymal chondrosarcoma affecting the popliteal fossa

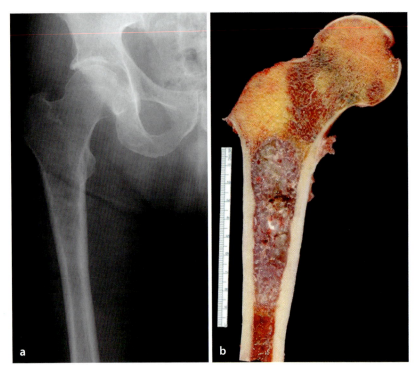

Fig. 8.89 a, b Radiograph (**a**) and gross specimen (**b**) of a low-grade chondrosarcoma in the proximal femur

8.1.12.3 Dedifferentiated

Radiographically, there will be areas that resemble a chondroid lesion juxtaposed with more aggressive, lytic, or permeative areas. Cortical breakthrough and soft-tissue mass are universally present.

Microscopically, there will be areas similar to lower-grade chondrosarcomas as well as components of higher-grade, spindle cells (Figs. 8.90–8.92).

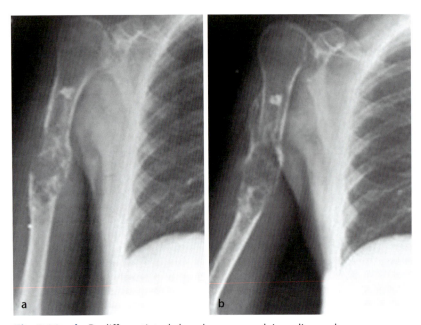

Fig. 8.90 a, b Dedifferentiated chondosarcoma plain radiographs

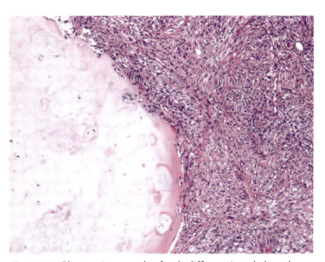

Fig. 8.91 Photomicrograph of a dedifferentiated chondrosarcoma. Note the juxtaposed area of Grade 1 chondrosarcoma

8.1.13 Clear Cell Chondrosarcoma

Clear cell chondrosarcoma is a rare varient of chondrosarcoma low malignant chondrosarcomas which tend to occur in the third and fourth decades. These are often indolent, slow-growing lesions that can cause pain for many years. Most patients present with some level of discomfort. Joint irritability is the most common finding on physical examination.

Lesions occur in the epiphysis of long bones. They may have characteristics of more benign processes, like chondroblastoma or chondromyxoid fibroma both clinically and with different imaging techniques. Approximately one-quarter of lesions will have intralesional calcifications (Figs. 8.93–8.97).

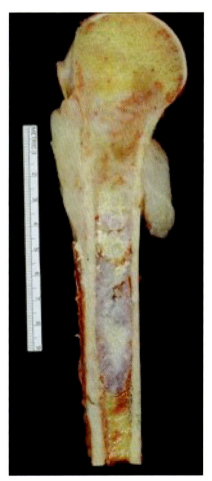

Fig. 8.92 Gross specimen of dedifferentiated chondrosarcoma and associated soft-tissue mass. Again, note the area of more normal-appearing chondroid tissue immediately adjacent to the higher-grade lesion

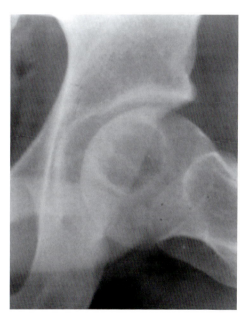

Fig. 8.93 This clear cell chondrosarcoma in the proximal femoral epiphysis presented as a lytic lesion with a sclerotic rim and a few punctuate calcifications. Its radiographic features simulate that of a benign chondroblastoma

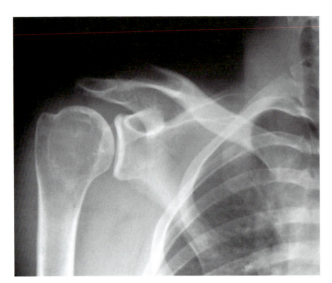

Fig. 8.94 In contrast, the clear cell chondrosarcoma in the proximal humerus shown here has more aggressive features with a lytic pattern of destruction and a wide zone of transition

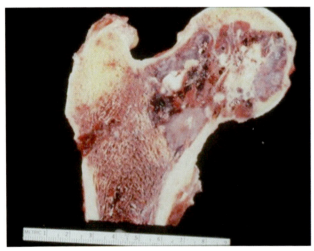

Fig. 8.96 Resected specimen showing clear cell chondrosarcoma involving the femoral head and neck

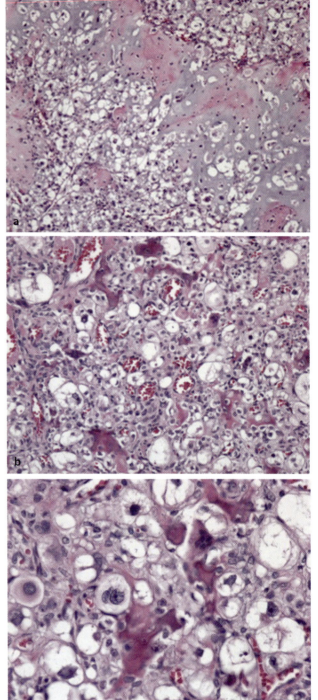

Fig. 8.95 a–c Pathologically, the tumor shows some lobular characteristics (**a**). With higher magnification (**b**), the cells typically have a large amount of clear cytoplasm. Bony trabeculae may also be present (**b, c**)

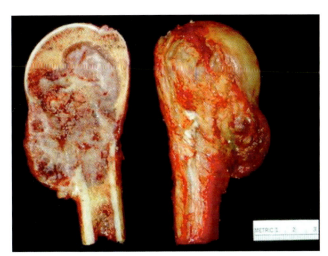

Fig. 8.97 Resected specimen of proximal humerus. Cortical destruction and soft tissue extension are clearly present

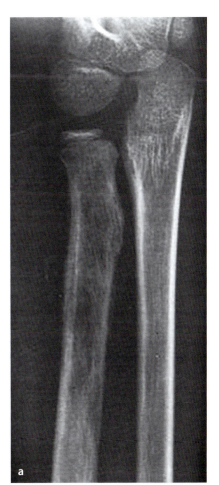

8.1.14 Ewing's Sarcoma/Primitive Neuroectodermal Tumor (PNET)

Ewing's sarcoma and PNET form a family of round cell sarcomas which show varying degree of neuroectodermal differentiation. These relatively rare malignant tumors most commonly present in the first three decades of life.

Most patients present with local or regional pain from the lesion. Swelling and a palpable mass may develop subsequently. Most patients will have pain at rest or at night; significant mechanical or activity-related pain may herald pathologic fracture. Many patients develop signs and symptoms of infection.

Lesions are often permeative with a broad zone of transition between the lesion and the surrounding bones. Lesions typically present in the diaphysis or metadiayphsis of long bones, although flat bones such as the pelvis and scapula may also be involved.

Histologically, tumors are composed of small, round, blue cells. By definition, Ewing's sarcoma is considered a high-grade lesion. Cells are typically uniform with little mitotic activity present (8.98–8.103).

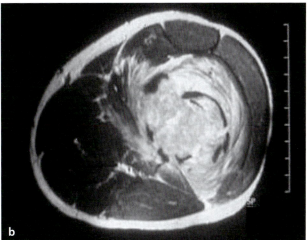

Fig. 8.98 a, b Proximal radial Ewing's sarcoma presented on radiograph (**a**). Note the permeative pattern, broad zone of transition, and periosteal reaction. MRI (**b**) showing bone destruction and large soft tissue mass

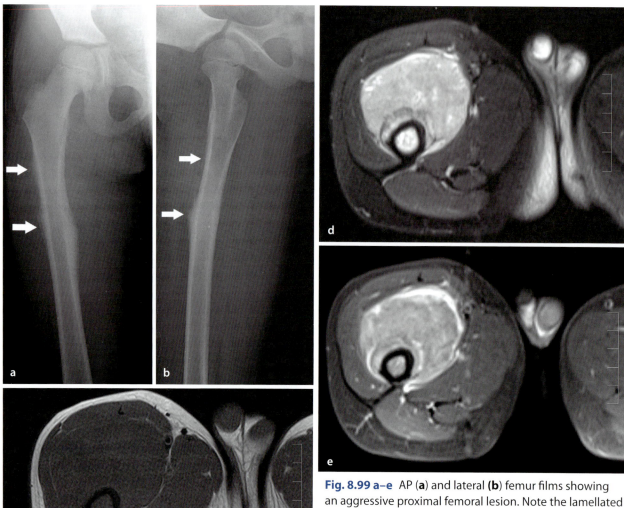

Fig. 8.99 a–e AP (**a**) and lateral (**b**) femur films showing an aggressive proximal femoral lesion. Note the lamellated periosteal reaction and broad zone of transition. MRI of the tumor: Note the large extraosseous component. Most patients with malignant bone tumors have extracompartmental (extraosseous) disease at presentation. Note the signal characteristics: low T1 (**c**) high T2 (**d**), and considerable enhancement with gadolinium (**e**)

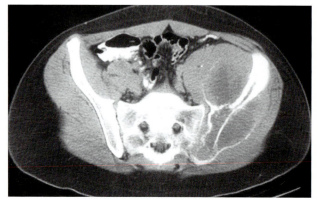

Fig. 8.100 CT scan demonstrating Ewing's sarcoma showing bone destruction and large intrapelvic mass

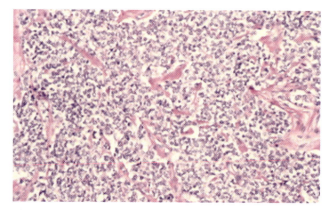

Fig. 8.101 Low-power photomicrograph. Note the uniform population of small, blue cells

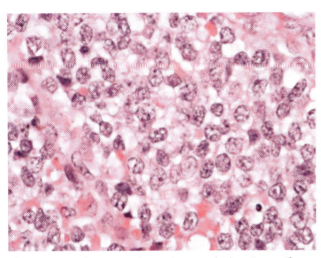

Fig. 8.102 High-power photomicrograph showing uniform cells and prominent nucleoli

8.1.15 Lymphoma

(Synonyms:reticulum cell sarcoma, non-Hodgkin lymphoma of bone). Lymphomas are lymphoreticular tumors that can arise from or spread to bones. Patients present at any age and any bone can be affected, but most often the femur is involved. The majority of bone lymphomas arise in nodal tissues and subsequently metastasize. Rarely, patients will present with a solitary osseous lesion. Patients usually complain of pain and swelling of the involved areas. Patients with multifocal bone involvement may complain of systemic symptoms such as malaise, night sweats, etc. Physical findings include a tender mass, lymphadenopathy and splenomegaly. Patients with spine involvement can have neurologic deficits (8.104–8.108).

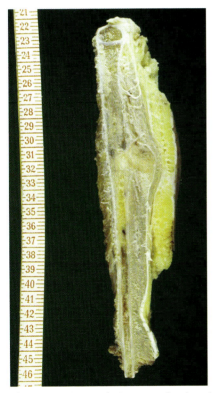

Fig. 8.103 Surgical photographs showing Ewing's sarcoma of the fibula

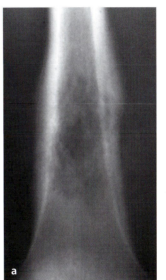

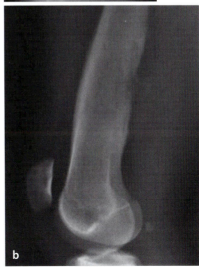

Fig. 8.104 a, b AP (**a**) and lateral radiographs (**b**) of a femoral lymphoma. Primary bone lymphomas tend to occur in the appendicular skeleton; metastatic lesions tend to occur in the axial skeleton. Note the poorly marginated, permeative pattern of bone destruction with associated cortical thickening and periosteal new bone formation

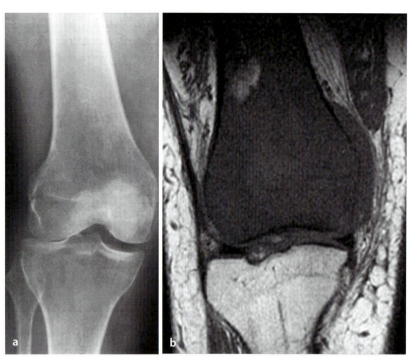

Fig. 8.105 a, b AP radiograph (**a**) of a woman with lymphoma of the distal femur. Radiographic findings may be subtle and easy to overlook. Coronal T1-weighted MRI (**b**) of the same lesion. The size of lesion detected on MRI with lymphoma is often for far greater than suggested on radiographs. There is a small soft tissue mass along the medial femoral condyle

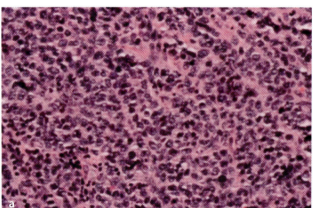
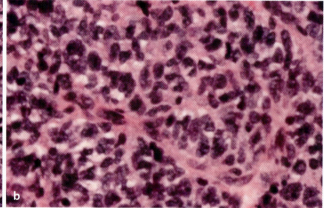

Fig. 8.106 a, b Low power view (**a**) of primary lymphoma of bone. Note the large cell size and the nuclear pleomorphism typically found in diffuse large B-cell lymphoma (the most common lymphoma of bone). The cytoplasm is generally moderately abundant, and may be pale or basophilic. Higher power view (**b**) of primary lymphoma of bone. Note the round or oval appearing nuclei, which appear vesicular, owing to the margination of chromatin at the nuclear membrane. Nucleoli may be single and central, or may number two or three and be located adjacent to the nuclear membrane. As these are mature B-cell tumors, they generally will stain positive for the immunohistochemical markers CD19 and CD20

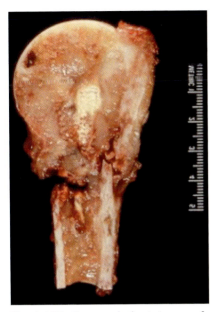

Fig. 8.107 Gross pathologic image of proximal humeral lymphoma. The lesion is permeative with poorly defined margins. Lymphoma often appears whitish and fleshy

8.1.16 Multiple Myeloma

Multiple myeloma is the most common primarily malignancy of bone. Multiple myeloma is a hematopoietic malignancy that typically affects patients older than 50. Pain is the most common patient complaint. A sudden increase in pain may indicate a pathologic fracture. A palpable mass may be present in patients with extraosseous extension. Many patients will also have systemic symptoms such as malaise and weight loss. Patients with osteosclerotic myeloma may develop peripheral neuropathy. In addition to a monoclonal gammopathy noted on serum electrophoresis, patients are often anemic (Figs. 8.109–8.115).

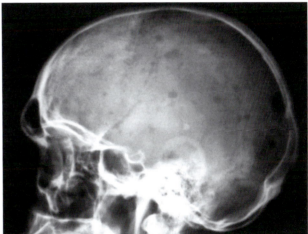

Fig. 8.109 Skull radiograph demonstrating multiple lytic lesions characteristic of myeloma with multiple small lesions with a "punched out" appearance

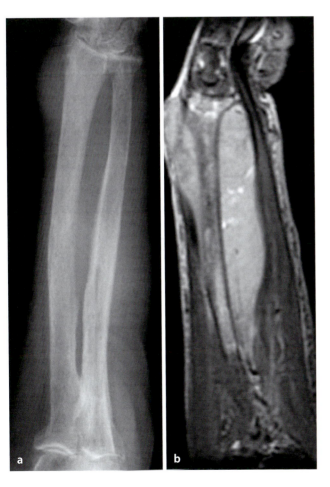

Fig. 8.108 a, b Lymphoma involving left forearm. Characteristically there is a soft tissue mass with minimal roenterographic changes (**a**). The MR picture (**b**) shows the large size of the tumor

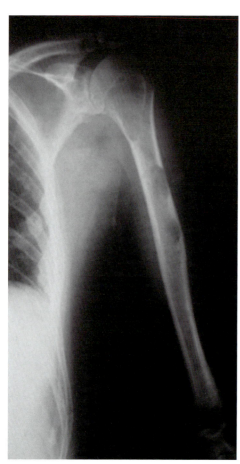

Fig. 8.110 AP radiograph of the left humerus shows multiple lytic lesions of multiple myeloma with associated endosteal scalloping

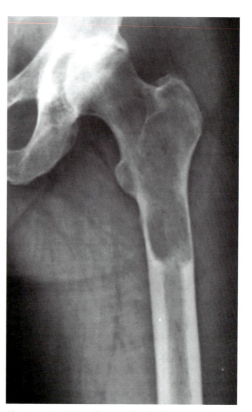

Fig. 8.111 AP radiograph of a lesion in the proximal left femur shows topical imaging features of multiple myeloma with purely lytic pattern of destruction with no evidence of host bone reaction in the form of medullary sclerosis or periosteal reaction

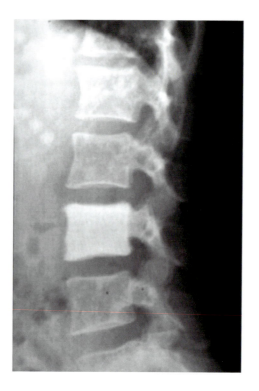

Fig. 8.112 Osteosclerotic vertebral lesion in a patient with the osteosclerotic variant of myeloma. These individuals typically have an associated peripheral neuropathy. Myeloma occurs most commonly in the axial skeleton

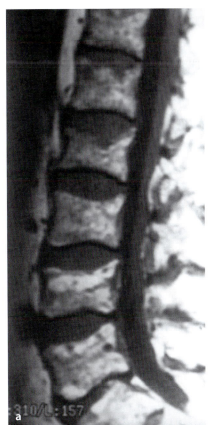

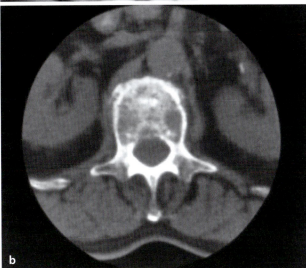

Fig. 8.113 a, b Diffuse involvement of the lumbar spine in a patient with myeloma presented on MR (**a**) and CT (**b**)

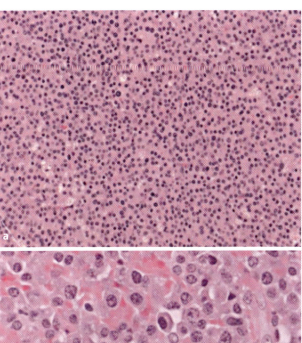

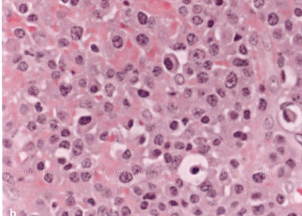

Fig. 8.114 a, b Low power photomicrograph of myeloma (**a**). Lesions are hypercellular without matrix production. Eccentric nuclei and prominent cytoplasm are evident on higher power (**b**). Myeloma cells are secretory and have well-developed golgi apparatus

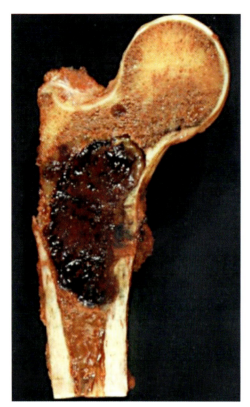

Fig. 8.115 Gross resection of a proximal femur. Note current jelly-appearance to tumor

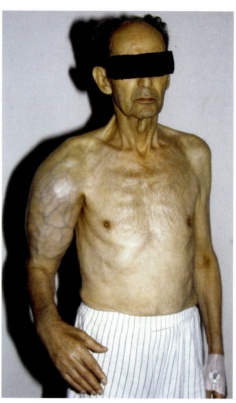

Fig. 8.116 Photograph taken from a cachectic patient suffering on a lung cancer. Note the enormous soft tissue extension of the metastasis in the right upper arm

8.2 Metastatic Bone Disease

Metastases are the most common malignant tumor in bones. Patients often present with local or regional pain. The pain is often at rest, while mechanical or activity-related pain may portend an impending pathologic fracture. Local tenderness or joint irritability may be present. Lesions are often contained in bone, although some patients will present with a palpable soft-tissue mass. Lung, breast, prostate, kidney, and thyroid cancers are the most frequent primary tumors associated with bony metastases. Patients may present with solitary or multiple lesions, often with a history of cancer. Sometimes, however, a bony metastasis will be the initial presentation of a tumor.

The radiographic appearance of metastases is highly variable. The appearance will vary from radiolucent to radiodense; some tumors have a mixed character. As these lesions tend to occur in an older age range than the primary tumors, the differential diagnosis includes myeloma and lymphoma (Figs. 8.116–8.125).

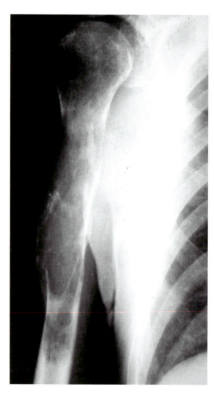

Fig. 8.117 Radiograph from the same patient. Lytic destruction of the entire bone

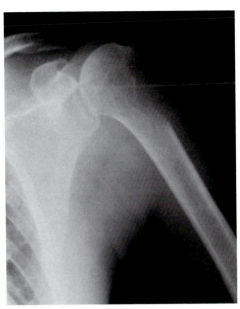

Fig. 8.118 Lytic proximal humeral lesion in a 53-year-old man with metastatic renal cell carcinoma

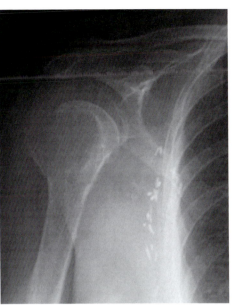

Fig. 8.120 84-year-old woman with a lytic metastasis to the proximal humerus. Note the surgical clips in the axilla. Pathology showed metastatic breast cancer

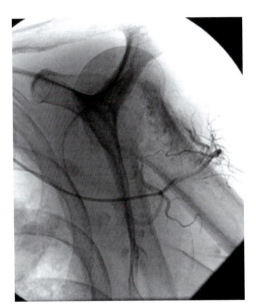

Fig. 8.119 Preoperative embolization showing abundant vascularity characteristic of renal cell tumors

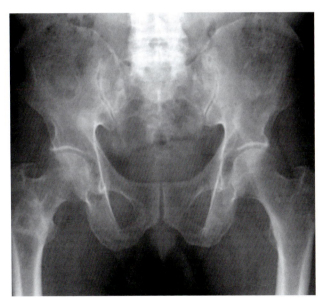

Fig. 8.121 Plain pelvis film of a 64-year-old man with multiple bony metastasis from prostate carcinoma

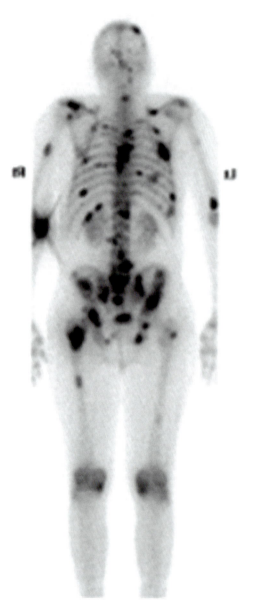

Fig. 8.122 Bone scan of multiple bony metastasis from prostate carcinoma

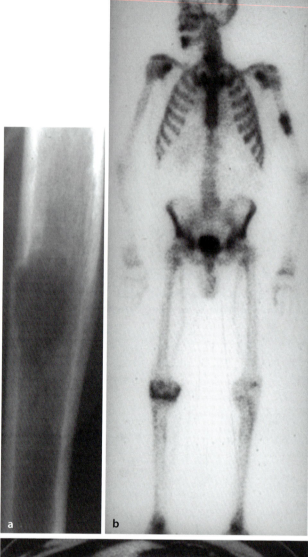

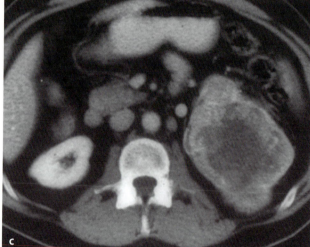

Fig. 8.123 a–c 57-year-old male presented with a lytic destruction of the shaft of the left humerus (**a**). Note the increased uptake in the bone scan (**b**). The CT abdomen showed the primary site in the kidney (**c**)

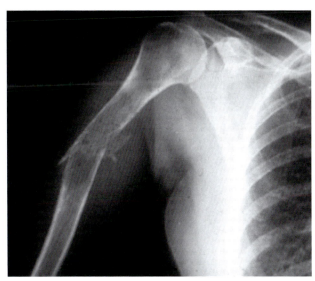

Fig. 8.124 Metastatic destruction with pathological fracture in a patient with breast cancer

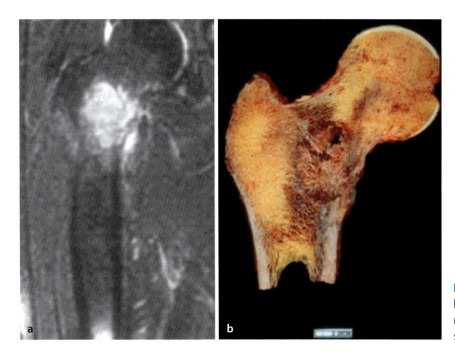

Fig. 8.125 a, b MRI demonstrating lytic destruction extent in the femoral neck (**a**). Resected specimen of metastatic bone disease (**b**)

Chapter 9

Soft Tissue Tumors

Contents

Chapter 9

Soft Tissue Tumors

F. Sim, R. Esther, and D. E. Wenger

Malignant mesenchymal tumors are rare (they amount to 1–1.2% of the overall human burden of malignant tumors); however, there is large variability in their histological subtypes with different clinical, prognostic, and therapeutic consequences. Most soft tissue tumors are benign, located in superficial soft tissue. About one-third of the benign tumors are lipomas, and another one-third are fibrohistiocytic tumors. Three-fourths of the soft tissue sarcomas are located in the extremities, one-third of them are superficial, and two-thirds are deep-seated. Most of them present as symptomless and painless mass that do not influence function or cause cachexia and are recognized accidentally. The superficially located sarcomas may persist for a long time, with same size leading both the patient and the doctor to misinterpret them as a benign condition. Deep-seated soft tissue sarcomas reach greater sizes (on average 8–10 cm) until they are recognized. The local recurrence rate and their capacity for metastasing differ widely according the histological subtypes; the primary filter for the metastases is, however, the lung, like in case of bone sarcomas.

9.1 Lipoma

Lipomas are an extremely common soft tissue tumor. Patients present with either a superficial or deep mass, which in most cases has been present for a considerable time. Lesions are almost uniformly asymptomatic. Subcutaneous lesions are soft and freely mobile, while subfascial tumors will feel more firm. Approximately 10% of patients will have multiple lipomas.

One can see a mass with the same density as fat on plain films. Magnetic resonance imaging (MRI) will show a well-circumscribed lesion with the same density as fat on all pulse sequences. Lipomas may contain a few scattered linear septations that have low signal intensity on T1 and low or high signal intensity on T2.

Gross examination reveals a lesion that looks like mature adipose tissue. Similarly, histologic studies will show mature adipocytes with no areas of increased cellularity or cellular atypia (Figs. 9.1–9.4).

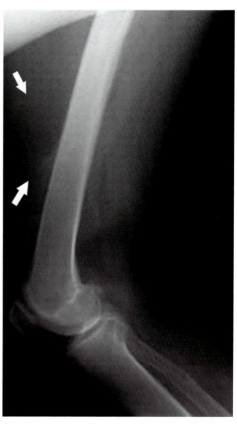

Fig. 9.1 Lateral radiograph of a patient with a mass in the anterior thigh showing a large mass in the soft tissues anteriorly that is less dense than muscle (*arrows*). This feature indicates that the lesion is composed, at least in part, of fat

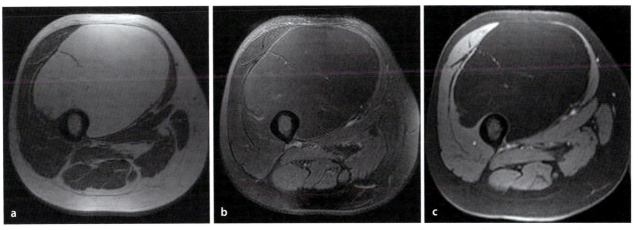

Fig. 9.2 a–c Axial T1 (**a**), T2 with fat saturation (**b**), and T1-weighted image with gadolinium and fat saturation (**c**) showing a large intramuscular lipoma with signal intensity of fat or all pulse sequences. These findings are characteristic of a benign lipoma

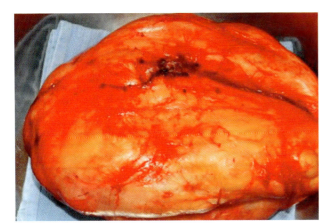

Fig. 9.3 Gross specimen of lipoma

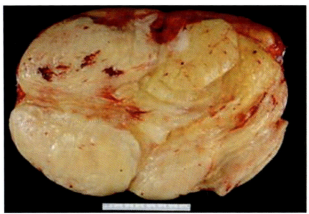

Fig. 9.4 Gross cross-section. Note the yellow appearance and similarity to normal fat

9.2 Atypical Lipoma

Atypical lipomatous tumors are fatty tumors that usually occur in deep tissues of the extremities. Patients are asymptomatic and notice a mass or asymmetry in the extremity, which may have been present for some time. The remainder of physical exam is usually unremarkable.

MRI shows a lesion that is composed predominantly of fat (greater than 75% of the tumor volume) in combination with nonlipomatous elements that can be in the form of thickened septations and/or scattered soft tissue nodularity. The latter features result in areas of hazy, decreased signal intensity in the background of a predominantly high signal intensity mass on T1-weighted images and create an appearance described as "dirty fat."

Grossly, lesions are more firm than lipomas and the tissue does not resemble mature fat. There is more atypia on histologic examination (Figs. 9.5–9.9).

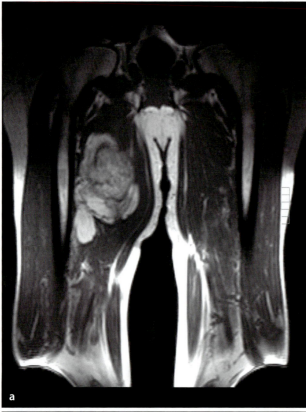

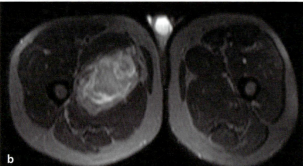

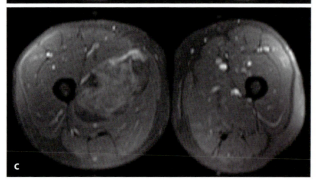

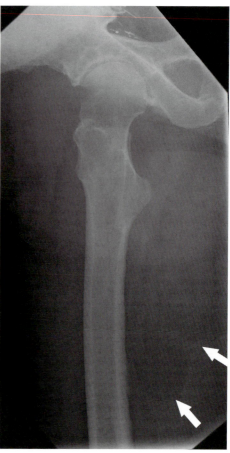

Fig. 9.6 Plain film of the thigh showing a large soft tissue mass consisting mostly of fat density (*arrows*)

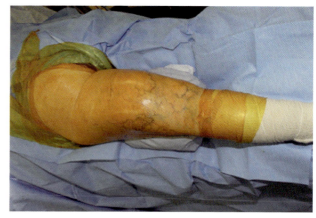

Fig. 9.5 a–c Coronal T1 (**a**) and axial T1 (**b**), and postcontrast image (**c**) of the thigh atypical lipoma seen on the plain radiograph above. While much of the lesion has signal characteristics of mature fat, there is a considerable amount of tissue that is not isointense with fat. Atypical lipomas will also have varying amounts of enhancement after contrast administration

Fig. 9.7 Clinical photograph of the posterior thigh demonstrating a large soft tissue mass and overlying varicosities

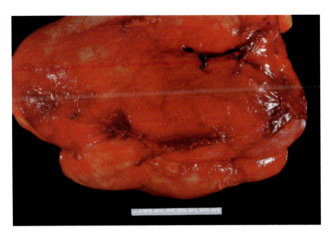

Fig. 9.8 Gross photograph of a resected specimen. The gross appearance is similar to normal mature fat

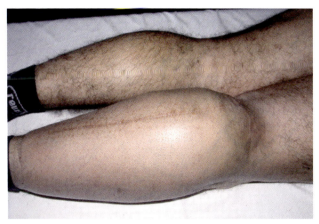

Fig. 9.10 Patient's photograph demonstrating the enlargement of his right leg due to recidive extra-abdominal fibromatosis. Note the scar from earlier operation

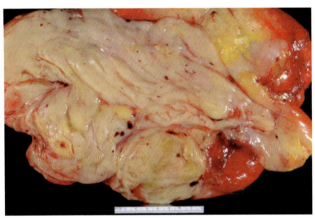

Fig. 9.9 Gross cross-section revealing firmer tissue than normal fat

9.3 Extra-abdominal Aggressive Fibromatosis

(Synonyms: desmoid, desmoid-type fibromatosis). Deep fibromatoses are less frequent than their superficial counterparts (palmar and plantar fibromatoses). These are clonal fibroblastic proliferations that arise from the musculoaponeurotic structures of the deep soft tissues. It may occur anywhere: it is observed, however, most frequently in the shoulder girdle, chest wall, upper arm, thigh, pelvis, and forearm. The peak age of occurrence is between puberty and 40 years, and it is more prevalent in women. The etiology is unknown, but the predisposing factors include trauma, rapid abdominal wall contraction after delivery, surgical procedure, scarring, and hormonal dysfunction (Figs. 9.10–9.13).

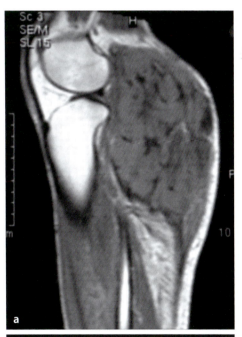

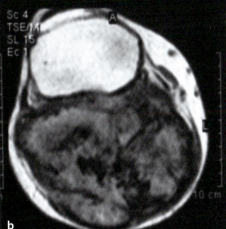

Fig. 9.11 a, b Sagital and axial MRI pictures presenting the enormous tumor that affects the whole popliteal region and the flexor muscles of the leg. It is attached to the dorsal part of the joint capsule and reaches the subcutis

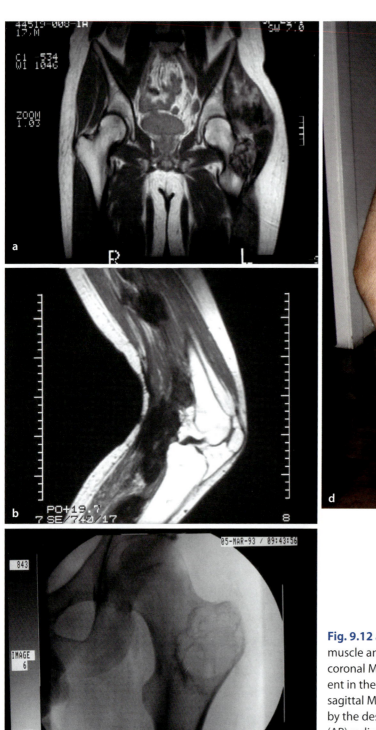

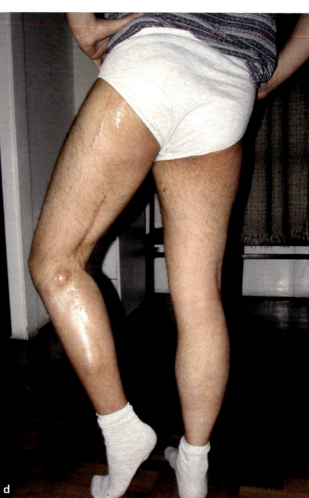

Fig. 9.12 a–d Multifocal desmoid affecting the left gluteal muscle and the greater trochanter of the left femur ((**a**): coronal MR picture), but another part of the tumor is present in the popliteal fossa and flexor muscles of the leg ((**b**): sagittal MR picture). The lytic lesion in the trochanter caused by the desmoid is also clearly seen on the anterioposterior (AP) radiograph (**c**). The extensive desmoid tumor caused contractures in the hip and knee joint in the patient (**d**)

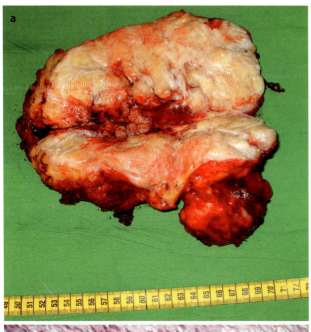

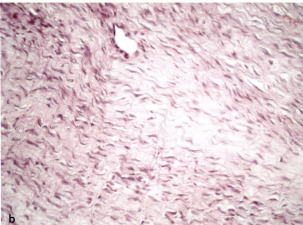

Fig. 9.13 a, b Whorled fibrous cut surface of a desmoid tumor (**a**). Characteristic histological picture of fibromatosis: ill-defined woven fascicles composed of spindle-shaped fibroblasts and abundant collagen fibers. No atypical mitosis is present (**b**)

9.4 Soft Tissue Sarcoma

Soft tissue sarcomas (malignant fibrous histiocytoma (MFH), liposarcoma, etc.) are uncommon soft tissue malignancies that most often occur in adults. Patients will note a firm mass that usually has been present for several months. Occasionally, patients will note a change in size over a fairly short time. Lesions are usually asymptomatic.

Although most often these lesions will occur in a deep, subfascial location, approximately one in three soft tissue sarcomas occurs in the subcutaneous tissues.

Radiographs are frequently negative, but may show a masslike area of soft tissue fullness. Most soft tissue sarcomas are isodense with the adjacent muscle. Many soft tissue sarcomas have nonspecific signal characteristics on MRI, with low to intermediate signal intensity on T1, heterogeneous primarily high signal intensity on T2, and variable enhancement with gadolinium. Areas of necrosis and/or hemorrhage are common in large lesions (Figs. 9.14–9.20).

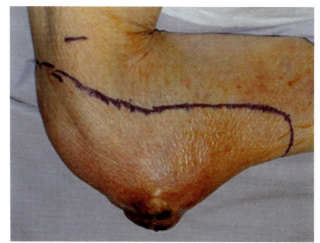

Fig. 9.14 Subcutaneous soft tissue sarcoma fungating through the skin near the elbow

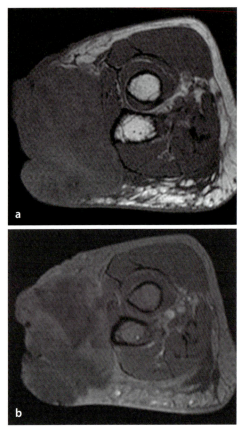

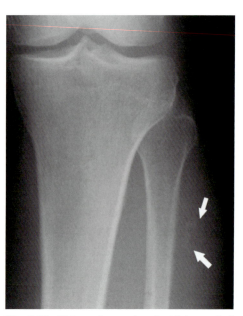

Fig. 9.16 Plain radiographs of a high-grade liposarcoma adjacent to the proximal fibula. Note the intralesional mineralization (*arrows*). The evaluation of all soft tissue masses should begin with a plain film

Fig. 9.15 a, b Axial T1- (**a**) and T2-weighted image with gadolinium and fat saturation (**b**) showing a heterogeneous soft tissue sarcoma in the proximal forearm that is predominantly in the subcutaneous tissues abutting the adjacent myofascial plane

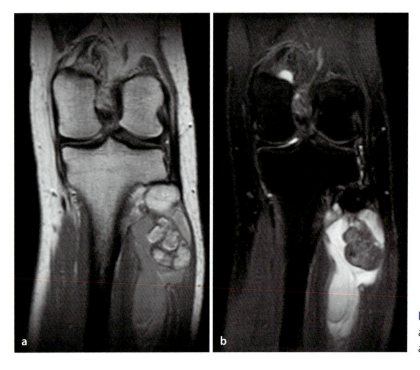

Fig. 9.17 a, b Proton density (**a**), T2 (**b**), images of the lesion. Note the heterogeneity and intimate association with the fibula

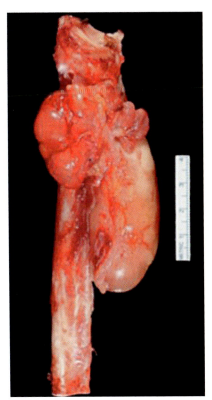

Fig. 9.18 Resected proximal fibula with adjacent liposarcoma

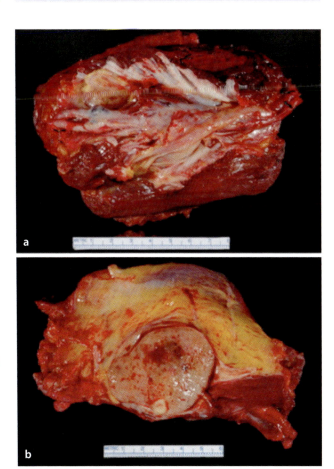

Fig. 9.20 a, b Gross specimen. The lesion encompassed the superficial femoral vascular bundle

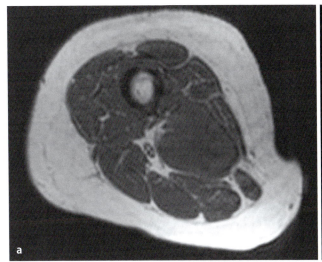

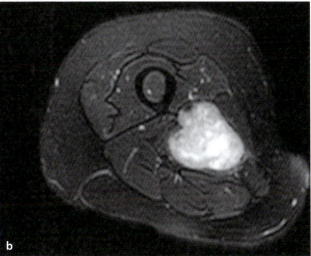

Fig. 9.19 a, b Axial T1- (**a**) and axial T2-weighted MRI with fat saturation (**b**) showing typical MRI features of a soft tissue sarcoma with intermediate signal intensity on T1 (isointense with muscle) and markedly heterogeneous pre-dominantly high signal intensity on T2. Note that the tumor originates within the deep muscular compartment of the thigh. The MRI nicely delineates the relationship between the mass and the adjacent neurovascular structures

Chapter 10

Synovial Neoformation and Tumors

Contents

Synovial Neoformation and Tumors

F. Sim, R. Esther, and D.E. Wenger

The rather rare synovial tumors and tumorlike lesions represent a distinct entity within the family of soft tissue tumors. Joints, bursae, and tendon seaths have the same type of synovial membrane, so similar tumors can develop from all of these structures. The clinical symptoms of synovial tumors and tumorlike lesions are uniform and present as swelling or visible and palpable masses within and/or around the joints. Synovial effusion, if any, can be blood stained or xanthochromic. Conventional radiographs are informative in only a minority of cases, such as synovial chondromatosis. More helpful are modern imaging methods such as computed tomography (CT) or magnetic resonance imaging (MRI); a definitive diagnosis can be obtained, however, after surgical intervention and histological examination of the removed tissue in most cases.

10.1 Synovial Chondromatosis

Synovial chondromatosis is a benign proliferation of cartilaginous tissue arising in the synovium of joints, tendon sheath, and bursae. It is a monoarticular process that most commonly affects the knee, hip, and elbow. Patients present with intermittent swelling, effusions, and progressive pain in the involved joint. Mechanical symptoms such as stiffness, joint locking, or catching may be present. Over time, patients may lose mobility and develop contractures.

Radiographs show intra- and periarticular soft tissue masses with varying amounts of calcification. Effusions may be present. Depending on the chronicity of the process, patients may develop secondary osteoarthritic changes.

Microscopially, nodules of hyaline cartilage are seen. There may be some degree of cytologic atypia. Surrounding synovium is hyperplastic (Figs.10.1 and10. 2).

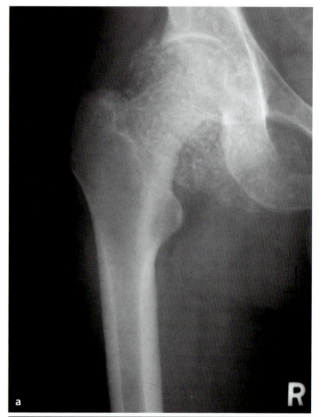

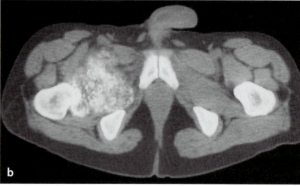

Fig. 10.1 a, b Plain radiographs (**a**) and CT scan (**b**) of synovial chondromatosis of the hip. Note the enlarged joint capsule filled by large mass of intra-articular calcified cartilaginous free bodies

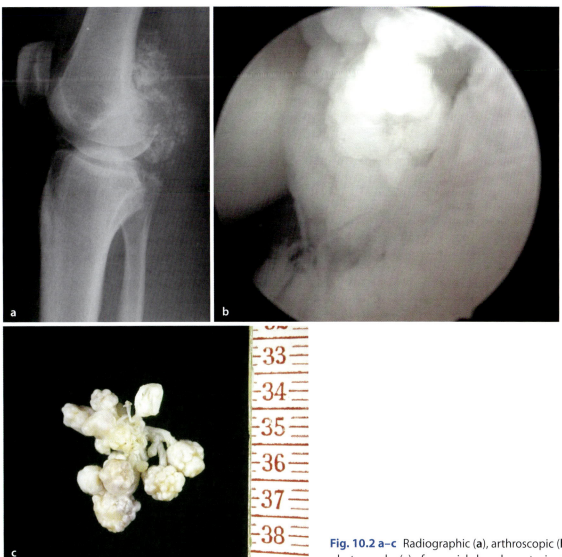

Fig. 10.2 a–c Radiographic (**a**), arthroscopic (**b**), and gross photographs (**c**) of synovial chondromatosis of the knee

10.2 Lipoma Arborescens

Lipoma arborescens is an extremely rare articular disease where there is fatty infiltration of a joint's synovial lining. Lesions are usually unilateral, but bilateral cases have been reported in the literature. The knee is the most commonly involved joint.

Clinically, patients present with nonspecific complaints and exam findings. Recurrent effusions and occasional pain flares are common. Patients usually report joint difficulties over a number of years, often decades.

Radiographs are often unremarkable, although swelling, effusions, and secondary degenerative changes may be present. MRI demonstrates characteristic imaging features with nodular masses within the joint that have signal intensity isointense with fat on all pulse sequences. There is usually an associated large joint effusion.

Grossly, lesions have fronds of fat. Microscopically, normal synovium is seen interspersed with mature adipocytes (Figs. 10.3 and 10.4).

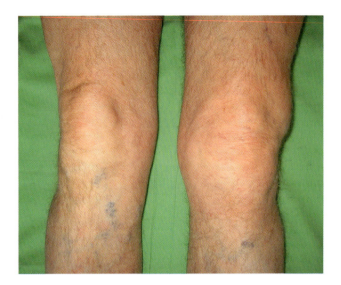

Fig. 10.3 Clinical photograph of lipoma arborescens of the knee. Note the considerable effusion of the left knee

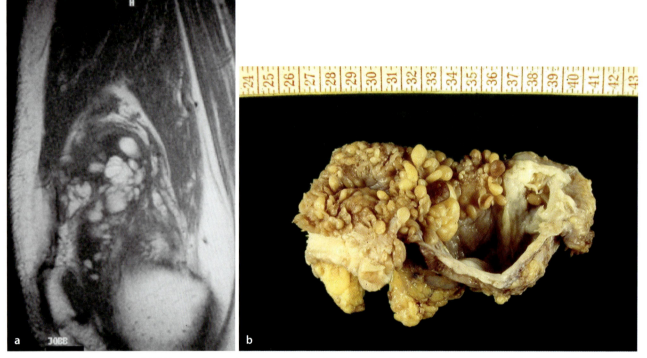

Fig. 10.4 a, b T1-weighted MRI image (**a**) and gross specimen (**b**). Note the frond-like appearance of the fatty villi corresponding to the areas of fat signal on MRI

10.3 Pigmented Villonodular Synovitis

(Synonyms: diffuse-type giant cell tumor, pigmented villonodular tenosynovitis). Pigmented villonodular synovitis (PVNS) is an idiopathic condition that most commonly affects the knee or hip in young adults (30s through 50s). The ankle may also be involved. Monoarticular swelling, loss of motion, recurrent effusions, hemarthrosis with intermittent flares of pain may all be present. In general, the clinical examination is nonspecific. Joint aspirates reveal fluid ranging from clear to bloody in appearance.

Radiographs often show periarticular lucencies, sometimes on both sides of a joint. At long duration, the destructive proliferation of synovial-like tissue can affect the adjacent bone. Secondary degenerative changes may also be present. There will often be considerable effusions present.

Lesions may be diffuse (villous) or localized (nodular). Grossly, the tissue is reddish brown in appearance, although some areas may appear more yellow because of the fat content. Lipid- or hemosiderin-filled macrophages are present. There will be occasional multinucleated giant cells (Figs 10.5–10.10).

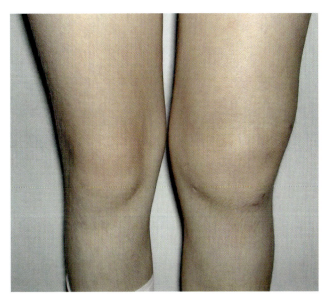

Fig. 10.5 Clinical photograph of a patient with pigmented villonodular synovitis (PVNS) of the left knee

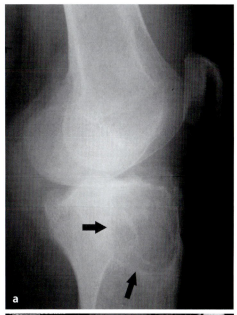

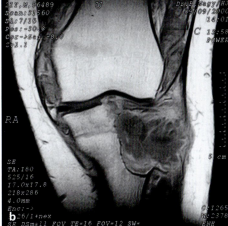

Fig. 10.6 a, b Lateral radiograph (**a**) of the knee demonsrating extensive erosive changes in the proximal tibia in a patient with PVNS. T1-weighted MR image (**b**) of the same patient. PVNS characteristically has low signal characteristics because of the hemosiderin present in the lesion

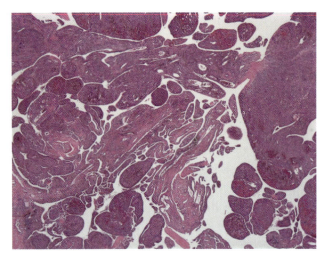

Fig. 10.7 Low-power micrograph showing villous finger-like and rounded masses underlying the synovial membrane

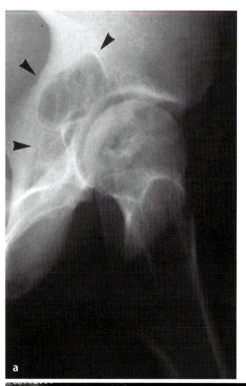

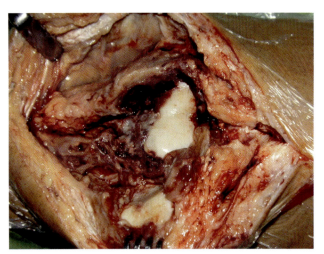

Fig. 10.8 Knee arthrotomy demonstrating intra-articular extent of the diffuse form of PVNS

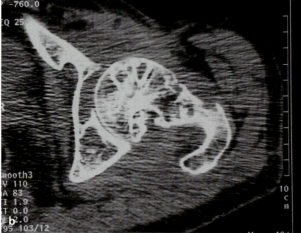

Fig. 10.9 a, b Extensive erosive changes, lytic lesions in the acetabulum (*arrows*), and femoral head caused by an aggressive, growing PVNS as demonstrated on radigraph (**a**) and CT (**b**)

10.4 Synovial Hemangioma

Synovial hemangiomas are unusual lesions. They arise from the synovial lining around joints. Patients present with local swelling, pain, joint irritability, and effusions. Most patients are in the first or second decade of life.

Radiographs may show an effusion and intralesional phleboliths. MRI demonstrates an intra- or periarticular soft tissue lesion with signal characteristics of hemangioma.

Histologically, lesions often resemble cavernous hemangiomas. Septations and hemosiderin deposition are present (Figs.10.11 and 10.12).

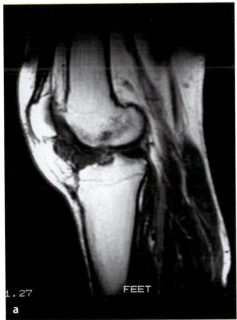

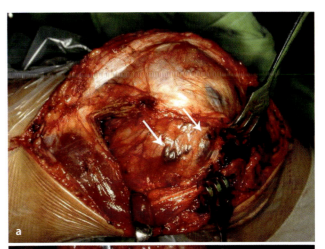

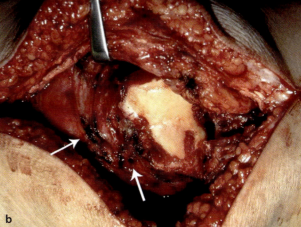

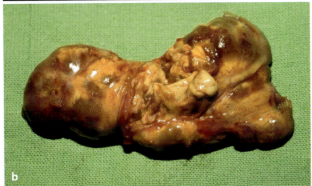

Fig. 10.11 a, b Intraoperative photographs of synovial hemangioma of the knee. Note the diffuse dark-colored areas present in the synovial lining

Fig. 10.10 a, b Sagital MR picture presenting nodular form of PVNS in the Hoffa's fat body (**a**). Gross specimen of this nodular PVNS (**b**)

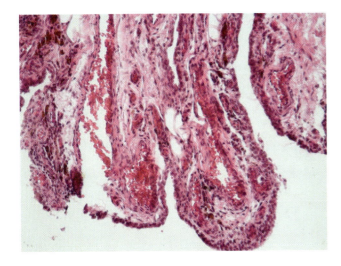

Fig. 10.12 Histology of synovial hemangioma displaying blood-filled spaces interspersed with bland stroma. There is no cellular atypia present

Chapter 11

Tumor-like Lesions
of Bone

Contents

Chapter 11

Tumor-like Lesions of Bone

F. Sim, R. Esther, and D.E. Wenger

The significance of the tumor-like bony lesions is that their radiographical appearance may mimic that of malignant bone tumors, which gives rise to differential diagnostic problems, since they are much more common than bone sarcomas. Regarding their progress, tumor-like bone lesions can be latent like nonossifying fibroma, active like juvenile bone cyst, or aggressive like some aneurysmal bone cysts, which later can destroy the bone and cause pathologic fracture. According to the type and progress of the lesions, they can be symptomless, or cause pain and tenderness in the affected limb.

11.1 Unicameral Bone Cyst

These lesions may be noted incidentally mostly in the first two decades of life. Local deformity may be present, especially with a prior pathologic fracture. Patients with pathologic fractures through bone cysts have the expected findings of inhibited motion and local tenderness.

These lesions typically occur in the metaphyses of the proximal humerus or less frequently the proximal femur and tibia. They will often abut, but not cross, the epiphyseal plate. These lesions appear benign, with a sharp, narrow zone of transition between the cyst and surrounding bone. Bony expansion is present but not to the extent seen in aneurysmal bone cysts. As a general rule, the cortex does not expand beyond the width of the adjoining physis.

There is a rim of fibrous connective tissue at the cyst's periphery. Multinucleated giant cells may also be present. There is no cytologic atypia (Figs. 11.1–11.6).

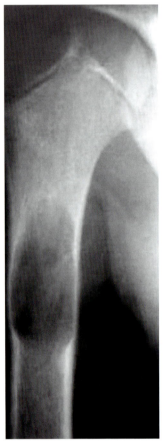

Fig. 11.1 Unicameral bone cyst (UBC), proximal humerus. Note multilocular nature of lucency with thinning of the cortices. The bony enlargement will not be wider than the physis (active)

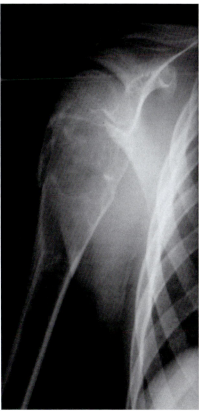

Fig. 11.2 UBC of proximal humerus with cortical thinning. Note the uninvolved area distal to the physis (latent cyst)

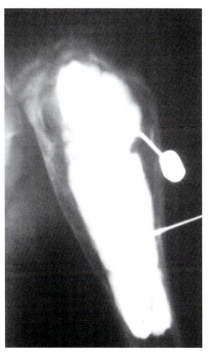

Fig. 11.3 UBC of proximal humerus with injection of dye at the time of prednisolone injection therapy

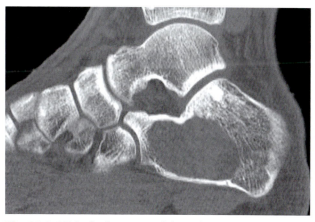

Fig. 11.4 UBC of calcaneus with large lucent area and cortical thinning

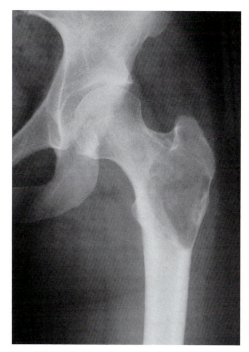

Fig. 11.5 UBC involving the femoral subtrochanteric area. The risk of fracture may necessitate bone grafting and internal fixation

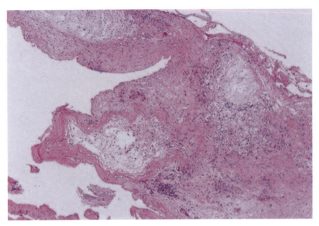

Fig. 11.6 Photomicrograph of fibrous lining of the solitary cyst

11.2 Aneurysmal Bone Cyst

Aneurysmal bone cysts are benign, locally aggressive cystic lesions that usually occur in the first two decades of life. They are slightly more common in women. Patients typically present with pain and swelling of the involved area. Physical findings include local tenderness, swelling, and limited range of motion. Aneurysmal bone cysts can occur de novo or as secondary phenomena in other conditions such as giant cell tumor, fibrous dysplasia, and chondroblastoma. It tends to recur in high percentage following curettage (20–50%) (Figs. 11.7–11.15).

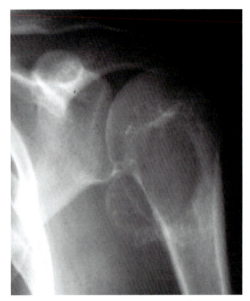

Fig. 11.8 Aneurysmal bone cyst of the proximal humerus. Again, note the eccentric metaphyseal location with expansion medially with an intact shell of bone

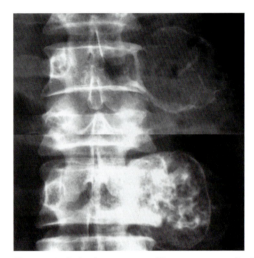

Fig. 11.9 Spinal aneurysmal bone cysts typically involve the posterior elements. Patients may present with neurologic symptoms

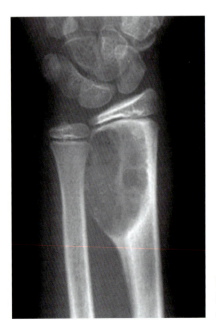

Fig. 11.7 Aneurysmal bone cyst of the distal radial metadiaphysis. This lesion illustrates the typical radiographic features of an aneurysmal bone cyst with an eccentric, lytic lesion with marked associated expansion and no intralesional matrix

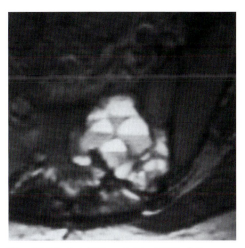

Fig. 11.10 Axial T2-weighted MRI of the sacrum shows typical MR imaging features of an aneurysmal bone cyst with multiple round, fluid-filled levels indicative of intralesional hemorrhage

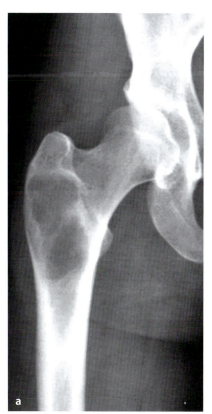

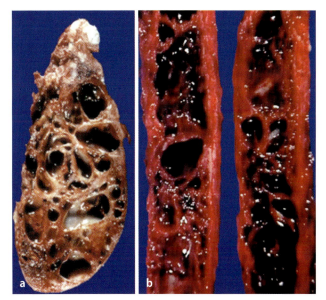

Fig. 11.12 a, b Gross appearance of aneurysmal bone cyst (**a, b**). Tissue can range in color from brownish to more hemorrhagic. Note the intralesional septations

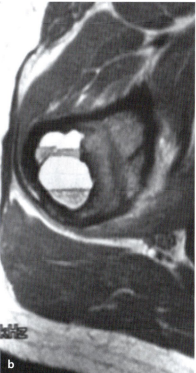

Fig. 11.11 a, b Conditions such as fibrous dysplasia can develop secondary aneurysmal bone cyst. This patient had fibrous dysplasia of the proximal femur (**a**). The MRI shows the fluid levels of the components of secondary aneurysmal bone cyst (**b**)

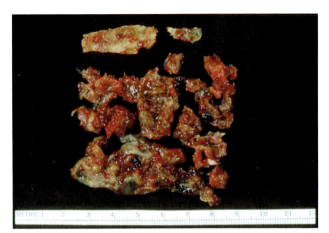

Fig. 11.13 Tissue from within an aneurysmal bone cyst is usually friable and brownish-red in color

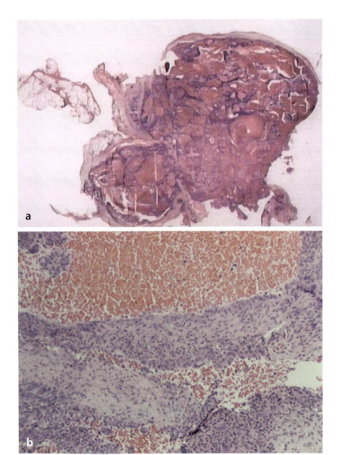

Fig. 11.14 a, b Photomicrographs show blood-filled cystic spaces with lining. Giant cells are often present

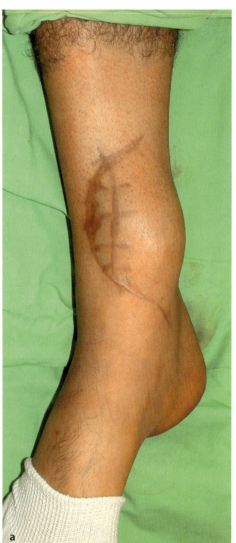

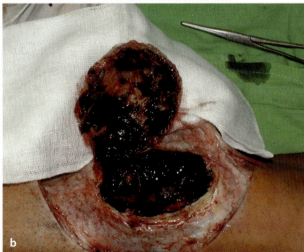

Fig. 11.15 a, b Clinical (**a**) and intraoperative (**b**) photographs of a lower-extremity aneurysmal bone cyst (ABC). Note the scars from prior surgery for recurrences. Intraoperative photo shows multiple septations and blood-filled spaces

11.3 Nonossifying Fibroma

(Synonym: Metaphyseal fibrous defect)These lesions most commonly are detected incidentally as part of an evaluation for other reasons, for example, knee pain. Peak age is the second decade. As they are asymptomatic, there are no common findings on physical examination. For large lesions occupying more than half of the bone diameter, patients may present with a pathologic fracture and have local tenderness.

Histology shows a variable pattern of fibrous stroma with occasional clusters of giant cells and macrophages. There is no nuclear atypia, although mitotic figures may be present (Figs. 11.16–11.18).

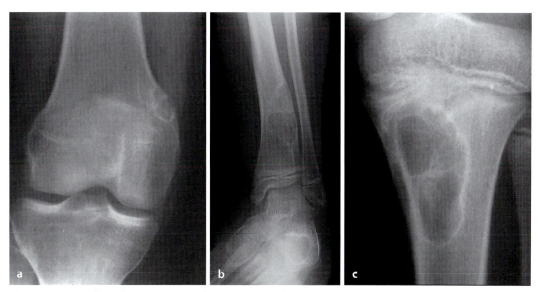

Fig. 11.16 a–c These lesions are usually eccentric and metaphyseal, often occurring in the long bones of the lower extremity, including the distal femur (**a**) and distal (**b**) and proximal (**c**) tibia. The overlying cortex may be thinned and/or expanded. Lesions may have a lobular or septated appearance and are usually sharply marginated

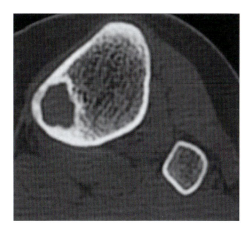

Fig. 11.17 CT scan: These lesions are benign-appearing with a narrow zone of transition

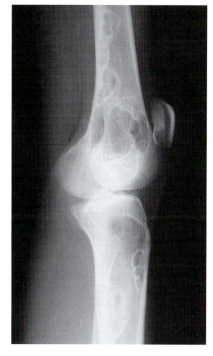

Fig. 11.18 Nonossifying fibroma appear often as multiple lesions around the knee

11.4 Osteofibrous Dysplasia

(Synonyms: Campanacci's tumor) Osteofibrous dysplasia is a benign, self-limited fibro-osseous lesion of bone that occurs exclusively in the tibia or fibula. Patients usually present in the first two decades of life. Patients may present with lower-extremity bowing, limb-length discrepancy, or gait abnormalities. These lesions are often painless (Figs. 11.19–11.22).

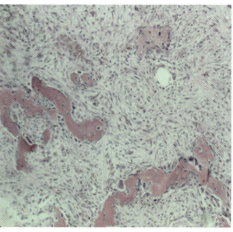

Fig. 11.20 Photomicrograph demonstrating irregular trabeculae in a fibrovascular stroma with osteoblastic rimming

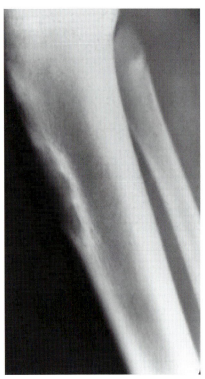

Fig. 11.19 Lateral radiograph of the tibia shows typical features of osteofibrous dysplasia with a lytic, mildly expansile intracortical lesion with a sclerotic rim. These lesions frequently involve the anterior cortex of the metadiaphysis of the tibia. Patients may have multiple radiolucencies in the involved bone

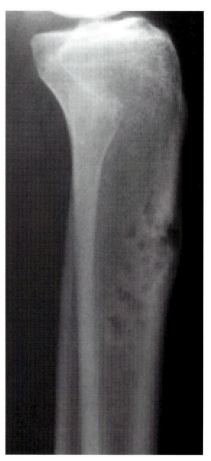

Fig. 11.21 Lateral roenterogram of tibia in 7-year-old boy. The mother noted enlargement of his leg. Note the multiple lucent areas with multiple lucent areas and cortical erosion typical for osteofibrous dysplasia. Similar appearance may be seen in adamantinoma

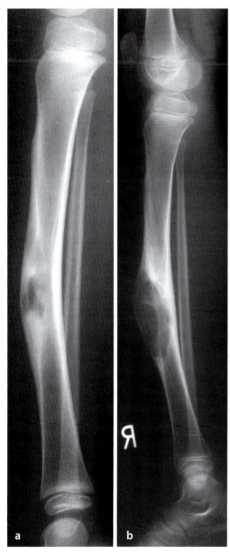

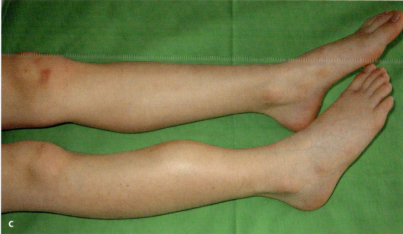

Fig. 11.22 a–c Typical osteofibrous dysplasia in the tibia at the age 4 (**a**) and 6 (**b**) in a girl. Note the progressive bowing of the bone very characteristic for the disease. Photograph of the patient's bowed leg (**c**)

11.5 Fibrous Dysplasia

Fibrous dysplasia is a fibro-osseous benign lesion. Clinically, patients are often asymptomatic but may present with pain, limp, or pathologic fracture. Fibrous dysplasia may be monostotic or polyostotic. Polyostotic fibrous dysplasia may be associated with syndromes. Patients with McCune–Albright's syndrome have abnormal cutaneous pigmentation, endocrine abnormalities, and multiple bone involvement. These patients may present with precocious puberty.

Mazabraud's syndrome is an association of fibrous dysplasia with soft tissue myxomas.

Lesions can occur in the ribs, skull and jaw, and the long and flat bones. Skull and facial lesions can cause significant deformity, exopthalmos, etc.

Histologically, these lesions demonstrate bland-appearing fibrous areas with interspersed trabeculae of woven bone (Figs. 11.23–11.29).

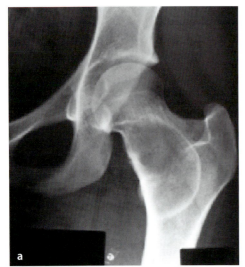

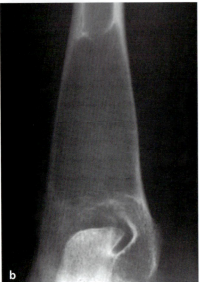

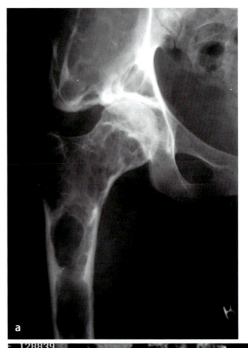

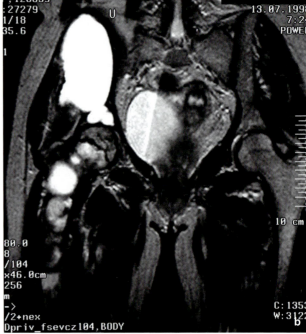

Fig. 11.23 a, b Radiographically, lesions originate in the medullary canal and may be metaphyseal or diaphyseal in location. The fibrous tissue may impart areas of hazy increased density within the lesion that have been described as "ground glass" density. Well-circumscribed lesion with sclerotic rim in the femoral neck (**a**) and less defined lesion in the distal humerus (**b**)

Fig. 11.24 a, b The lesions are usually benign-appearing, presenting a bubbly lytic or mixed lytic and sclerotic lesions with a narrow zone of transition and a sclerotic margin as seen in this patient with polyostotic disease affecting both the femur and pelvic bone as presented on the radiograph (**a**) and MR imaging (**b**)

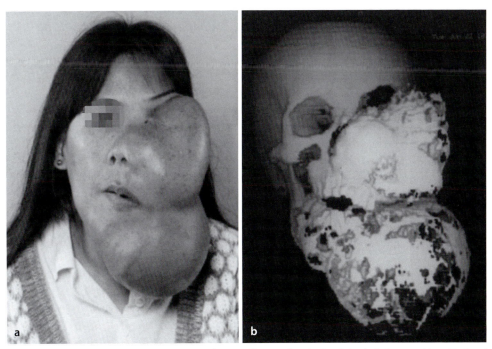

Fig. 11.25 a, b Massive deformity secondary to fibrous dysplasia of the left face and jaw. Patient's photograph (**a**) and 3D CT (**b**)

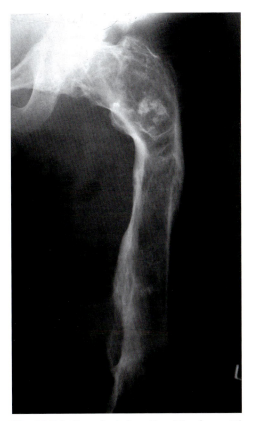

Fig. 11.26 Chronic deformity of the femur(the character-istic "shepherd's crook" deformity) in a patient with polyos-totic fibrous dysplasia

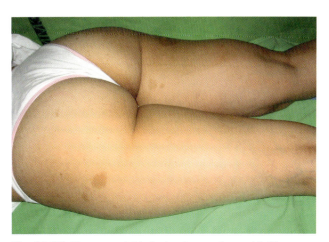

Fig. 11.27 Pigmented skin lesion in a patient with fibrous dysplasia and precursor puberty (Albright's disease)

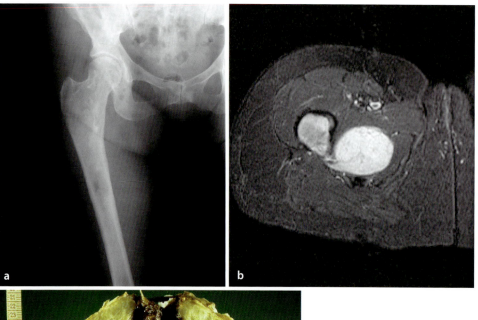

Fig. 11.28 a–c Maz-abraud's syndrom: Radiograph of the patient's proximal femur, and pelvis demonstrating characteristic polyostotic fibrous dysplasia (**a**). MR picture from the tigh (**b**) presents large myxoid soft tissue tumor. Cross-specimen of intramuscular myxoma (**c**)

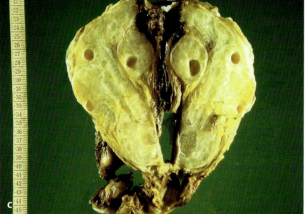

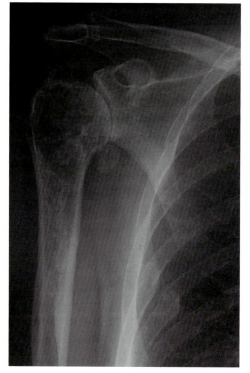

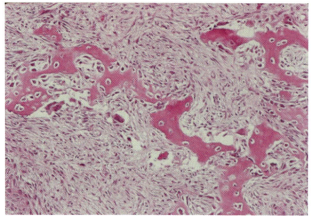

Fig. 11.29 Histologically, one will see a combination of benign, proliferating fibroblastic cells, and islands of woven bone. The bony trabeculae area arranged in an erratic pattern sometimes referred to as "an alphabet soup"

Fig. 11.30 Anterioposterior (AP) shoulder radiograph of a man with long-standing bone infarct of the proximal humerus and concomitant glenohumeral arthritis. Note the serpiginous mineralization pattern extending through the diaphysis

11.6 Bone Infarcts

As opposed to patients with osteonecrosis of the proximal humerus or femur, patients with bone infarcts of the long bones often are asymptomatic. These lesions may be noted incidentally when studies are initiated for other reasons.

Lesions often occur in the diaphysis and metadiaphyseal regions of long bones. Bone infarcts are medullary lesions.

Radiographically, medullary infarcts present with patchy areas of increased density or sclerosis in the metaphysis or diaphysis of long bones. They may have somewhat angular margins demarcating the boundary of the necrotic and adjacent normal trabecular bone.

Histologically, the bone will show marrow necrosis and empty bony lacunae. Various amounts of reparative fibrous tissue may be present.

Secondary malignancies can occur in bone infarcts as a consequence of the chronic reparative process. These malignancies are very rare but should be considered in a patient with new onset of pain or areas of extensive radiolucency and cortical destruction (Figs. 11.30–11.32).

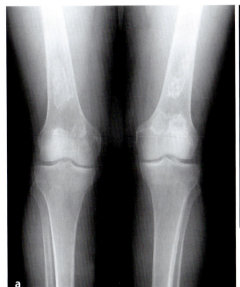
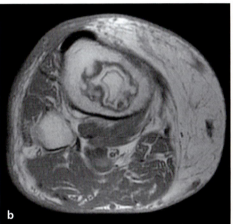
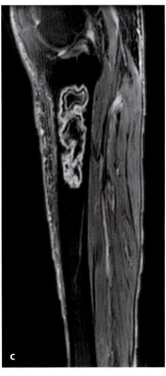

Fig. 11.31 a–c Partly mineralized bone infarct presented on radiograph of the knee (**a–c**) and MRI pictures. Calcified enchondromas can have a similar appearance

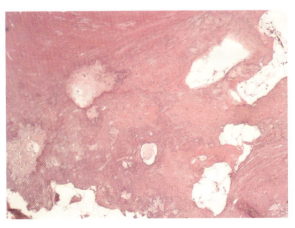

Fig. 11.32 Histological picture shows dense calcified bony trabecules with empty canals; no cellular elements are seen

11.7 Heterotopic Ossification

(Synonym: myositis ossificans) Heterotopic ossification is a benign ossifying process that most commonly occurs in muscle bellies. The etiology is almost universally traumatic, with affected individuals developing pain and tenderness. Subsequent findings include swelling and reduced range of motion of the involved extremity. Common locations include the quadriceps, brachialis, and gluteal muscles. These extensively mineralized lesions may be mistaken for malignancies (extraskeletal or parosteal osteosarcoma), but their characteristic appearance on radiographs usually means a biopsy is not necessary (Figs. 11.33–11.38).

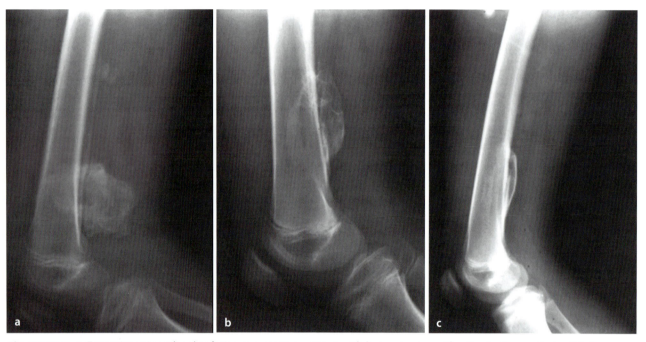

Fig. 11.33 a–c Extensive mineralized soft tissue mass in a patient with heterotopic ossification in the posterior thigh. Note the zonal pattern of ossification with more mature bone at the periphery of the lesion (**a**). Serial radiographs showing gradual reduction in size of mass (**b**). Eventual fusion to posterior cortex (**c**)

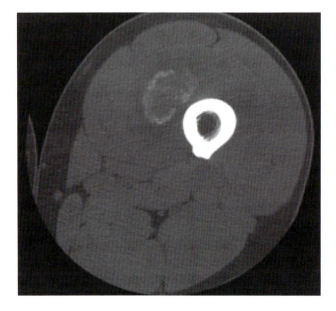

Fig. 11.34 CT scan of the thigh demonstrating characteristic pattern of heterotopic ossification, with a mature shell of bone at the periphery of the lesion

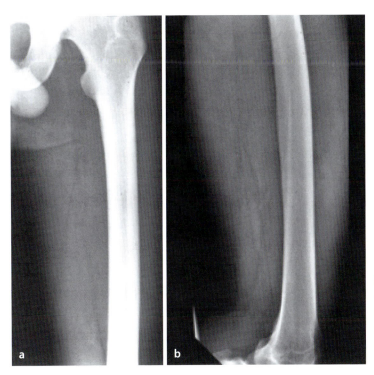

a   b

Fig. 11.35 a, b Plain radiographs of a 28-year-old man taken shortly after he developed painful swelling in the thigh. Although there is considerable soft tissue swelling, early in the course there is no visible mineralization on the a–p (**a**) and lateral (**b**) radiographs

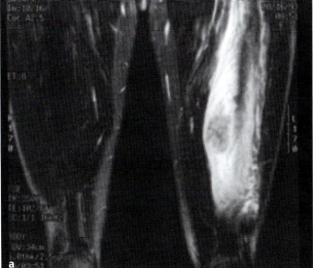

a

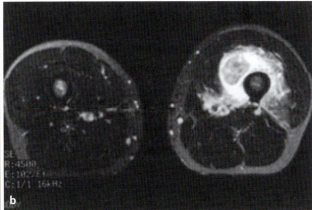

b

Fig. 11.36 a, b Coronal (**a**) and axial (**b**) T2-weighted images with fat saturation shows a large region of abnormal signal primarily confined to the vastus intermedius muscle that extends almost the entire length of the thigh. There is a rounded focus of lower signal intensity at the epicen-ter of the process, which represents the mass of myositis ossificans. The signal change around the mass represents extensive edema and reactive change. These findings are characteristic of myositis ossificans

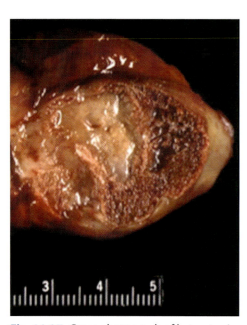

Fig. 11.37 Gross photograph of heterotopic ossification. Again, note the zonal phenomenon where there is more mature bone at the periphery and immature bone at the center

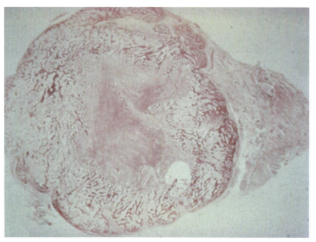

Fig. 11.38 Low-power photomicrograph demonstrating immature central bone and mature peripheral bone

11.8 Langerhans Cell Histiocytosis

This is a hematopoietic condition that can affect a variety of ages, although most patients are under age 30. Pain and swelling of the involved bone are the most common clinical findings. Any bone may be affected, but there is a predilection for the skull, femur, ribs, and ilium. Patients may develop diabetes insipidus. Those with mastoid involvement may have hearing loss. Lesions tend to be symptomatic (pain, swelling) and only rarely will an area of histiocytosis be discovered incidentally (Figs. 11.39–11.44).

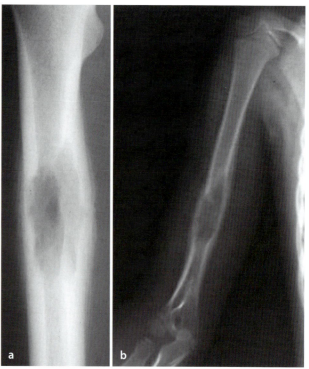

Fig. 11.39 a, b Plain radiograph demonstrating lesions in the femur (**a**) and humerus (**b**). These lesions are typically lytic or mixed lytic sclerotic with variable degrees of sclerosis, expansion, and cortical reaction. Benign periosteal new bone formation is common

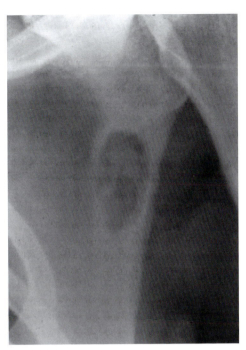

Fig. 11.40 Radioluceny lesion in the scapula showing the appearance of Langerhans cell histiocytosis in flat bones. Note hole in appearance

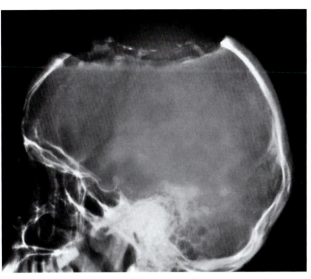

Fig. 11.42 Destruction of skull secondary to Langerhans cell histiocytosis

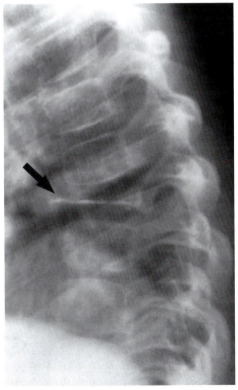

Fig. 11.41 Calve's disease, thoracic vertebrae. Flattening of vertebral body (*arrow*) is typical for Langerhans cell histiocytosis

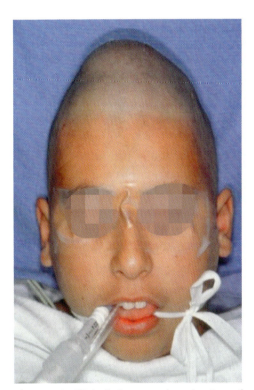

Fig. 11.43 Clinical photograph at the time of surgery showing enlargement of the skull

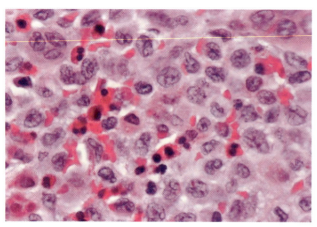

Fig. 11.44 Histologically, lesions are composed of many cell types, including histiocytes, plasma cells, eosinophils, and other inflammatory cells. Langerhans cells usually have an indented nucleus and small nucleoli. There may be many eosinophils present

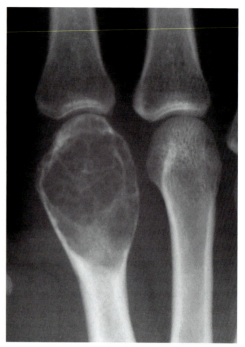

Fig. 11.45 Plain radiograph of a giant cell reparative granuloma of the distal metacarpal. The lesion is expansile and associated with cortical thinning

11.9 Giant cell Reparative Granuloma

(Synonyms: giant cell reaction) Often seen in the skull and small tubular bones of the hands and feet, giant cell reparative granuloma (giant cell reaction) is a benign lesion. Although local recurrence is possible, these lesions do not have metastatic potential.

Lesions are often asymptomatic, although local swelling from bony deformation, pain, and pathologic fracture may be present.

Lesions are typically radiolucent with variable degrees of associated cortical thinning and expansion. In the tubular bones, lesions often extend to the epiphysis and may mimic giant cell tumor (Figs. 11.45 and 11.46).

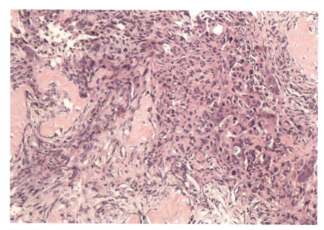

Fig. 11.46 Histology of the lesion demonstrates bland fibrous stroma with clusters of giant cells. Reactive bone is also present. Areas of hemorrhage or secondary aneurysmal bone cyst may also be identified

11.10 Avulsive Cortical Irregularity

Avulsive cortical irregularity is a benign, reactive process located in the posteromedial aspect of the distal femur. This lesion also has been called fibrous cortical defect or periosteal desmoids. Patients are asymptomatic, and lesions are discovered incidentally when radiographs are taken following an injury. The lesions are self-limiting and pose no long-term issues for the patient (Figs. 11.47–11.52).

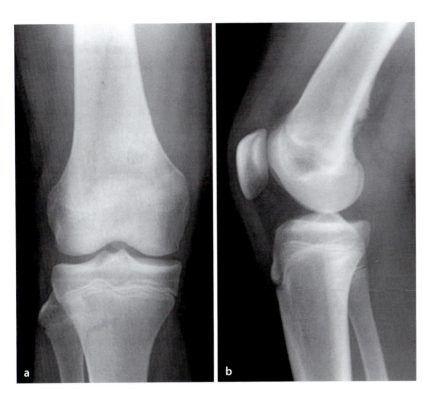

Fig. 11.47 a, b AP and lateral radiographs of a 15-year old with an incidentally discovered avulsive cortical irregularity. The AP radiograph (**a**) shows a subtle area of lucency and sclerosis in the supracondylar region medially. The lateral view (**b**) shows focal periosteal reaction along the posterior aspect of the distal femur at a similar level

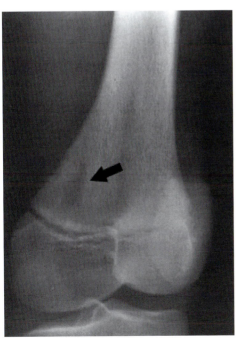

Fig. 11.48 Avulsive cortical irregularity demonstrated as a subtle area of lucency along the posteromedial aspect of the distal femur on an oblique radiograph. Lesions that are not clearly seen on AP and lateral images may be seen to better advantage on an oblique view

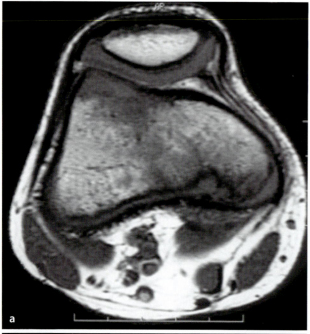

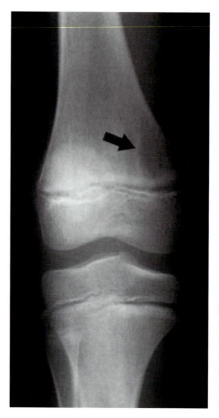

Fig. 11.50 AP radiograph in 9-year-old patient. Note the radiolucency in the posteromedial aspect of the distal femur

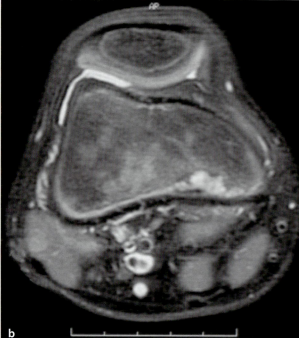

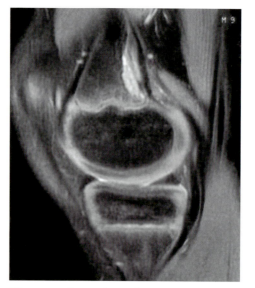

Fig. 11.49 a, b Axial T1- (**a**) and axial T2-weighted image with fat saturation (**b**) show typical features of avulsive cortical irregularity with an elliptical focus of abnormal signal involving the cortex along the medial aspect of the distal femur with associated bone marrow edema

Fig. 11.51 Sagittal MRI shows typical features of avulsive cortical irregularity involving the posteromedial cortex. Associated bone marrow edema is seen

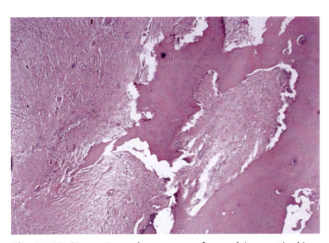

Fig. 11.52 Biopsy is rarely necessary for avulsive cortical irregularity. Histologically these lesions are hypocellular with considerable collagen and no nuclear atypica

Chapter 12

Connective Tissue Disorders

Contents

12.1 Scleroderma (Systemic Sclerosis)

Scleroderma is a syndrome in which genetic factors appear to predispose, and is characterized by inflammation associated with fibrosis and pathological remodeling of connective tissues. Pathological deposition of extracellular matrix in systemic sclerosis is most probably caused by changes in the regulation of dermal fibroblasts. The prevalence is 15/100,000. Affected patients are female in 80% of the cases. Early signs can appear under age of 3, but skin signs generally present in the forties.

Obliteration of arteries and arterioles, arterial hypertension, myocardial involvement, and glomerulonephritis can appear as late complications. In serious generalized forms, calcification in the subcutaneous soft tissues and contractures can be observed. Rare but serious neurological complications are also known in cases of spinal involvement and spinal cord compression by calcinosis (Figs. 12.1–12.4).

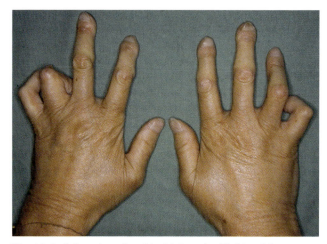

Fig. 12.2 Sclerodactyly with thick and stiff skin of fingers. On radiograph, resorption of distal phalanx is possible. Joint pain and tendon friction rub are common because of subcutaneous calcinosis, which is usually located on the extensor surface of the phalanges, periarticular tissue, and over the bone prominences. Myositis and Raynaud's phenomenon are also often seen

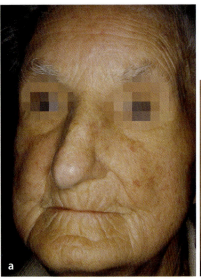

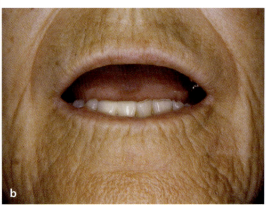

Fig. 12.1 a, b Face of a 67-year-old woman with scleroderma (**a**). Note the skin pigmentation disturbance with acrosclerosis (**b**). It is often associated with reduced saliva and tear secretion

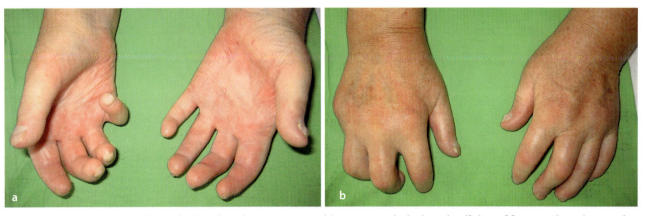

Fig. 12.3 a, b More severe form of sclerodactyly in a 36-year-old woman with thick and stiff skin of fingers. Clinical view of the palmar (**a**) and dorsal (**b**) surfaces

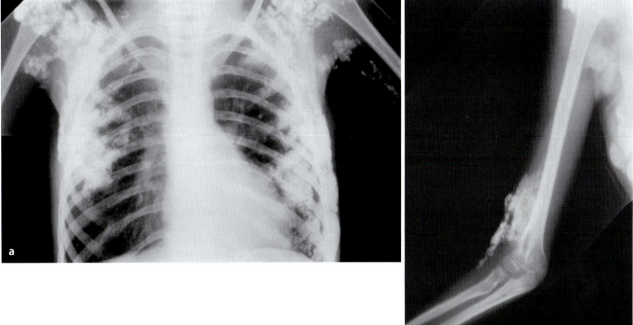

Fig. 12.4 a, b Radiograph of severe calcinosis of the chest (**a**) and elbow (**b**). On the radiograph of the elbow, linear scleroderma is also seen. It is called also "en coup de sabre"

12.2 Ehlers–Danloss's Syndrome

This syndrome is a heritable disorder of connective tissue (collagen fibers and mucopolysaccharides), which is characterized by skin hyperextensibility, generalized joint hypermobility, fragile and soft skin, delayed wound healing with formation of atrophic scars, and easy bruising. Ehlers–Danloss's syndrome is caused by a mutation, leading to a nonfunctional COL5A1 allele, and resulting in a functionally defective type V collagen protein. Inter- and intrafamilial phenotypic variability is observed, but no genotype–phenotype correlations have been made so far.

Other extraskeletal manifestations are also known, such as respiratory and cardiac complications due to pulmonary hypertension, heart dilatation, and particular aortic dissection. Neurologic complications are sensorineural deafness, chorea and cerebellar ataxia, and percussion myotonia (Figs. 12.5–12.8).

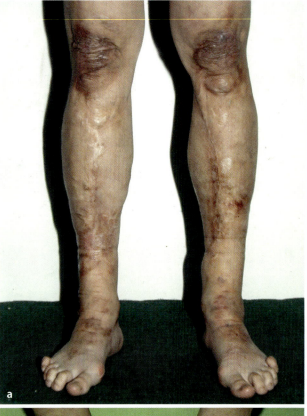
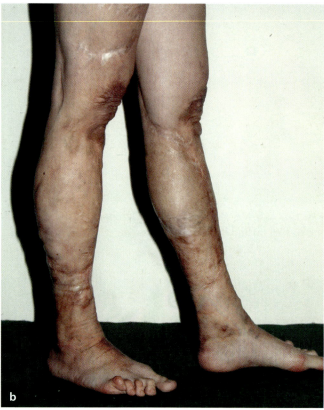
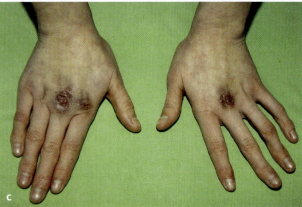

Fig. 12.5 a–c Photographs taken from the lower extremities of a 24-year-old woman with cicatrix formation and loss of subcutaneous fat above the knee joints. Varicosity and flat foot are also frequently present (**a**, **b**). The skin on the extensor site of the joint has a tendency to split easily and leave pigmented tissue-paper-like scar demonstrated here above the metacarpophalangeal (MP) joints of the hands (**c**)

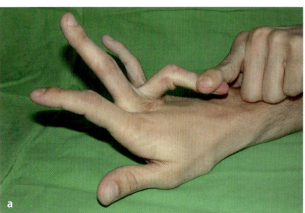
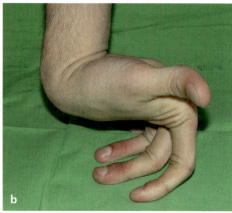

Fig. 12.6 a, b Excessive mobility of the joints (**a**, **b**)

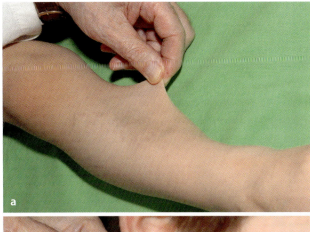

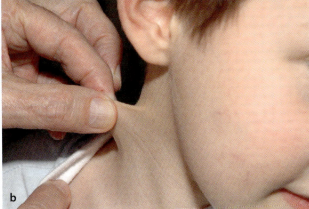

Fig. 12.7 a, b Skin hyperelasticity of a 4-year-old boy in lower extremity (**a**) and in the neck region (**b**)

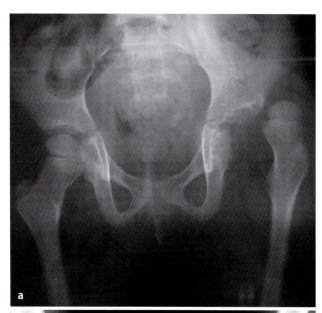

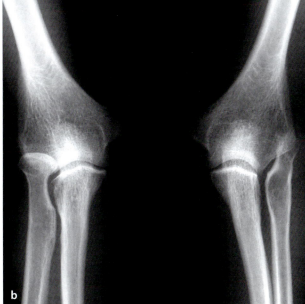

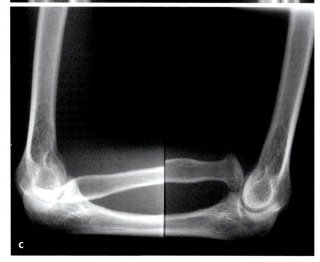

Fig. 12.8 a–c Radiograph of dislocated hip (**a**) and elbow (**b, c**) joints (note the radial head) in Ehlers–Danloss's disease

12.3 Fibrodysplasia Ossificans Progressiva

Fibrodysplasia ossificans progressiva (synonyms: progressive osseous heteroplasia, myositis ossificans progressiva, Münchmayer's disease) is a rare autosomal dominant disorder in which there are variable defects on the great toes with progressive ectopic ossification of the large striated muscles, leading to gross and progressive disability. The prevalence is 1:2,000,000, and the disease occurs world-wide without racial, ethnic, or geographic predilection. The characteristic skeletal malformations are the painful swelling and fibrosis of muscles, leading to ossification. The onset of this disease is between age 0 and 15 years. There is no efficient treatment; the patients are confined to a chair by the age of 30 because of the serious contractures and decreased range of movement of the joints (Figs. 12.9–12.14).

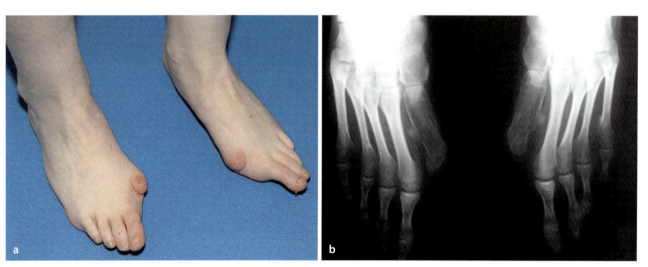

Fig. 12.9 a, b Photograph (**a**) and radiograph (**b**) of a 15-year-old girl with typical short great toes with "hallux valgus-like" malformations and absent phalanges

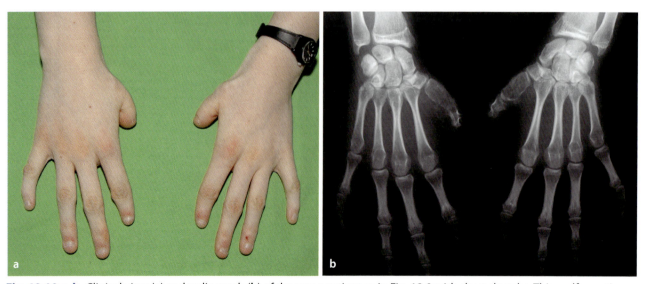

Fig. 12.10 a, b Clinical view (**a**) and radiograph (**b**) of the same patient as in Fig. 12.9 with short thumbs. This malformation is not always present

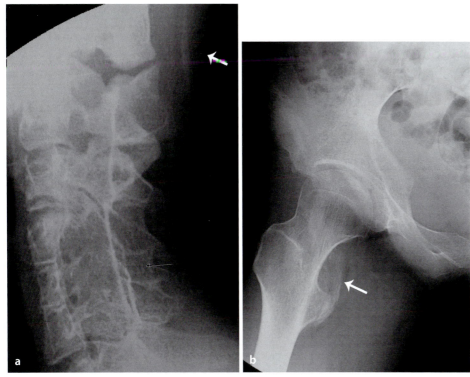

Fig. 12.11 a, b The disease begins with a distinct ossification line in the upper paraspinal muscles of the neck (**a**, *arrow*) and later spreads from axial to appendicular, cranial to caudal, and proximal to distal, also involving the muscles around the hips (**b**, *arrow*) and other major joints. The bony growths involve tendons, ligaments, fibrous muscle tissue, and connective tissue. In affected areas the bone slowly replaces the fibrotic muscles

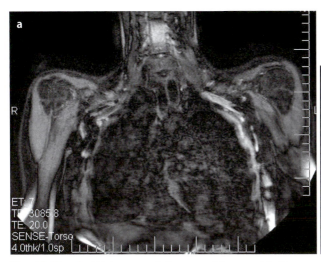

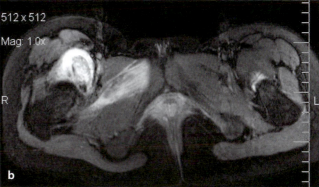

Fig. 12.12 a, b MR images of the same 15-year-old girl as in Fig. 12.9. On MR images the high signal intensity means the ongoing process of the progressive myositis ossificans. On the frontal plane of the chest (**a**) and on the horizontal MRI picture of the pelvis (**b**) high signal intensity is visible in intercostal muscles on the left, as well as in the obturator ex-ternus and iliopsoas muscles on the right side. The terminal phase of this disease provoke just ossification and calcification in muscles, and does not cause any edema. That is why the terminal phase of fibrodysplasia ossificans progressiva is less clearly visible on MR images

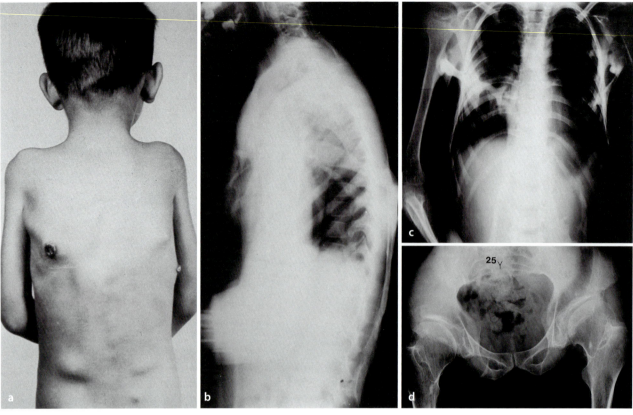

Fig. 12.13 a–d Photograph of a 4-year-old boy (**a**, archive). Note the exulcerations of the skin caused by the ossifications of the dorsal muscles of the back. Lateral (**b**) and anteroposterior (**c**) radiographs of the chest of the same child present severe deforming ossifications both in abdominal and dorsal muscles. Radiograph of the pelvis and deformed hip joints of the same patient at age 25 years (**d**)

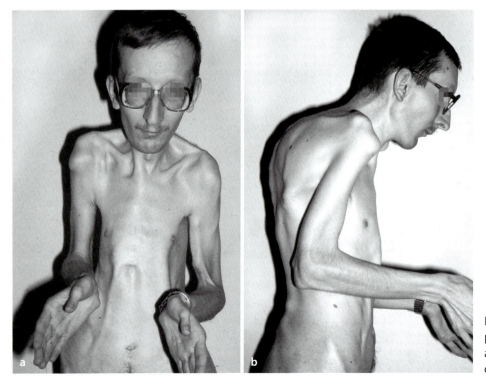

Fig. 12.14 a, b The same patient as in Fig. 12.13 at the age of 46 years with myositis ossificans progressive (archive)

12.4 Systemic Lupus Erythematosus (SLE)

SLE is an archetypal autoimmune disease, given its complex clinical and molecular manifestations. The disease with inflammation of organs has genetic and environmental origins. The prevalence is 30/100,000. The affected patients are women in 90% of cases. First signs are fever, weakness, weight loss, which appear between age of 20 and 60 years. Glomerulonephritis in 40% of patients with proteinuria (>0.5 g per day) and cylinders in urine called also "lupus nephritis" can develop. Cardiac manifestations are common, as premature coronary heart disease and pericarditis in 30–60% of patients. Types are subacute cutaneous lupus erythematosus (SCLE), neonatal LE, drug-induced lupus, and secondary antiphospholypid syndrome (Figs. 12.15–12.17).

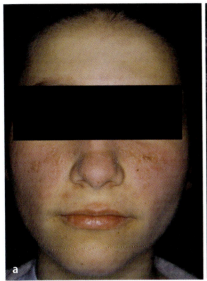
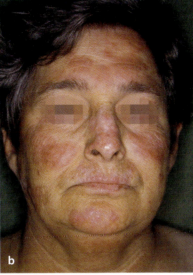

Fig. 12.15 a, b Specific cutaneous manifestations appears in 80% of patients: pink rash over the face in acute case of a 16-year-old girl (**a**) and of a 40-year-old woman (**b**). Urticaria or purpura and atopic eczema are often seen

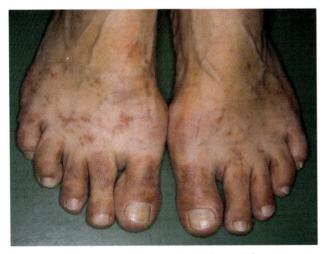

Fig. 12.16 Symmetrical nonerosive and nondeforming arthritis of small joints with joint pain, as is well known. Primary aseptic bone necrosis is frequently seen in femoral and humeral head

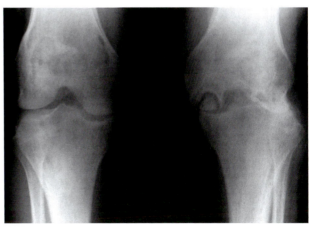

Fig. 12.17 Severe secondary arthrosis of the left knee joint due to systemic lupus erythematosus (SLE) and steroid therapy

12.5 Dermatomyositis

This syndrome is a systemic immune disorder, a primary inflammatory myopathy with autoimmune pathogenesis. It is associated with substantial muscle weakening in its course, especially proximally in the extremities. The prevalence is 1:100,000. Women are affected twice more than men. First skin signs can appear during childhood as well as in adults. In 7–66% of cases of adult dermatomyositis, different malignant tumors can develop. Other extraskeletal differences are pulmonary fibrosis, conduction abnormalities and arrhythmias, myocarditis and coronary artery disease, calcifying myonecrosis, pericarditis and pulmonary hypertension, dysphagia, and retinopathy (Figs. 12.18–12.20).

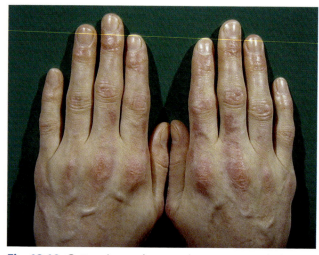

Fig. 12.19 Gottron's papules over the metacarpophalangeal joints (violet-colored skin pigmentation on the extensor surface of small joints) of a female patient. It is often complicated with cutaneous ulcers and poor wound closure or poor healing

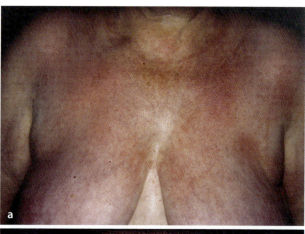
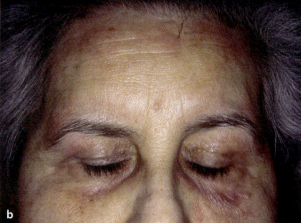

Fig. 12.18 a, b A 62-year-old patient with rash over the breast (**a**), and heliotrope rush and heliotrope edema of the eyelids and lipodystrophy (**b**)

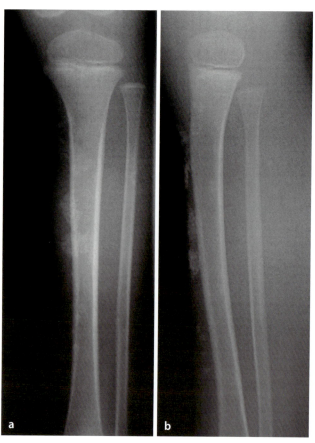

Fig. 12.20 a, b Calcareous deposits in subcutis of an 8-year-old boy in anteroposterior (**a**) and lateral (**b**) radiograph. In some cases symmetrical, proximal muscle weakness or severe and debilitating calcinosis can be observed because of calcification of muscles with contractures

Chapter 13

Pediatric Orthopedics

Contents

Pediatric Orthopedics

G. Szőke, S. Kiss, T. Terebessy, and G. Holnapy

13.1 Congenital and Developmental Disorders

13.1.1 Congenital Muscular Torticollis

Torticollis (wry neck) is a congenital or acquired condition of limited neck motion in which the child holds the head to one side with the chin pointing to the opposite side. It is the result of shortening of the sterno-cleidomastoid muscle. In most cases, the shortening is a consequence of injury during birth. In early infancy, a firm, nontender mass may be felt in the mid portion of the muscle. The mass usually disappears and is replaced with fibrous tissue. If untreated, there can be permanent limitation of neck movement. There may be flattening of the head and face on the affected side (Figs. 13.1 and 13.2).

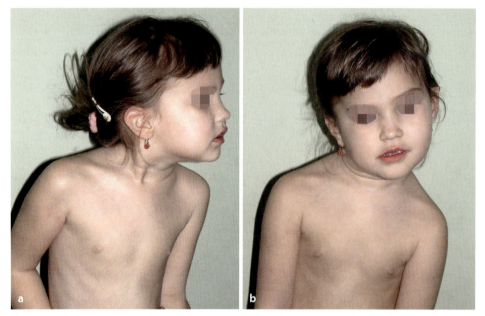

Fig. 13.1 a, b Three-year-old girl with congenital torticollis, presenting itself in the shortening of mainly the sternal portion of the right sternocleidomastoid muscle (**a**). Anterior–posterior view presenting the typical asymmetry of the face (**b**)

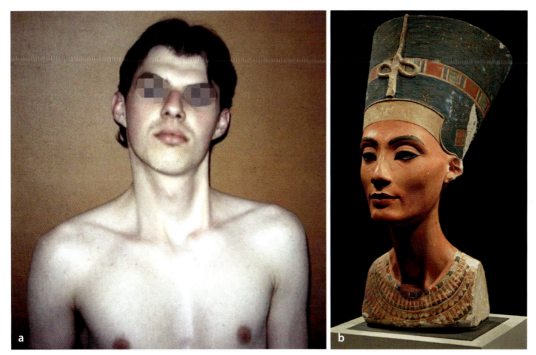

Fig. 13.2 a, b Rare form of muscular torticollis is when both sternocleidomastoids are affected (**a**). It makes an appearance of the face like Nofertiti's famous half-length-portrait (**b**)

13.1.2 Sprengel's Deformity

Sprengel's deformity (congenital high scapula) is defined as a congenital abnormal elevation of one or both scapulas from the normal anatomic scapula position. This anomaly is often associated with other anomalies of the skeletal system and other organs. The possibilities of pathogenesis of the deformity are: first, that it is a failure of descent caused by (a) great intrauterine pressure, due to either an increased or a diminished amount of amniotic fluid; (b)

abnormal articulations of the scapula with the vertebral column, named as omovertebral bone, may be attached to the vertebral border of the scapula in a number of ways: by bony continuity, by cartilaginous union, or by a fibrous band; (c) a defective musculature, unable to draw the scapula caudally; or (d) a normal musculature, which is unable to draw the scapula caudally too. Second possible etiology is that the changes in the shape and size of the scapula are an arrest of development due to improper or defective muscular tension (Figs. 13.3–13.5).

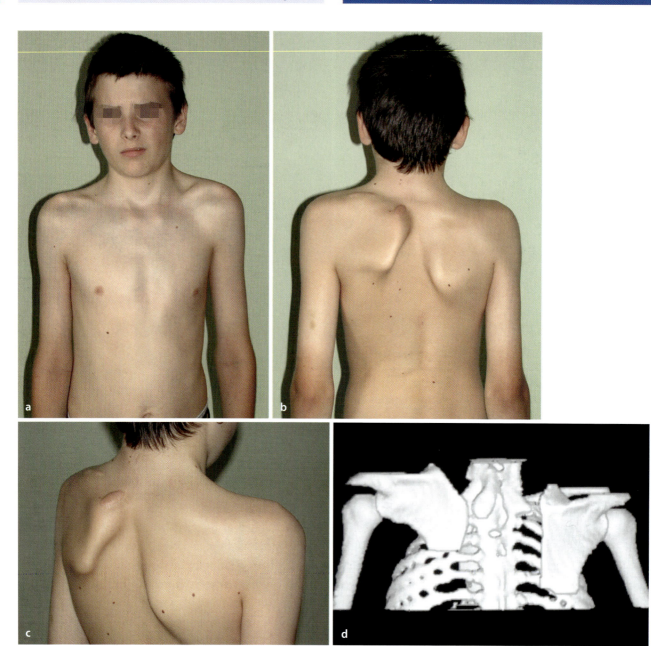

Fig. 13.3 a–d The asymmetry of the shoulder is caused by the upward and forward displacement of the scapula (**a**) The left scapula is elevated, and its size is smaller than that at the opposite side (**b**) The scapula is rotated about the sagittal axis, bringing the upper medial angle away from the spinal column and the lower angle close to it (**c**) 3D CT of the left omovertebral bridge. One third of patients has omovertebral bone. This is a trapezoid-shaped structure of cartilage or bone. It usually lays in a strong fascia sheath extending from the superomedial border of the scapula to the spinous processes, lamina, or transverse processes of the cervical spine, most commonly the fourth to seventh cervical vertebrae (**d**)

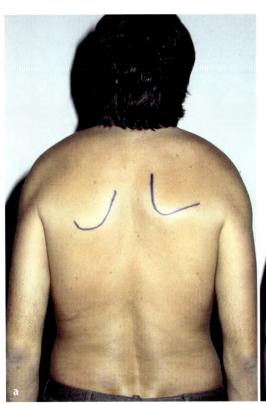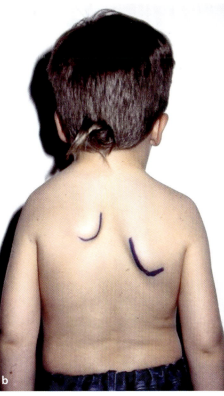

Fig. 13.4 a, b The condition usually is sporadic, rarely it may run in families at autosomal dominant pattern of inheritance. The father has bilateral high scapula (**a**) while his son has left side deformity (**b**)

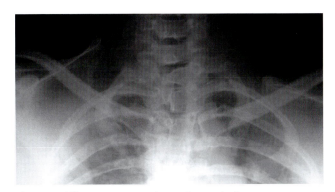

Fig. 13.5 The anteroposterior radiograph demonstrates a high standing scapula on the right site. Associated malformations are often present. These can include anomalies in the cervicothoracal vertebrae or the thoracic rib cage. The most common anomalies are absent or fused ribs, chest-wall asymmetry, Klippel–Feil's syndrome, cervical ribs, congenital scoliosis, and cervical spina bifida

13.1.3 Idiopathic Acetabular Protrusion

Idiopathic protrusion of the acetabulum is a displacement of the acetabular medial wall towards the intrapelvic space. Two-thirds of the cases are classified as primary forms without any recognizable cause, also referred to as Otto pelvic (Otto, 1824) or arthrokatadysis. The secondary form of the disease most frequently accompanies Marfan's syndrome, rheumatoid arthritis, spondylitis ankylopoetica, septic arthritis, degenerative joint diseases.

Acetabular protrusion is more frequent in women than in men, can be mono or bilateral (Fig. 13.6).

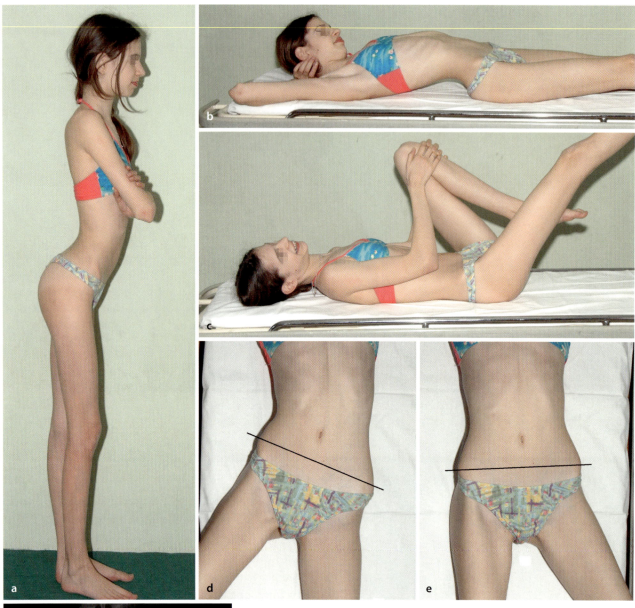

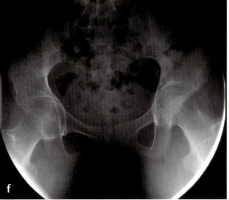

Fig. 13.6 a–f A 15-year-old girl with bilateral acetabular protrusion. Hip pain and decreased range of motion are the main complaints. The increased lumbar lordosis due to the flexion contracture of both hips is well recognizable (**a**). The lack of flattening of the increased lumbar lordosis can be observed also in declined position (**b**). The flexion contracture of the hip can be visualized by the Thomas test (**c**). No femoral abduction can be performed on the right side due to adduction contracture. Note the tilting of the pelvis during the abduction maneuver (**d**, **e**). Anteroposterior radiograph, of the pelvis of the same patient. The protrusion accompanied by both sides chondrolysis is apparent. The Köhler's sign is not visible (**f**)

13.1.4 Syndrome of Seven Symptoms

This syndrome contains: scoliosis, lumbodorsal kyphosis, inclined position of the head (e.g., torticollis), asymmetry of the skull, dysplasia of the hip, asymmetry of the pelvis, foot deformity (e.g., clubfoot or calcaneal deformity) (Fig. 13.7).

individuals, but racial background (50-fold increase in the frequency in Laplanders, higher prevalence in Central Europe and in Native Americans), genetical factors (tenfold increase in frequency in the case of DDH of parents), intrauterine positioning (breech), female sex and being the first-born child are all associated with an increased prevalence of DDH (Figs. 13.8–13.10).

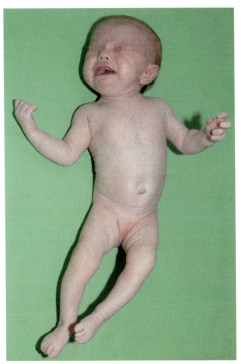

Fig. 13.7 Syndrome of seven symptoms of a 3-month-old child: you can observe all the deformities described above

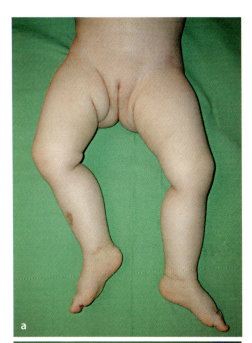

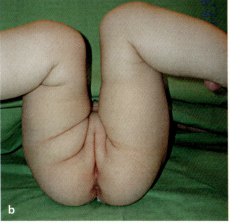

13.1.5 Congenital Dislocation and Dysplasia of the Hip

The congenital dislocation of the hip is also known, as hip dysplasia or developmental dysplasia of the hip (DDH). The etiology is not clear, but hip dysplasia does appear to be related to a number of different factors (polygenic inheritance). The developmental disorder of the hip, involve not just the osseous structures, such as the acetabulum and the proximal femur, but also the labrum, capsule, and other soft tissues. This problem may occur at any time, from conception to skeletal maturity. Bilateral involvement is frequent. The overall frequency is 1/1,000

Fig. 13.8 a, b Findings in late dislocation (right side of this 12-month-old female) include asymmetry of the gluteal thigh or labral skin folds (a), decreased abduction on the affected side, standing or walking with external rotation, and leg length inequality, examined by Galeazzi's sign (b). Note that proximal femoral focal deficiency can masquerade as hip dysplasia and often manifests similarly

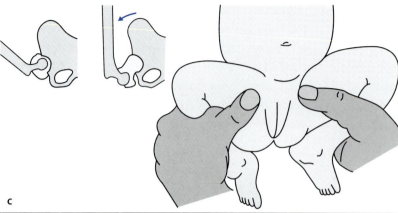

c

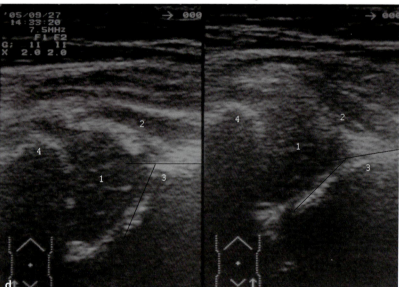

d

Fig. 13.8 c, d In a newborn child Ortolani's sign is referred to as a clunk, felt when the hip reduces into the acetabulum, with the hip in abduction (**c**). Barlow described a test that is performed with the hips in an adducted position in which slight gentle posterior pressure is applied to the hips. A clunk should be felt as the hip dislocates out of the acetabulum. 2-month-old girl's (**d**) ultrasound image of the right hip, which is well developed and healthy (alpha angle 62°, beta angle 50°), femoral head (1), cartilaginous acetabular rim (2), osseous acetabular corner (3), greater trochanter (4). Hip dysplasia is seen in the left hip (Type III according to the classification of Graf, alpha angle 34°, beta angle 80°)

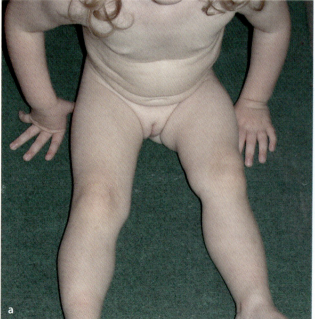

a

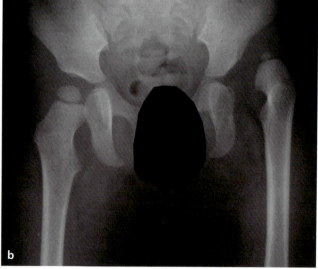

b

Fig. 13.9 a, b 26-month-old girl untreated case of DDH at the left side, note the shortening of the left thigh (**a**). Radiograph of the same patient (**b**)

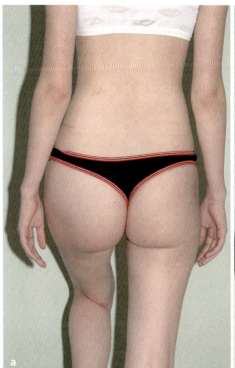
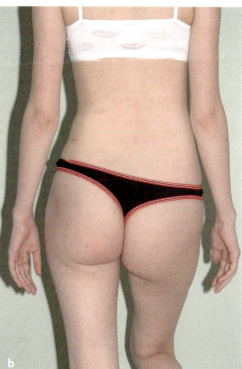
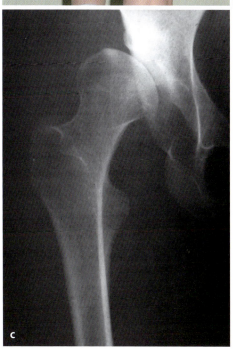

Fig. 13.10 a–c Trendelenburg's test: When the patient stands on the leg at the site of her normal healthy hip, due to the normal gluteus muscles function and anatomical hip joint the hip remains stable at the same level (or rises slightly) (**a**). The Trendelenburg's test is positive at her left affected side (**b**), when she is standing upon it. Due to the insufficient gluteus muscles strength and/or dislocated position of the femoral head (e.g., DDH) the muscles are unable to keep the hip at the same level, the buttock droops downwards, the hip is unstable. In bilateral case a waddling gait with hyperlordosis is present. Radiographic finding underline this: dislocated hip on the left side (**c**)

13.1.6 Pes Equinovarus Congenitus

Clubfoot, also known as talipes equinovarus, is a congenital deformity of the foot that occurs in about 1 in 1,000 births. The affected foot and lower limb tends to be smaller than normal, with the heel pointing upward and varus and forefoot turning inward. Most commonly it is an isolated congenital birth defect and the cause is idiopathic. Clubfoot is about twice as common in males, and occurs bilaterally in about 50% of cases. If both parents are normal with an affected child, the risk of the next child having a clubfoot is 2–5% (Figs. 13.11–13.14).

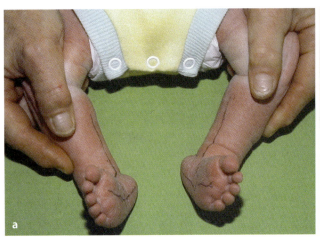
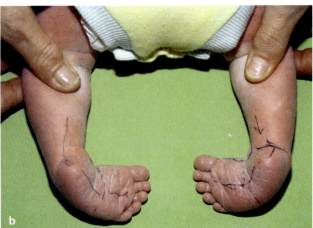

Fig. 13.11 a, b Fixed plantar flexion (equinus) of the ankle, characterized by the drawn up position of the heel and inability to bring the foot to a plantigrade position. The heel is in varus position, adduction of the forefoot and midfoot giving the foot a kidney-shaped appearance. The navicular is displaced medially, as is the cuboid. Contractures of the medial plantar soft tissues are present

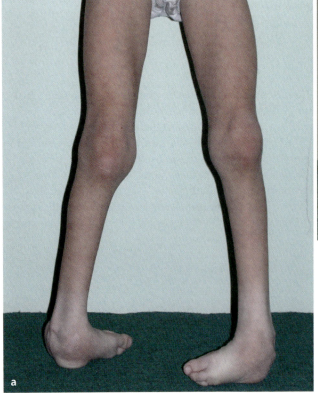
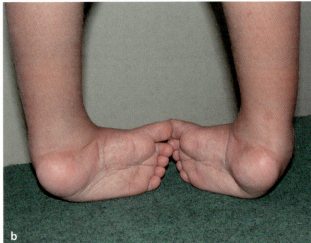

Fig. 13.12 a, b If left untreated, the deformity will not go away. It will continue to get worse over time, with secondary bony changes developing over years. An uncorrected clubfoot in the older child or adult is very disabling. Because of the abnormal development of the foot, the patient will walk on the outside of his foot, which is not designed for weight-bearing

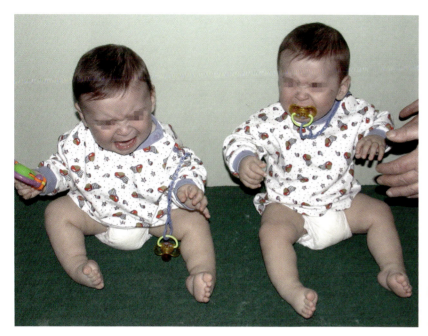

Fig. 13.13 If one monozygotic twin has a clubfoot, the second twin has approximately a 32% chance of having a clubfoot

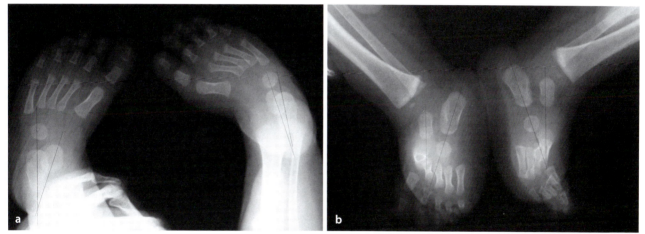

Fig. 13.14 a, b The AP (**a**) and the lateral talocalcaneal lines (**b**) are almost parallel in clubfeet. Mild clubfoot is on the left (AP = 18°, lat = 20°), severe on the right side (AP = 8°, lat = 19°). AP lines in normal feet subtend an angle of 25–40°, talocalcaneal angle on lateral view is usually 35–50°

13.1.7 Vertical Talus

Congenital vertical talus is an uncommon disorder of the foot, clinically manifested as a rigid flatfoot with a rocker-bottom appearance of the foot with irreducible and rigid dorsal dislocation of the navicular on the talus. In untreated case, it results in a painful and rigid flatfoot with weakness in push-off power. This disease is frequently associated with neuromuscular disorders, but it can appear due to genetic or idiopathic disorder. The incidence of talus verticalis is approximately one tenth that of congenital clubfoot (Figs. 13.15 and 13.16).

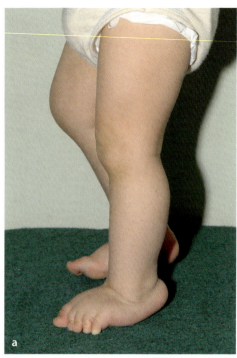

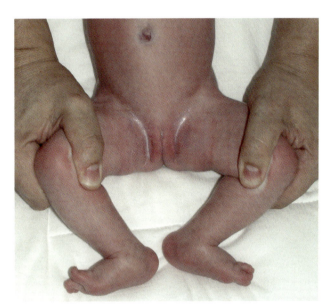

Fig. 13.15 Photo of a 2-month-old child with bilateral involvement of talus verticalis

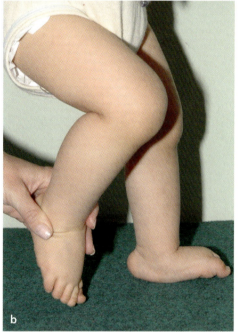

Fig. 13.16 a–c The characteristic photograph taken from a 1-year-old child with talus verticalis at the left side. Note that the calcaneus is in fixed equinus, and the Achilles tendon is very tight and the hindfoot is also in valgus. The forefoot is abducted and dorsalflexed (**a**, **b**). The radiographic finding reveals (**c**) the dorsal dislocation of the navicular bone on the talus. The head of the talus is found medially in the sole, creating the rocker bottom appearance

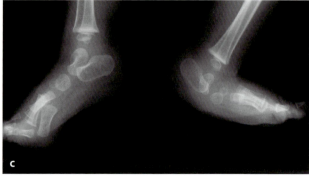

13.2 Osteochondroses and Related Diseases

13.2.1 Legg–Calvé–Perthes Disease

Legg–Calvé–Perthes disease is the avascular necrosis of the femoral head resulting from compromise of the tenuous blood supply to this area. The necrosis is followed by the removal of necrotic bone and replacement with new bone, with remodellation of femoral head. The adequacy of bone replacement depends on congruity of the involved joint and the age of the patient, so the new bone formation can result in a normal bone. This disease generally occurs unilaterally in children aged 4–10 years, approximately 4 of 100,000 children, predominantly in males (male-to-female ratio of approximately 4 · 1). The cause is unknown, but the affected children have delayed bone age, disproportionate growth, and a mildly shortened stature.

Earliest clinical sign is an intermittent limp with pain in the anterior part of the thigh, and antalgic gait with limited hip motion. Limited range of passive and active motions especially internal rotation and abduction are common, resulting in adduction flexion contracture with quadriceps muscles atrophy (Figs. 13.17–13.20).

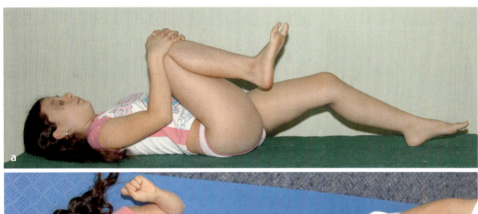

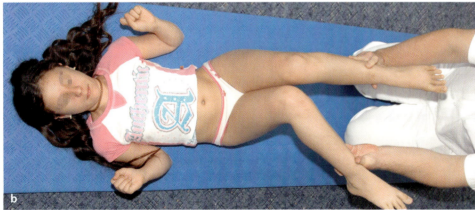

Fig. 13.17 a, b 11-year-old girl with Legg–Calvé–Perthes disease at the left side. Note the 25° flexion contracture at the left side (**a**) and maximal internal rotation in both hips: on the left side the range of internal rotational motion decreased, here almost 0° (**b**)

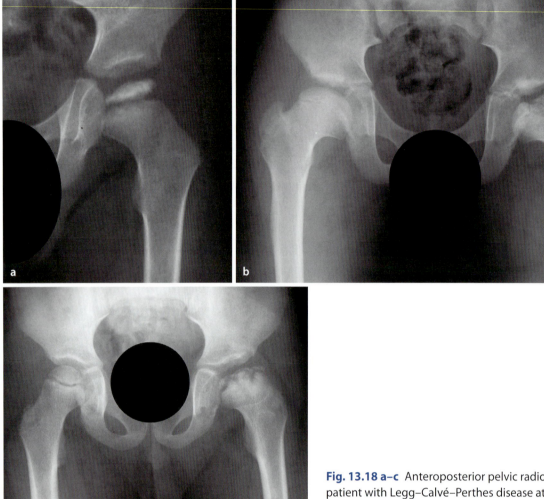

Fig. 13.18 a–c Anteroposterior pelvic radiograph of a patient with Legg–Calvé–Perthes disease at the left side in sclerotic phase (**a**), in early fragmentation phase (**b**), and late fragmentation phase with beginning hinge sign (**c**)

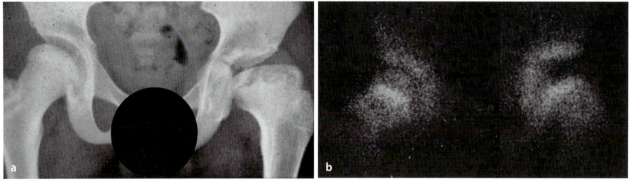

Fig. 13.19 a, b End stage of Legg–Calvé–Perthes disease. Note the depressed and flat femoral head after it's remodellation, with beginning hinge sign (**a**). Bone scan of the same patient. Note the hypoperfusion on left femoral head (**b**)

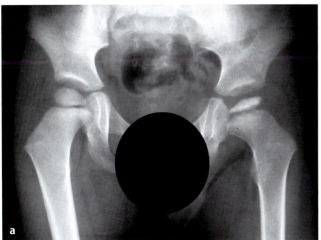 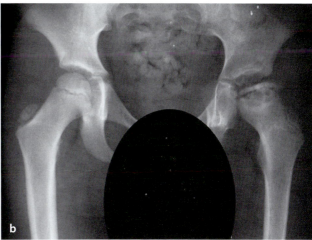

Fig. 13.20 a, b Recently the most frequently used classification for the disease is the Herring's lateral pillar classification. In Herring's group A the height of the lateral pillar of the femoral head at the fragmentation phase is normal. In Herring group B the height of the lateral pillar is between 50 and 100% of the original height compared to the unaffected side (**a**). In group C the height of the lateral pillar is less than 50% of the original height (**b**). The classification helps to predict the later flattening of the femoral head during remodellation

13.2.2 Osgood–Schlatter's Disease

Osgood–Schlatter's disease is the most frequent cause of knee pain in children aged 10–15 years, but the real cause is unknown. They presented with pain at the insertion of the patellar tendon, which improved with rest and worsened with activity. The onset of the disease is gradual, and after skeletal maturity the patients may rarely have persisting knee problems. The disease is more appropriately described as a disorder or a condition. The apophysis is subject to traction during the adolescent years due to repetitive quadriceps contraction through the patellar tendon, which can result in microfractures, avulsion fractures of portions of the distal tibial tubercle (Fig. 13.21).

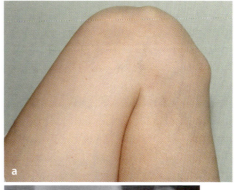

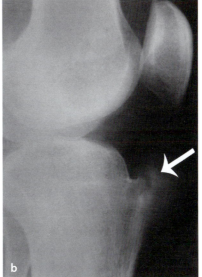

Fig. 13.21 a, b Clinical photo and radiograph of a 16-year-old boy, with a visible and well palpable prominence and soft tissue swelling over the tibial tubercle (**a**). Note the unusual fragmentation of tibial tubercle on radiograph (**b**)

13.2.3 Köhler's Disease I

Köhler's disease I is the rare avascular necrosis of the navicular bone. This disease occurs in children aged 5–10 years and is more common in boys, but because of the ossification onset, girls with Köhler's disease I often are younger than boys. The etiology is unknown, but the vascular incident and a retarded bone age have been implicated, as the navicular is the last tarsal bone to ossify in children. Navicular bone might be compressed between the already ossified talus and the cuneiforms when the child becomes heavier. Compression involves the vessels in central spongy bone leading to ischemia (Figs. 13.22 and 13.23).

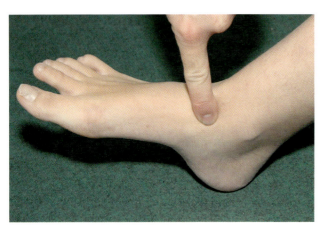

Fig. 13.22 Ischemia causes clinical symptoms, like antalgic limp and local tenderness of the medial aspect of the foot over the navicular

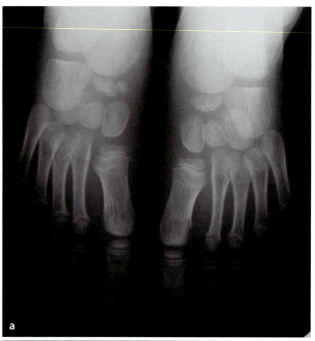

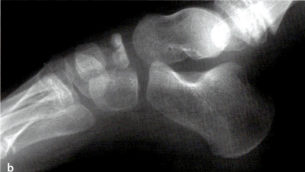

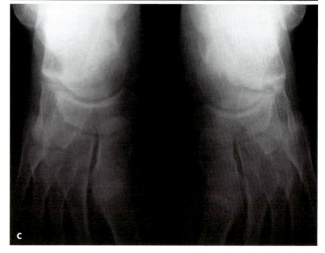

Fig. 13.23 a–c Anteroposterior (**a**) and lateral (**b**) view radiographs of the foot of a 6-year-old boy. The child can walk with an increased weight on the lateral side of the foot. Note the fragmentation of navicular bone on right side, especially in lateral view. Seven years later at age 13 a complete rebuilding of the navicular bone is demonstrated on radiograph (**c**)

13.2.4 Köhler's Disease II

Köhler's disease II is characterized by the painful collapse of the articular surface of the second metatarsal head – called also Freiberg's infraction or Freiberg's disease. Of all the osteochondroses, Freiberg's disease is reported to be the fourth most common. Any of the metatarsals may be involved, but in the 95% of the cases the disease affects the second or third metatarsal, with the second metatarsal being affected more often. Bilateral involvement is rare. Freiberg's disease can occur at any age, but most commonly is seen in younger age, predominantly in females (male-to-female ratio 1:5).

Etiology of this disease is unknown, the cause seems to be multifactorial with no single etiology responsible for all cases (Fig. 13.24).

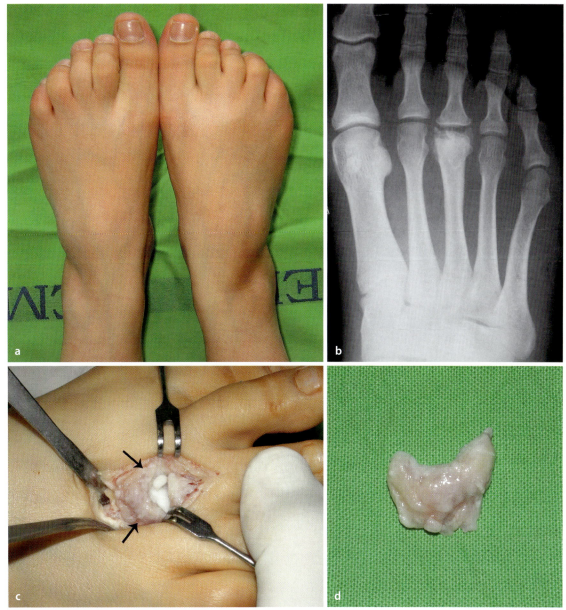

Fig. 13.24 a–d Painful limp and discomfort with swelling over the second metatarsophalangeal joint of the right foot of a 17-year-old female (**a**). The range of motion is decreased in the MP joint. Some cases are asymptomatically with changes noted only on radiographs. X-ray (**b**) and intraoperative picture (**c**) of Köhler II disease: subchondral collapse and fragmentation of the joint surface of the second metatarsal head is visible (**c**). The removed fragment (**d**)

13.2.5 Vertebra Plana

Vertebra plana – also called "Calvé's disease" – is a kind of juvenile osteochondroses involving only one vertebral body. Disease damaging the primary ossification center of the vertebral body affects the thin and depressed vertebra. During the remodelation phase, the height of vertebral body can reconstruct almost its normal size. The intervertebral discs cranially and distally attached to the vertebral body are not damaged. This disease occurs in children around 6 years. The etiology could be avascular necrosis of the ossification center, or eosinophil granuloma. In some cases painful angular kyphosis can develop with limited range of motion on thoracic spine, but the patients are frequently without complaint (Figs 13.25 and 13.26).

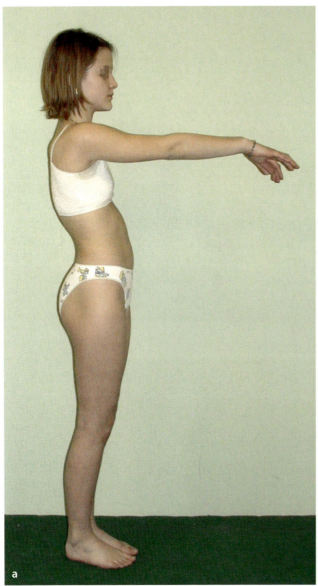

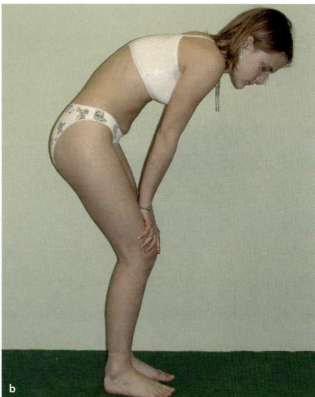

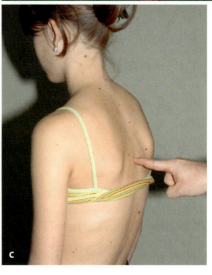

Fig. 13.25 a–c Lateral clinical view of a girl with vertebra plana. Note, there is nothing observed in standing position (**a**), but the range of motion in flexion of dorsal spine is limited, and painful (**b**), the area of the affected vertebra is usually sensitive for pressure (**c**)

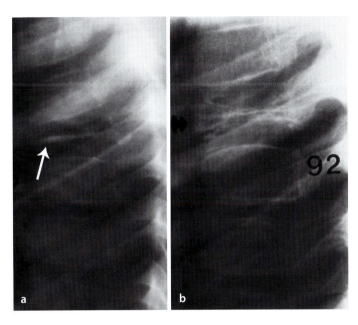

Fig. 13.26 a, b The lateral view radiograph of the sixth thoracic vertebral body's osteochondrosis (**a**), and after 3 years following the remodellation. Note that the height of the affected vertebral body reached almost that of the adjacent vertebras (**b**)

13.2.6 Scheuermann's Disease

Scheuermann's disease (juvenile kyphosis) refers to osteochondrosis of the secondary ossification centers of the vertebral bodies. The lower dorsal and upper lumbar vertebrae are involved initially. The process may be limited to several bodies or may involve the entire dorsal and lumbar spine. The prevalence rate of Scheuermann's kyphosis is 1–5%. Males are affected more frequently than females, aged 10–16 years. Patients have an increased kyphosis in the thoracic or thoracolumbar spine, with hyperlordosis in the lumbar region. There is high association between scoliosis and Scheuermann's disease, and increased incidence of spondylolysis and spondylolisthesis is described too. Backache is characteristic especially in patients with lumbar localization of the disease. After the skeletal maturity the pain decreases, and if the residual kyphosis is less than 60° the prognosis is good for minimal problems in adult life. This disease is heterogeneous, including mechanical, metabolic, and endocrinologic causes and also an autosomal dominant pattern of inheritance is published (Figs. 13.27–13.31).

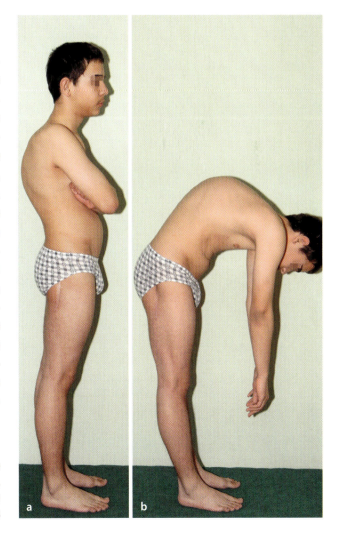

Fig. 13.27 a, b 16-year-old patient with typical juvenile kyphosis (**a**). Decreased flexibility of the spine is noted (**b**), indicating the structural nature of the kyphotic deformity, in contrast to patients with flexible postural kyphosis

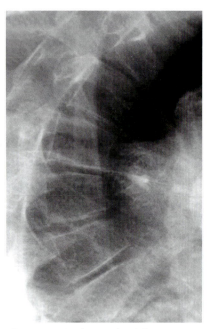

Fig. 13.28 Radiograph of the same patient: the osteochondrosis of the secondary ossification centers of the vertebral bodies are seen

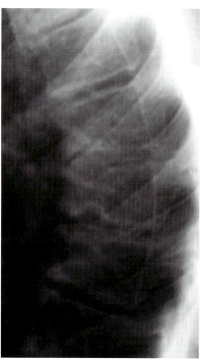

Fig. 13.30 Lateral view radiograph with typical signs of Scheuermann's disease: Schmorl's herniation on vertebral bodies

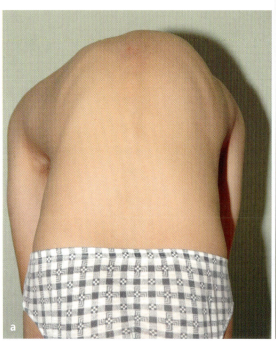

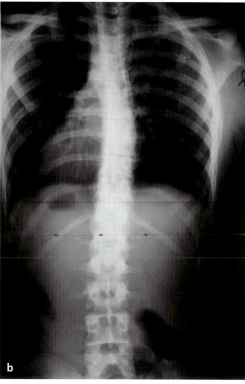

Fig. 13.29 a, b The disease involve the entire dorsal spine, where mild secondary scoliosis also presents (**a**, **b**)

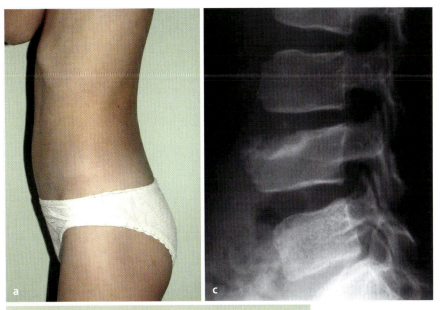

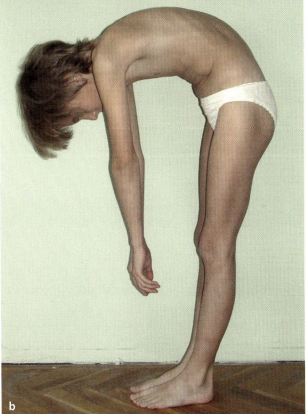

Fig. 13.31 a–c Thirteen-year-old girl with lumbar Scheuer-mann's disease straightening of the lordosis, decreased mobility and an increased kyphotic curve can be seen on the lumbar spine.(**a**, **b**). Lateral view radiograph of the same patient. Apophysitis of the fourth lumbar vertebral body is well recognizable (**c**)

13.2.7 Schintz–Sever's Disease

Schintz–Sever's disease is a relatively common nonarticular osteochondrosis, the painful inflammation of the calcaneal apophysis, caused by decreased resistance to shear stress at the bone growth–plate interface. Characterized by the heel pain in a growing active child, improved with rest and worsened with activity. This disease occurs in children aged 10–12 years and is more common in boys, but because of the ossification onset, girls with Schintz–Sever's disease often are younger than boys (male-to-female ratio is approximately 2:1). Bilateral involvement is present in approximately 60% of the cases. The etiology of pain in Schintz–Sever's disease is believed to be repetitive trauma to the weaker structure of the apophysis, induced by the pull of the Achilles tendon on its insertion (Fig. 13.32).

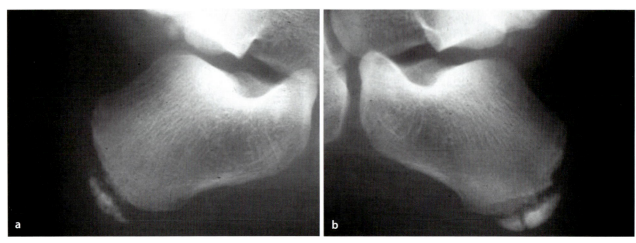

Fig. 13.32 a, b Osteochondroses of the right calcaneal apophysis. The radiographic appearance of resorption, fragmentation, and increased sclerosis leading to eventual union (**a**). Radiograph showing fragmentation of the apophysis is not diagnostic because multiple centers of ossification may exist in the normal apophysis (**b**)

13.2.8 Osteochondritis Dissecans (Patella, Femur, Talus)

Osteochondritis dissecans (OCD) is characterized by separation of an osteochondral fragment from the articular surface. OCD occurs in the knee in 75% of the cases, the elbow in 6% of them , and the ankle in- 4%. In the knee it can involve the medial and lateral condyle as weight-bearing surfaces and the patella too. The prevalence of OCD in femoral condyles is 4/10,000, wherein males are twice more affected than females. The onset of this disease in knee is in the third–fourth decade of life, in ankle and elbow in second decade. The etiology of OCD is described as traumatic (repetitive impingement), ischemic, idiopathic, and hereditary, so a result of multifactorial elements. In physical examination, intermittent limitation of range of motion of the joint, varying pain and swelling, catching, locking, and giving-way often occur. The stages in progression are:

Stage I consists of a small area of compression of subchondral bone. Fissuras may present.

Stage II consists of a partially detached osteochondral fragment. A radiograph of the bone may reveal a well-circumscribed area of sclerotic subchondral bone separated from the remainder of the epiphysis by a radiolucent line.

Stage III lesions are the most common and consist of a completely detached fragment that remains within the underlying crater bed.

Stage IV lesions consist of a completely detached fragment that is completely displaced from the crater bed. This is also termed a loose body (Figs. 13.33–13.35).

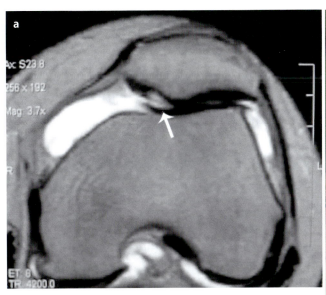

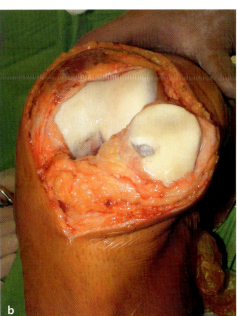

Fig. 13.33 a, b Osteochondritis dissecans of the patella in a horizontal scan of MRI (**a**), and intraoperatively (**b**)

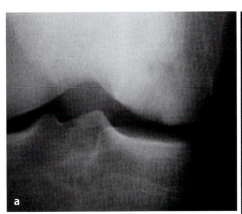

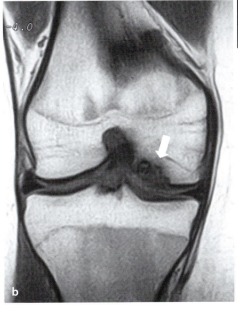

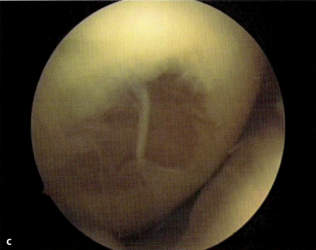

Fig. 13.34 a–c Osteochondritis dissecans of the medial femoral condyle. Radiograph (**a**), MRI (**b**) and arthroscopic (**c**) view. Note: the underlying bone from which the fragment separates has normal vascularity. It distinguishes OCD from osteonecrosis, in which the underlying bone is avascular

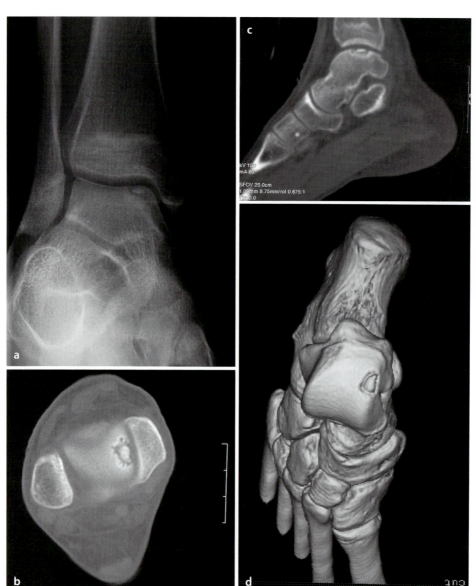

Fig. 13.35 a–d Osteochondritis dissecans of the talus in the posteromedial aspect. Radiograph (**a**), horizontal CT scan (**b**) and sagittal reconstruction (**c**) and 3D CT (**d**) of the affected region. The OCD can occur also in the anterolateral aspect of the talus

13.3 Slipped Capital Femoral Epiphysis

Slipped capital femoral epiphysis (SCFE) is characterized by the posteroinferior displacement of the femoral head due to shear stresses across the physis. This disease occurs in obese or excessively tall children aged 11–15 years and more common in boys, but because of the onset of ossification, girls with slipped capital femoral epiphysis often are younger than boys (male-to-female ratio of approximately 2–5 : 1). Prevalence has been reported to be 0.2–10 cases per 100,000. Bilateral involvement is present in more than 50% of cases. The etiology is unknown in majority of cases, but there is a high association between the disease and the combination of both biomechanical (extended femoral retroversion, deeper acetabulum, obesity) and biochemical (hypothyroidism, acromegaly, adiposogenital syndrome, hyperparathyroidism) factors, due to increased stresses across a weakened physis. Acute, chronic, and acute on chronic forms of SCFE can be identified. Complicated and untreated slipped capital femoral epiphysis lead to deformity and early osteoarthrosis of the hip (Figs. 13.36–13.39).

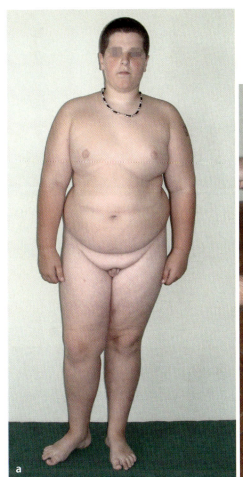
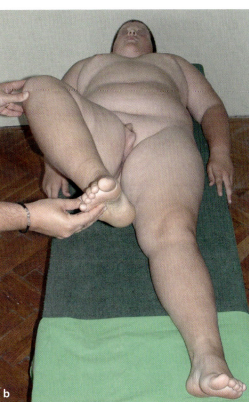

Fig. 13.36 a, b A 13-year-old boy presenting limping and hip and knee pain on the right side due to SCFE. Externally rotated attitude of the affected right lower limb can be seen (**a**). Positive Drehmann's sign: spontaneous external rotation in flexion (**b**)

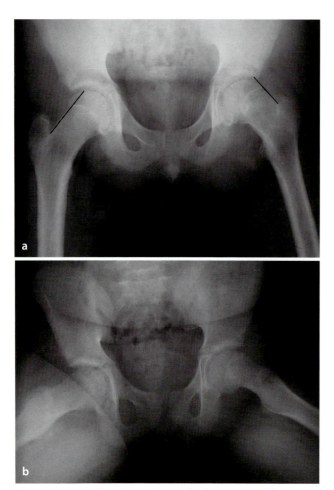

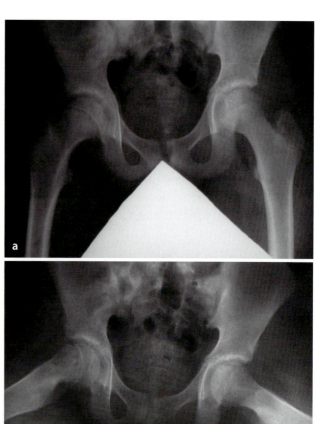

Fig. 13.37 a, b AP pelvic radiograph of a 11-year-old patient with mild slipped capital femoral epiphysis. Almost no deformity is recognizable on the AP radiograph. The physeal plate is widened on the left side. The Klein's line (along the femoral neck) does not intersects the lateral portion of the femoral head on the left side that shows a suspicion for SCFE (**a**). Even the mild slipping is apparent on the frog lateral radiograph (**b**)

Fig. 13.38 a, b AP (**a**) and frog lateral (**b**) view radiograph of a 13-year-old boy with moderate slipping of the right capital femoral epiphysis

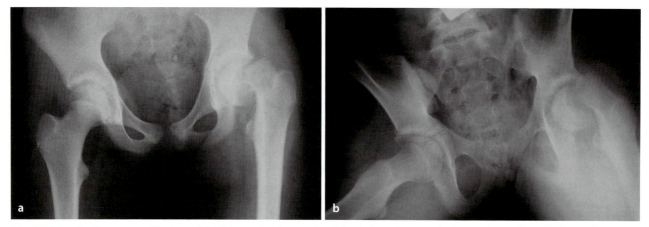

Fig. 13.39 a, b The severe slipping of the left capital femoral epiphysis is well recognizable on both the AP (**a**) and frog lateral (Lauenstein) view radiographs of a 12-year-old girl (**b**)

13.4 Neuromuscular Diseases

13.4.1 Cerebral Palsy

Cerebral palsy is a neuromuscular disease with diverse manifestations. The damages of the developing brain that can be prenatal (infections, malformations, drugs, etc.), perinatal (prematurity, anoxia), or postnatal (injury, infection) lead to clinical signs. Depending on the area of cerebral lesions different movement disorders such as hemiplegia, di/paraplegia, or quadriplegia can be caused. Physiologically three forms of the disease can be distinguished: spastic, athetotic, and ataxial types. Only the spastic group may be treated by orthopedic surgical techniques. Muscle-length shortening, contractures, acetabular dysplasia, hip subluxation or dislocation, scoliosis and walking inability are the most common causes to visit an orthopedic surgeon (Figs. 13.40–13.46).

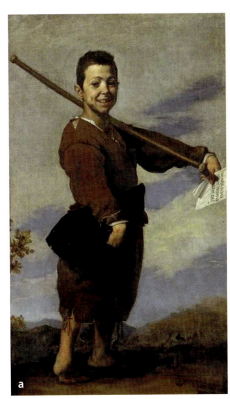
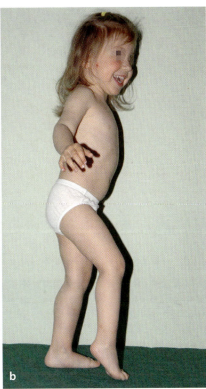

Fig. 13.40 a, b Although the title of this picture is the "The Beggar (The Clubfoot)," hemiplegia spastica would be a better diagnosis for the young man on the painting. Flexion contracture of the right wrist and equinus contracture of the right ankle are well recognizable. The Beggar (The Clubfoot) 1642; Jusepe de Ribera (Spanish 1591–1652); Musée du Louvre, Paris (**a**). A 3-year-old girl with cerebral palsy having very similar deformity (**b**)

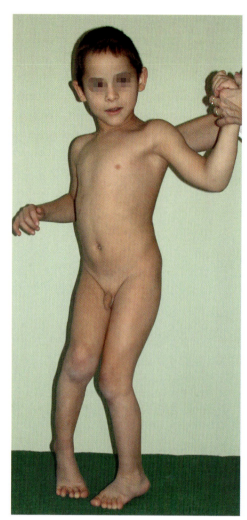

Fig. 13.41 A 6-year-old boy with diplegia. Typical signs of flexion-, adduction- and internal rotational contracture of the hips, flexion contracture of the knees and equinus contractures of the ankles can be observed

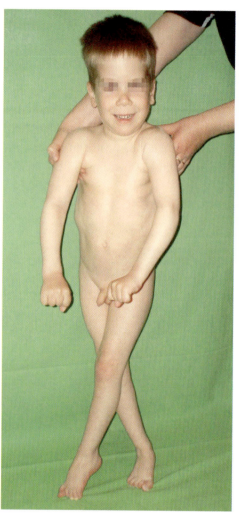

Fig. 13.42 A 4-year-old tetraplegic patient with the signs of "crossing legs" phenomenon (severe adduction contracture of the hips) and also flexion contracture in both upper limb

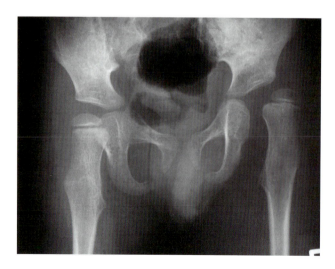

Fig. 13.43 Hips are well developed at birth but due to the adduction contracture coxa valga, mild dysplasia, subluxation may occur (*left side*)

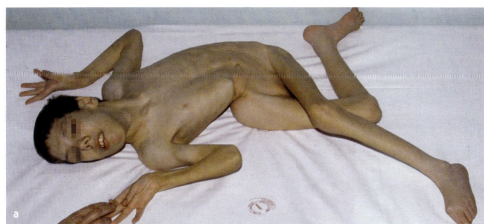

Fig. 13.44 a, b In case of severe spastic contraction of the flexor and adductor muscles of the hip fixed hip dislocation can also develop (a). Pelvic radiograph of the above 14-year-old boy with fixed dislocation of both hips (b)

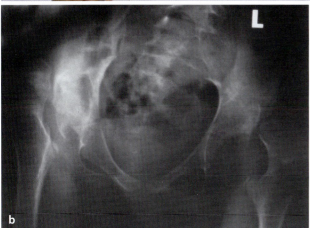

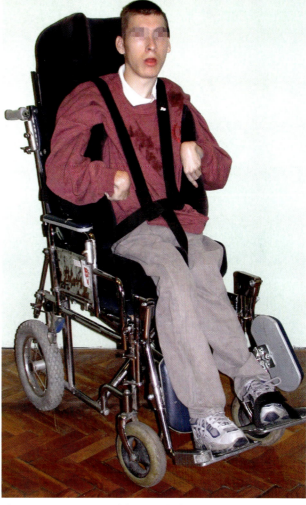

Fig. 13.45 A 21-year-old nonambulatory patient with severe spastic tetraparesis

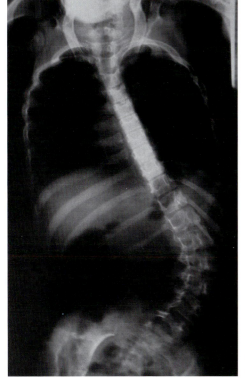

Fig. 13.46 Because of the imbalance of the paravertebral muscles, scoliosis is a frequent accompanying sign to cerebral palsy

13.4.2 Myelomeningocele

Myelomeningocele is the most frequent subgroup of neural tube defects with plenty of orthopedic complications. The abnormal neural elements take part in the formation of myelomeningocele, resulting in different types of paralysis mainly on the lower limbs. Orthopedic treatment is given only following neurosurgical interventions (closure of the meninx and the skin, ventriculo–peritoneal shunt) (Figs. 13.47–13.49).

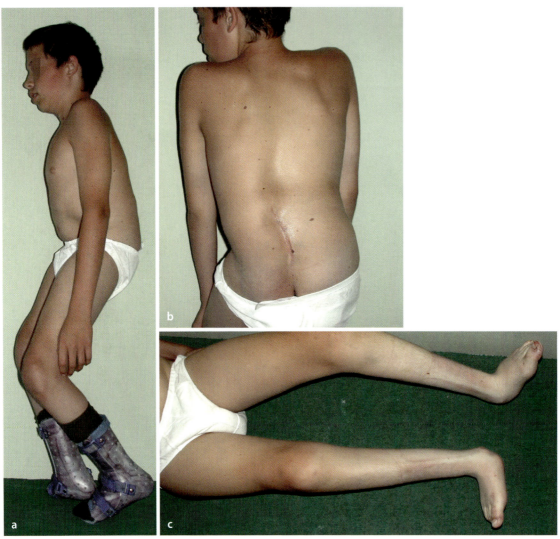

Fig. 13.47 a–c A 15-year-old boy with meningomyelocele. Weakness of the muscles of the lower limb, are detectable. A foot and ankle orthesis is needed for standing and walking to strengthen the power of the calf muscles and to correct foot deformity (**a**). The scar of the initial operation, in which closure of the meninx was done, and secondary left lumbar scoliosis are visible. The boy needs to wear nappy because of the accompanying incontinentia (**b**). Bilateral flatfeet and calcaneovalgus feet were developed in the above patient, but also secondary clubfoot and pes cavus may be present in myelomeningocele (**c**)

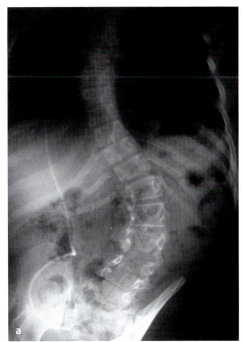

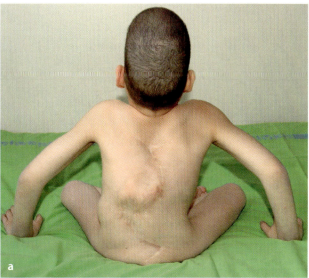

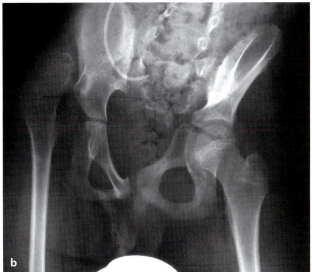

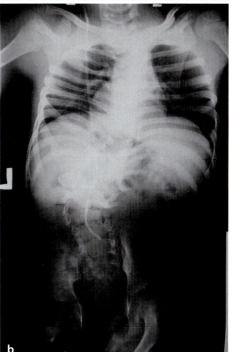

Fig. 13.48 a, b Secondary left lumbar scoliosis the unclosed vertebral arches and the ventriculo–peritoneal shunt can be seen on the AP spine radiograph of the above patient (**a**). Secondary valgus position of the femoral neck, dysplasia of the acetabulum and high, fixed dislocation of the right hip is present (**b**)

Fig. 13.49 a, b Eight-year-old boy with meningomyelocele. The primary defect was closed surgically in age of newborn. Bilateral clubfeet were also treated surgically. The patient is able to stand up in orthesis. Posterior view (**a**), and radiograph (**b**) of him. On radiograph, note the severe scoliosis and the ventriculo–peritoneal shunt

13.4.3 Poliomyelitis

Poliomyelitis is an infectious disease that used to be the most common cause of paralysis in young people. The worldwide prevalence of this infection has decreased significantly since then because of aggressive immunization programs.

Complications of polio infection may include life-long severe muscle weakness, often in the leg, causing the foot to drop and making walking difficult.

Patients who have recovered from poliomyelitis occasionally develop a postpoliomyelitis syndrome, in which recurrences of weakness or fatigue are observed and usually involve groups of muscles that were initially affected. This postpolio syndrome may develop 20–40 years after infection with poliovirus (Figs. 13.50–13.53).

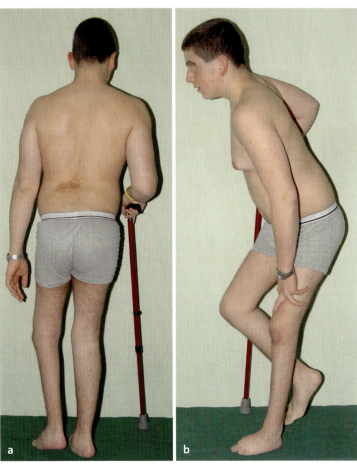

Fig. 13.50 a, b The affected paralyzed left leg has atrophied calf muscles and a 3 cm shortening (**a**). The patient has to hold the left thigh during walking because of the weakness of quadriceps muscle (**b**)

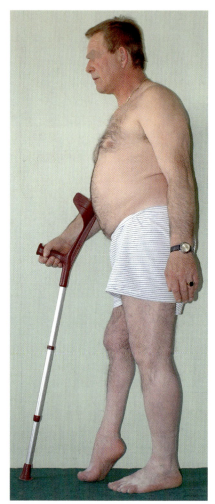

Fig. 13.51 Very common symptom is the drop foot because of the weakness of extensor muscles of the lower leg

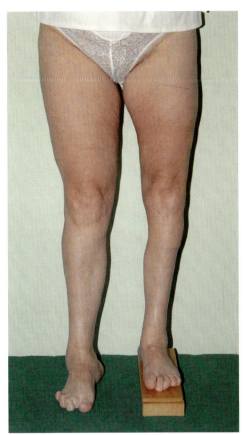

Fig. 13.52 Poliomyelitis during childhood frequently causes leg length discrepancy. The woman has 4 cm shortening of the paralyzed left leg

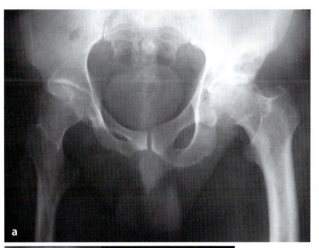

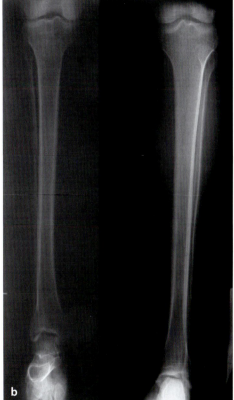

Fig. 13.53 a, b Radiograph picture of a 49-year-old man. The hypoplasia and osteopenia of the right pelvic bones and right femur are well detectable, the secondary osteoarthritis of the unaffected hip due to overload may often occur (**a**). Tibia and fibula of the affected side are also shortened (**b**)

13.4.4 Peroneal Muscular Atrophy (Charcot–Marie–Tooth)

Charcot–Marie–Tooth disease is one of the most common inherited neurological disorders, affecting approximately 1 in 2,500 people. It is also known as hereditary motor and sensory neuropathy (HMSN) or peroneal muscular atrophy, comprises a group of disorders caused by mutations in genes that affect the normal function of the peripheral nerves.

Some patients experience mild to severe pain.

The patients slowly loose normal use of their feet and legs, and later hands and arms as nerves to the extremities degenerate and the muscles in the extremities become weak because of the loss of stimulation by affected nerves. Many patients also loose sensory nerve function (Figs. 13.54 and 13.55).

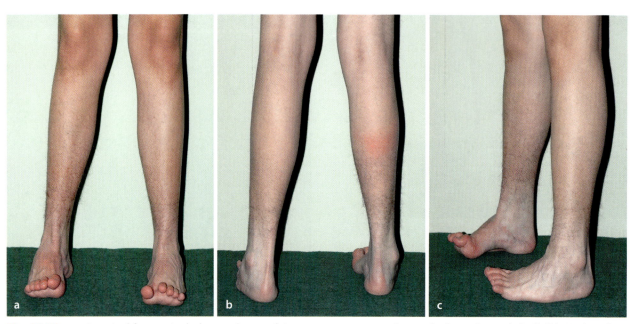

Fig. 13.54 a–c A typical feature includes weakness of the foot and lower leg muscles, which may result in foot drop and a high-stepped gait with frequent tripping or falls (**a**). The lower legs may take on an "inverted champagne bottle" appearance due to the loss of muscle bulk (**b**). High arches and hammertoes are also characteristic due to weakness of the small muscles in the feet, presented in the lateral clinical view (**c**)

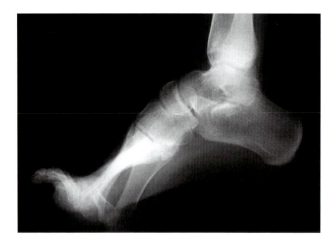

Fig. 13.55 Lateral view radiograph of the excavated right foot

13.4.5 Arthrogryposis Multiplex Congenita

Arthrogryposis multiplex congenita is a nonprogressive congenital neuromuscular syndrome characterized by severe joint contractures, muscle weakness, and fibrosis.

The etiology of arthrogryposis is unknown. Restriction of intrauterine movement is probably responsible for the severe joint stiffness. The contractures and muscle loss correlate with specific segmental neurological motor deficits and decreased anterior horn-cell populations.

The primary joints involved (in order of decreasing prevalence) include the foot, hip, wrist, knee, elbow, and shoulder. Other associated conditions include scoliosis, lung hypoplasia leading to respiratory problems, growth retardation, midfacial hemangioma, facial and jaw deformities, respiratory problems, and abdominal hernias.

Cognition, intelligence, and speech are usually normal (Figs. 13.56–13.61).

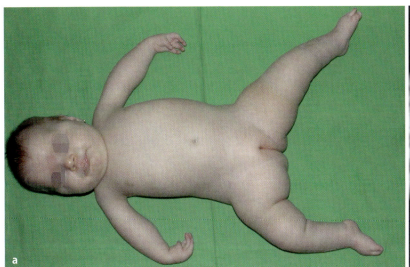 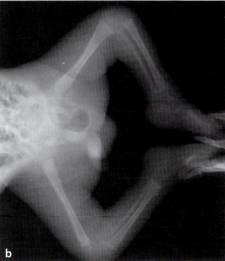

Fig. 13.56 a, b AMC is typically symmetrical and involves all four extremities with some variation seen as presented on photograph (**a**) and radiograph (**b**). Flexion creases are often absent, suggesting an early intrauterine onset. This type presents with abducted and externally rotated hips, flexed knees, clubfeet, internally rotated shoulders, extended elbow, pronated forearm, and flexed and ulnarly deviated wrists ("waiter's tip")

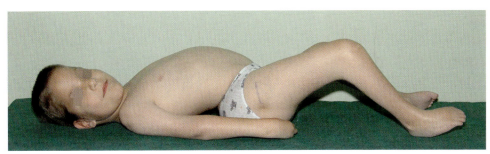

Fig. 13.57 Flexion contracture in the hip and knee joints

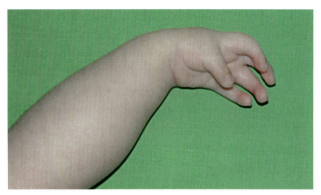

Fig. 13.58 The hand in flexion contracture in the wrist joint

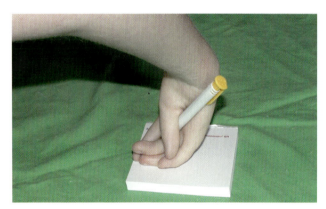

Fig. 13.59 Children usually learn using pen even in extreme hand position

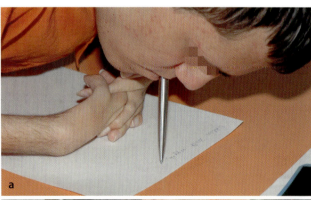

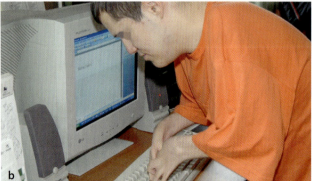

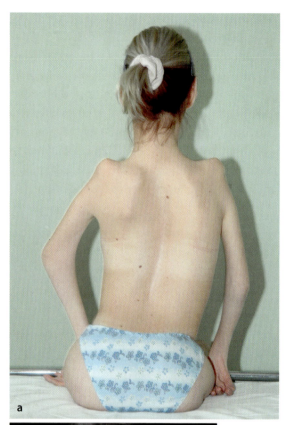

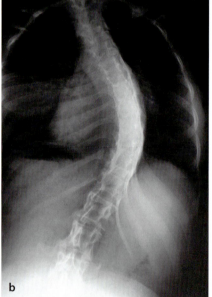

Fig. 13.61 a, b Photograph (**a**) and radiograph (**b**) of a 21-year-old nonambulatory woman with right thoracic scoliosis

Fig. 13.60 a, b Another patient would rather take the pen in his mouth to write (**a**), but can use his hands for manipulating the keyboard (**b**)

13.4.6 Progressive Muscular Dystrophy

Progressive muscular dystrophies are a group of disorders with ongoing muscular weakness and progressive degeneration of the muscles. The disorders have been classified on clinical severity and the pattern of genetic inheritance. The most well-known sex-chromosome-linked muscular dystrophies are the severe Duchenne's type and the rather benign Becker's type. The facioscapulohumeral type is the most frequent among the autosomal inherited muscular dystrophies (Figs. 13.62–13.66).

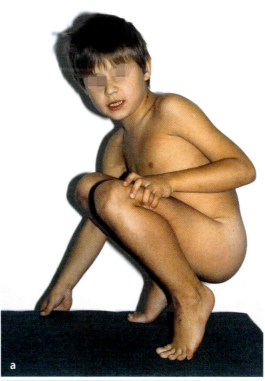

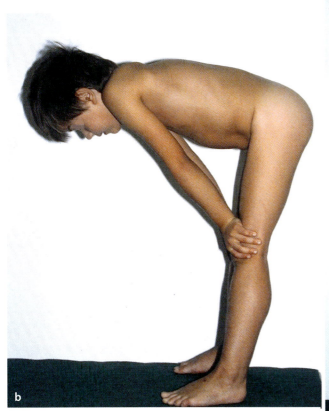

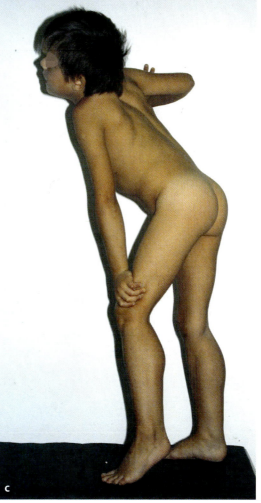

Fig. 13.62 a–c Nine-year-old boy with Duchenne's type muscular dystrophy. The child uses special maneuvers to stand up from cowering (**a–c**)

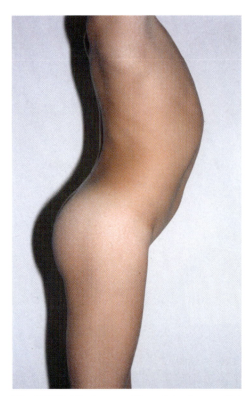

Fig. 13.63 Weakness of the gluteal musculature causes a specific posture in muscular dystrophy. Dorsal shift of the trunk, increased lumbar lordosis and anterior tilt of the pelvis can be observed

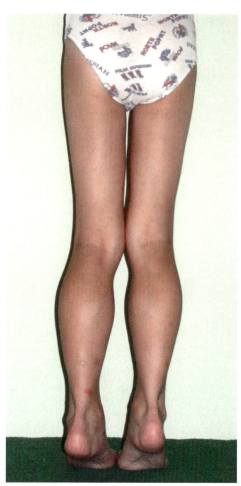

Fig. 13.64 Pseudohypertrophy of the calf muscles is apparent in Duchenne's dystrophy due to the degeneration of muscle tissue and accumulation of fat

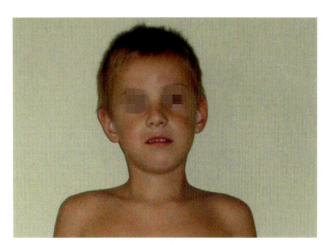

Fig. 13.65 First the facial muscles are involved in the facioscapulohumeral muscular dystrophy. Lack of mobility, pouting lips can be seen

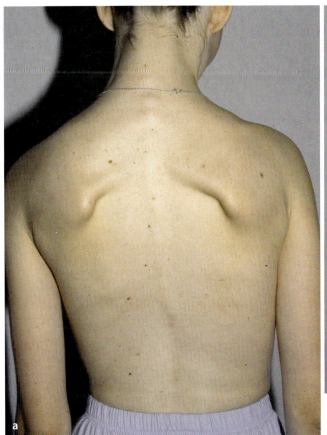

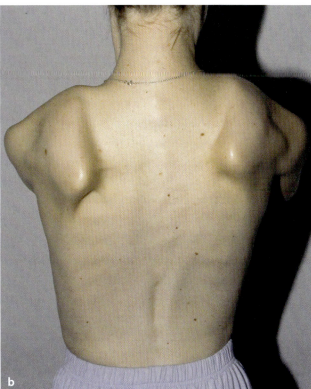

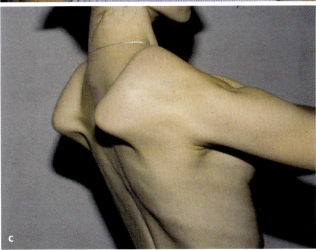

Fig. 13.66 a–c The weakness of the shoulder girdle muscles results in bilateral winging scapula (**a**). The winging of the scapula is more pronounced by elevating the arms (**b**, **c**)

13.5 Scoliosis

13.5.1 Scoliosis, Congenital

Congenital deformity of the spine may lead to deviation even in the sagittal (kyphoses) and frontal (scoliosis) planes. Deformities are usually acquired during pregnancy mainly due to toxic damage. Hereditary factors are the cause only in 1% of the cases. The prevalence of vertebral abnormalities is very high of about one in thousand, but many of the deformities do not produce any symptoms. The male-to-female ratio for congenital scoliosis is 1:1.4. The vertebral abnormalities are present at birth, but clinical deformity may not be evident until later in childhood, when progressive scoliosis is evident.

Classification according to MacEwen:

- Failure of formation (wedge vertebra: partial failure of formation, hemivertebra: complete failure of formation)
- Failure of segmentation (unilateral unsegmented bar: unilateral failure of segmentation, block vertebra: bilateral failure of segmentation)
- Mixed (elements of both failure of formation and segmentation) (Figs. 13.67–13.69)

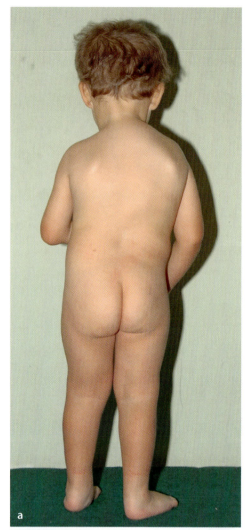

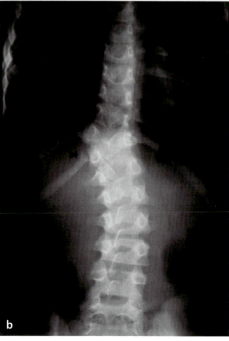

Fig. 13.67 a, b A 2,5-year-old boy with congenital deformity of the spine. No significant trunk asymmetry or scolioses are present in younger age (**a**) radiograph image of the same patient shows a hemivertebra formation at Th 11 vertebral level (**b**)

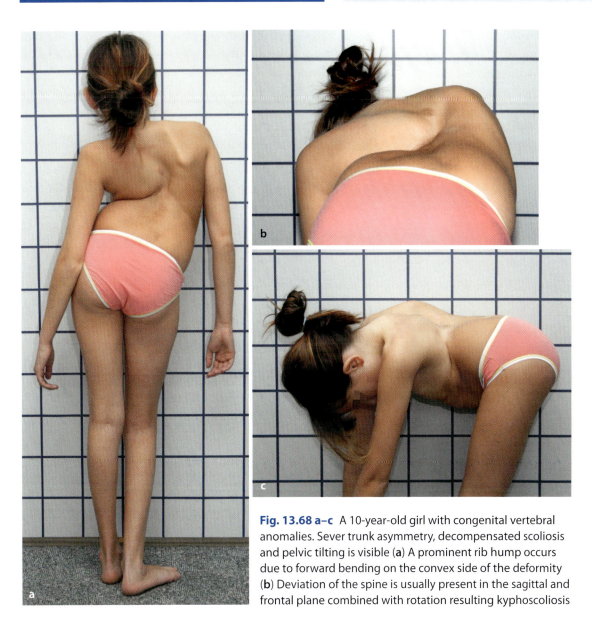

Fig. 13.68 a–c A 10-year-old girl with congenital vertebral anomalies. Sever trunk asymmetry, decompensated scoliosis and pelvic tilting is visible (**a**) A prominent rib hump occurs due to forward bending on the convex side of the deformity (**b**) Deviation of the spine is usually present in the sagittal and frontal plane combined with rotation resulting kyphoscoliosis

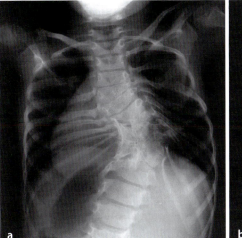
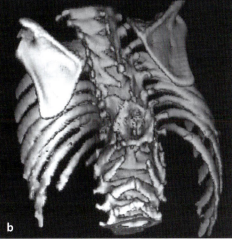

Fig. 13.69 a, b (a) Radiograph of the same patient shows unilateral unsegmented bar at dorsal level of the spine. (b) 3D CT image shows more detailed picture of the deformity. Note the fusion of the ribs on the concave side

13.5.2 Scoliosis, Idiopathic

Idiopathic scoliosis is the lateral bending of the spine combined with vertebral rotation and torsion. There are many theories for the cause of this problem. Most of the authors suppose a genetic origin for idiopathic scoliosis but other theories such as the vestibular imbalance or trunk muscle imbalance are also reported. Classification according to the American Scoliosis Research Society describes infantile (0–3 years), juvenile (4–10 years) and adolescent (over 10 years) forms.

The infantile and juvenile forms are rare without difference in the incidence among boys and girls. The curves are usually progressive and located at the thoracic level with left side convexity and combined with kyphosis.

The adolescent form is more frequent and occurs 3.5 times more in girls. The prevalence is 1.2% at the age of 14 years. The most common types of curve patterns are the right thoracic, the right thoracic and left lumbar, the thoracolumbar, the double thoracic and the isolated left lumbar. The most frequent curves are at the thoracic level with right side convexity. The deformity occurs less frequently at the thoracolumbar or lumbar level and in about 10% is S shaped (Figs. 13.70–13.73).

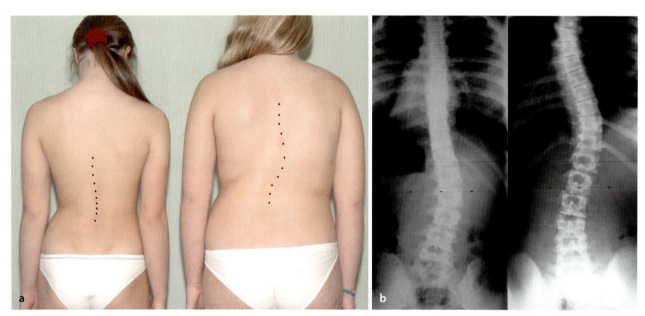

Fig. 13.70 a, b The clinical manifestation of a lumbar (*left side*) and thoracic (*right side*) scoliosis may be very similar. The asymmetry of the trunk and the curve of the spine are well appreciable (**a**). radiographs of the above two 12-year-old girls (**b**)

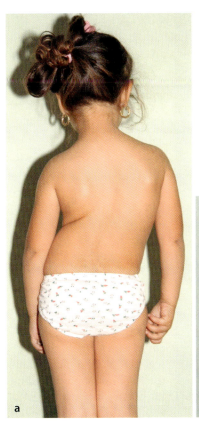

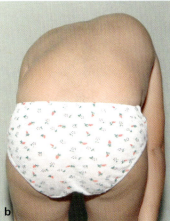

Fig. 13.71 a, b Infantile right thoracic noncompensated scoliosis. The asymmetry of the trunk-arm triangles are well recognizable (**a**). Upon forward bending the deformity of the rib cage is apparent (**b**)

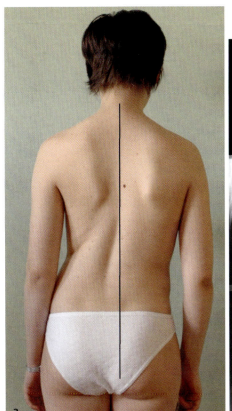

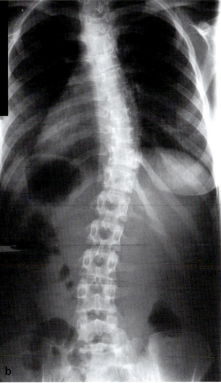

Fig. 13.72 a, b The posture often independent of the severity of scoliosis. A 13-year-old girl with 30° right thoracic scoliosis that resulted a non compensated posture (**a, b**)

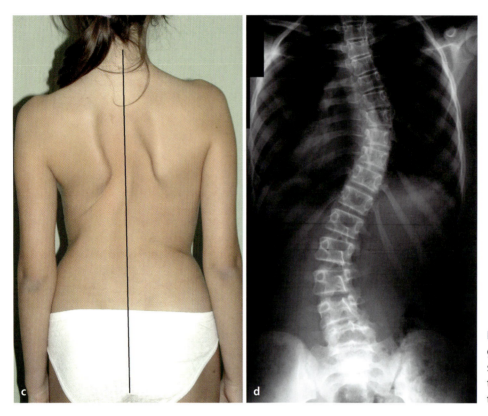

Fig. 13.72 c, d A 15-year-old girl (**c**) with 45° right thoracic scoliosis (**d**). Deformities of the trunk are well appreciable but the posture is compensated

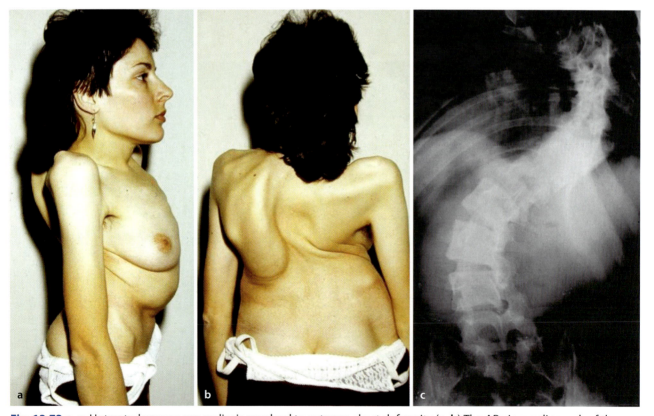

Fig. 13.73 a–c Untreated very severe scoliosis may lead to extreme chest deformity (**a, b**). The AP view radiograph of the 22-year-old women. The more than 90° left-sided thoracic and a bit smaller, compensatory right lumbar scoliosis are well detectable (**c**)

Chapter 14

Neck, Chest, Spine and Pelvis

Contents

Chapter 14

Neck, Chest, Spine and Pelvis

J. Lakatos, K. Köllő, G. Skaliczki, and G. Holnapy

14.1 Congenital and Developmental Disorders

14.1.1 Klippel–Feil Syndrome

Klippel–Feil syndrome is a rare condition characterized by a short neck, limited range of movement in the cervical spine and a low hairline. Its incidence is approximately 2 cases per 100,000 newborn. The etiology of the disease is unknown; however, fetal alcohol syndrome, genetic disorder and vascular disorder have been named among others as grounds for the disease. The syndrome is classified into three types: massive fusion of the cervical spine belongs to type I, fusion of one or two cervical vertebrae marks type II, and type III occurs when the lumbar or thoracic vertebrae are involved besides the cervical spine. Other anomalies are often presented together with Klippel–Feil syndrome, such as congenital scoliosis, Sprengel's deformity, renal disorders, congenital heart disease, abnormalities of the craniocervical junction, synkinesis, torticollis or loss of hearing (Figs. 14.1–14.4).

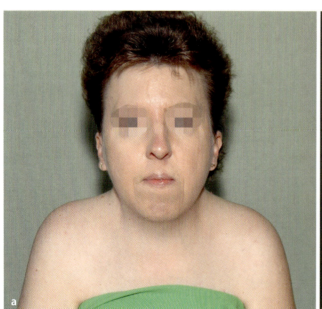
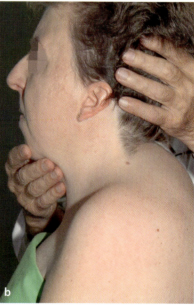

Fig. 14.1 a, b The typically short neck of a patient with Klippel–Feil syndrome (**a**) and her low hairline (**b**) can be seen

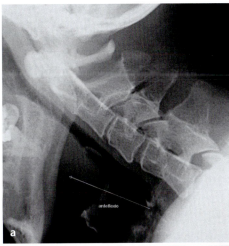

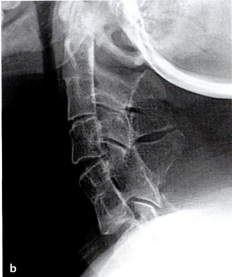

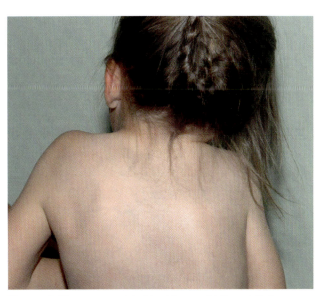

Fig. 14.3 Three-year-old girl with type II Klippel–Feil syndrome

Fig. 14.2 a, b Fusion of the C1–2–3 and C5–6 vertebrae is seen on the previous patient's radiograph, classifying her into type I Klippel–Feil syndrome. The limited range of movement of the cervical spine at anteflexion (**a**) and retroflexion (**b**) is also visible

Fig. 14.4 a, b Lateral radiograph of the cervical spine of the previous patient shows the fusion of C3–4–5 vertebrae (**a**). As a concomitant disease she has congenital scoliosis as well (**b**)

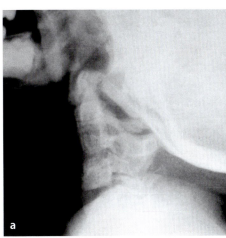

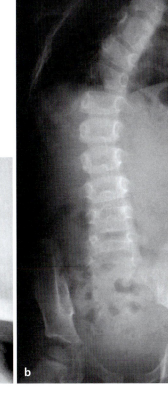

14.1.2 Cervical Rib

Above the normal first rib, a supernumerary rib can be observed, arising from the seventh cervical vertebra. The incidence of the cervical rib is about 0.5%. Compressing the neurovascular structures at the superior aperture of the thorax, it may cause thoracic outlet syndrome (TOS). In most of the cases (95%) the brachial plexus is affected, but the subclavian vein (4%), and the subclavian artery (1%) can also be involved (Fig. 14.5).

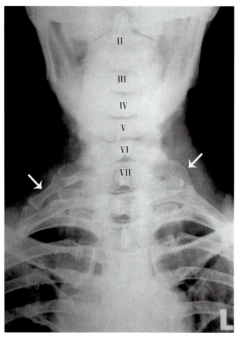

Fig. 14.5 Elongated transversal process on the left (*arrow*) and cervical rib arising from the 7th. cervical vertebra on the right (*arrow*)

14.1.3 Pectus Excavatum Congenitum, Pectus Carinatum Congenitum

Pectus excavatum is the most common chest deformity affecting males three times more frequently than females. The appearance of the abnormality varies from the mild to the severe, and worsens in the early teenage years. It can occur as a single disorder or as part of Marfan's and Poland syndromes. The aetiology of the disease is not known; however family occurrences can be observed in 35% of the cases. The condition is usually asymptomatic raising cosmetic questions mainly; however, restrictive pulmonary changes, mitral valve prolapse or decreased cardiac index could be the signs of cardiopulmonary impairment (Figs. 14.6–14.9).

Pectus carinatum, also known as bird chest, chicken breast, is a deformity of unknown origin representing the protrusion of the anterior chest wall. Males are affected four times as more frequently as than women. The disease can occur as a single deformity, or in association with other abnormalities such as congenital heart disease, scoliosis, Morquio's syndrome, kyphosis, etc. Although the deformity is usually asymptomatic, causing only cosmetic concerns, decreased lung compliance, progressive emphysema, and increased frequency of respiratory tract infections can be observed (Figs. 14.9 a–c).

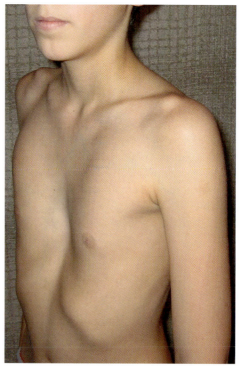

Fig. 14.6 Ten-year-old boy presenting with symmetric pectus excavatum congenitum causing cosmetic complaints only without any sign of respiratory or cardiovascular difficulties

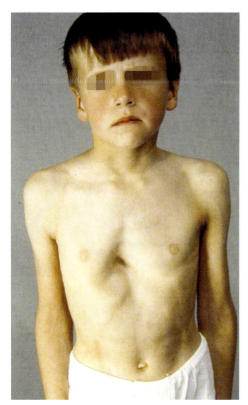

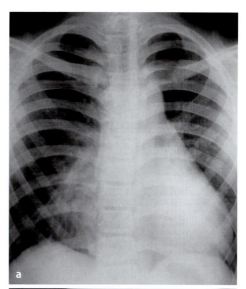

Fig. 14.7 The pit in the right side of the chest refers to asymmetric pectus excavatum congenitum

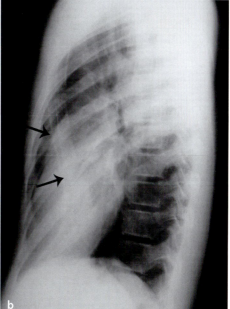

Fig. 14.8 a–c AP view-chest radiograph of a patient with symmetric pectus excavatum congenitus showing laterally displaced heart due to the chest deformity (**a**).Lateral view chest x-ray of the same patient shows the narrowing of the mediastinal space. The white line demonstrates the abnormal form of the sternum (**b**). According to the CT scan of the chest the retrosternal space is 21.11 mm narrow at its biggest diameter (**c**).

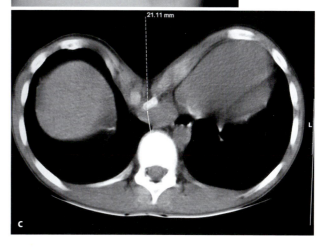

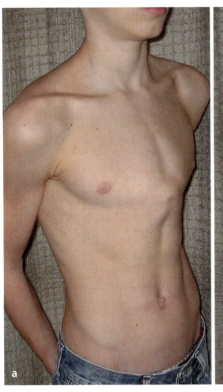
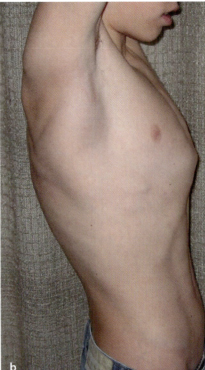
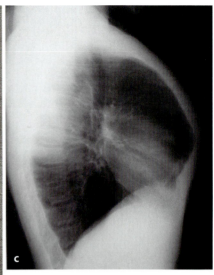

Fig. 14.9 a–c Twelve year-old boy presented with pectus carinatum (**a**, **b**). Lateral view radiograph of a patient's chest with pectus carinatum showing huge space between the sternum and the spine (**c**)

14.1.4 Pectoral Major Muscle Aplasia

The pectoralis major is a large, fanlike muscle that covers most of the upper front part of the chest. Its absence is a rare condition that is congenital. Affected individuals may have variable associated features, such as underdevelopment or absence of one nipple, forearm and hand deformities (Fig. 14.10).

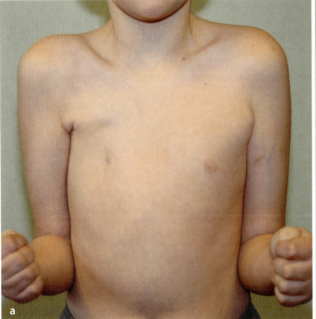
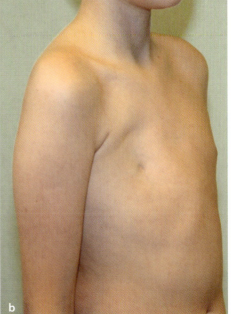

Fig. 14.10 a, b The photograph presents a 12-year-old boy with pectoralis major muscle aplasia on the right side

14.1.5 Spondylolysis, Spondylolisthesis, Spondyloptosis

The portion of the neural arch of the spine that connects the superior and inferior articular facets is rather narrow. Any defect in this narrow bony bridge results in *spondylolysis*. The incidence ranges from 5 to 8% depending on the sex, age and race. Some 80% of the cases develop at the L5–S1 level, another 10% at the L4–5 level, leaving the rest for the other parts of the spine. The most common classification of causes (Wiltse) defines five groups differentiating congenital, isthmic, degenerative, traumatic and pathologic spondylolysis. Being bilateral, spondylolysis can lead to forward slipping of the vertebra upon the one below it, causing a *spondylolisthesis*. The most popular grading system developed by Meyerding classifies the patients into five groups of increasing severity. The classification is based on the distance the slipped vertebra had moved relative to the adjacent vertebral body. In the most severe cases the slipped vertebra is practically subluxated and displaced ahead of the adjacent vertebral body. Although most patients with spondylolysis or spondylolisthesis are asymptomatic, those who have symptoms usually complain of pain in the lower back , and tenderness over the lower lumbar spine. On physical examination, gait, paraspinal muscle spasm, and "step-off" over the spinous processes at the level of displacement are the leading symptoms (Figs. 14.11–14.20).

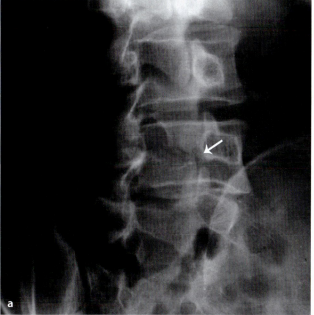
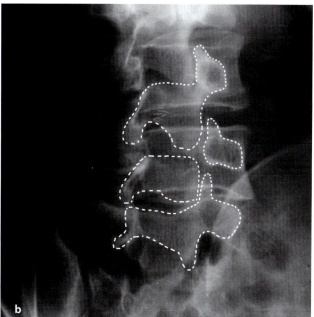
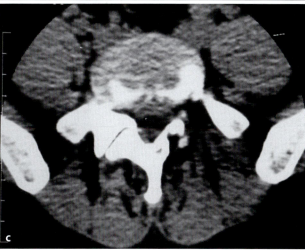

Fig. 14.11 a–c In this case a 12-year-old boy was presented with low back pain and the cause of this was a L4 spondylolysis. The white arrow points to the defective part of the neural arch (pars interarticularis) (**a**). Oblique radiograph (Dittmar's -view) – such as this- are important in the differentiation of spondylolysis and spondylolisthesis. The posterior facet joints and laminae imitate a series of "scottie dogs" in the lumbar region (**b**). Interruption of the neck of the "dog" without slipping represents spondylolysis. A wide interruption area with more or less forward shifting of the proximal vertebras refers to spondylolisthesis. CT scan reveals the defect of the arch (**c**)

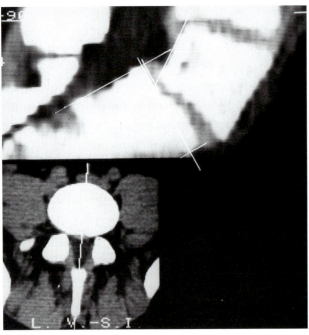

Fig. 14.12 Reconstruction CT picture presents a Meyerding's type I spondylolisthesis at L5/S1 level. The spinal canal is not narrowed

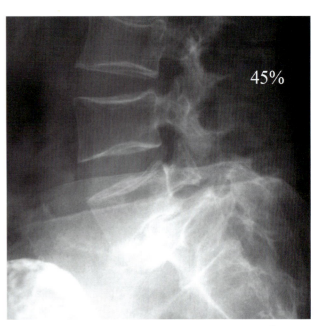

Fig. 14.14 Lateral view radiograph shows a Meyerding's type II spondylolisthesis with 45% forward slipping of the vertebra L5

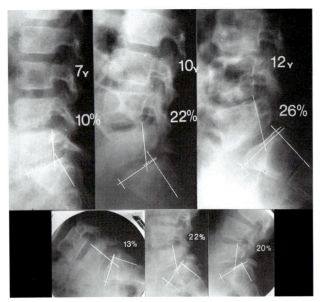

Fig. 14.13 Progression of Meyerding's type I spondylolisthesis to type II at lumbosacral level from the age of 7–12. Functional view of the spine can be seen in the lower images with the patient bending forward on the left side, standing straight in the middle and bending backward on the right. Note the instability of the lumbar vertebral column

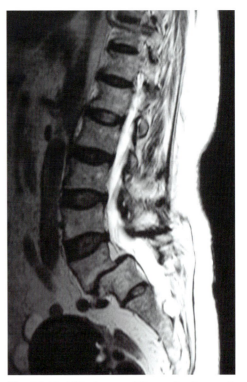

Fig. 14.15 MRI picture of Meyerding's type II spondylolisthesis with moderate stenosis of the spinal canal

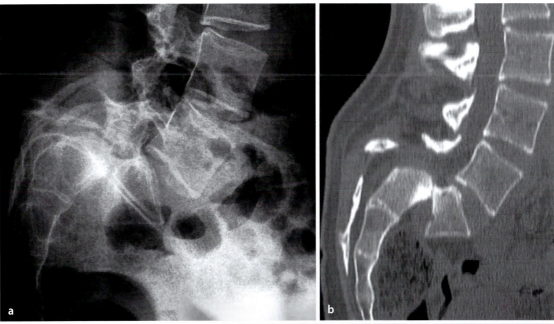

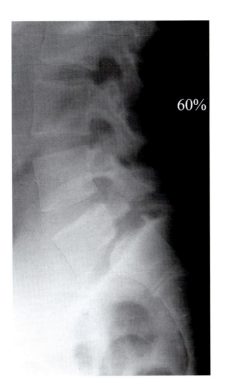

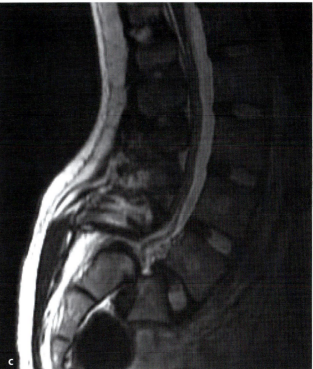

Fig. 14.16 Meyerding's type III. spondylolisthesis at L5/S1 level with 60% forward shift of the L5 vertebra

Fig. 14.17 a–c Meyerding's type IV spondylolisthesis (spondyloptosis). The affected vertebra (L5) is subluxated and articulates the anterior border of the endplate of the S1 vertebra as shown on the lateral view radiograph (**a**), reconstructive CT scan (**b**) and MR picture (**c**). Note the stenosis of the vertebral canal which did not caused significant neurological problems (courtesy of dr. P.P.Varga,Inst. of Spinal Surg. Budapest)

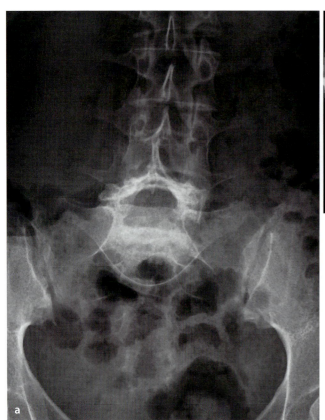

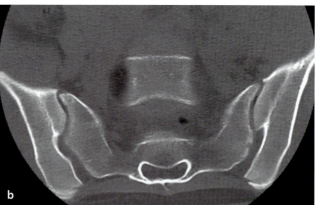

Fig. 14.18 a, b AP radiograph taken from the lumbosacral region of the previous patient with spondyloptosis. The body of the slipped L5 vertebra and its transverse processes are projected together with the shadow of the sacrum giving the appearance of the so called "inverted Napoleon hat" (**a**). On the CT scan (**b**) the horizontal cross section of the sacrum and the coronal cross section of the L5 vertebra can be seen on the same image referring to the serious deformity

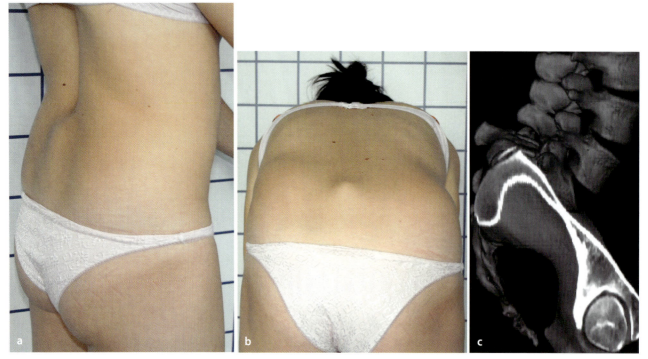

Fig. 14.19 a–c The forward shift of the L5 vertebra causes a step-off of the spinous processes, which occurs as a prominence at the level of the lumbosacral junction (**a**). Bending the patient anteriorly, the phenomenon can be better observed (**b**).The relative protrusion of the S1 spinous process is well demonstrated on the reconstructive CT scan (**c**)

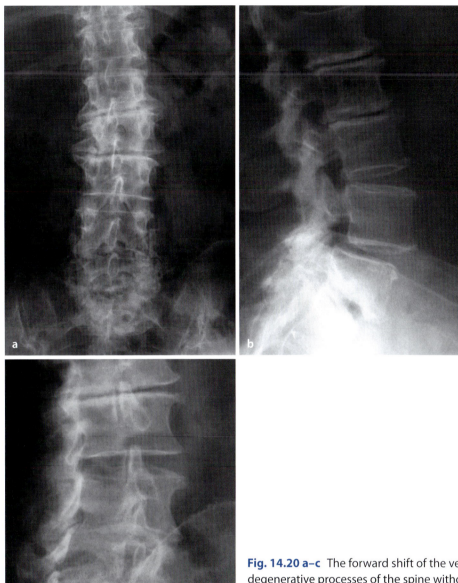

Fig. 14.20 a–c The forward shift of the vertebral column can occur in degenerative processes of the spine without spondylolysis – it is called pseudolisthesis. Note the degenerative changes of the lumbar vertebras on the a–p radiograph (**a**), the shifting phenomen of the fourths lumbar vertebral body (radiograph, lateral view, (**b**)) without a spondylolysis: the dog's neck is intact (radiograph, oblique view, (**c**))

14.1.6 Transient Lumbosacral Vertebrae

Vertebral segments at the lumbosacral transition are relatively often affected by developmental abnormalities, e.g., lumbalization, sacralization, hemilumbalization or hemisacralization. In case of sacralization the elongated and broadened transversal processes of the fifth lumbar vertebra are partially or totally fused or articulated with the sacrum. Patients with bilateral symmetric fusion are generally free of complaints, but the unilateral fusion can lead to low back pain due to spondylosis of the upper vertebral segments. Lumbalization occurs when the ossification of the sacrum with the first sacral segment is disturbed. It can be partial or total, turning the appearance of the first sacral segment similar to the fifth lumbar vertebra in the latter case. As it is at sacralization, bilateral deformity is usually asymptomatic, unilateral form can cause low back pain though (Figs. 14.21 and 14.22).

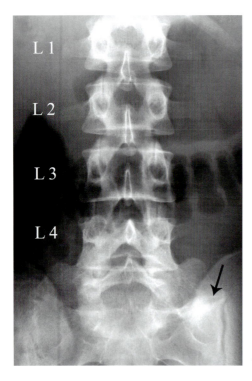

Fig. 14.21 Elongated and broadened transverse processes of the L5 vertebra are fused with the sacrum. Only four lumbar vertebrae are shown. Note the pseudoarthrosis on the *left* side (*arrow*)

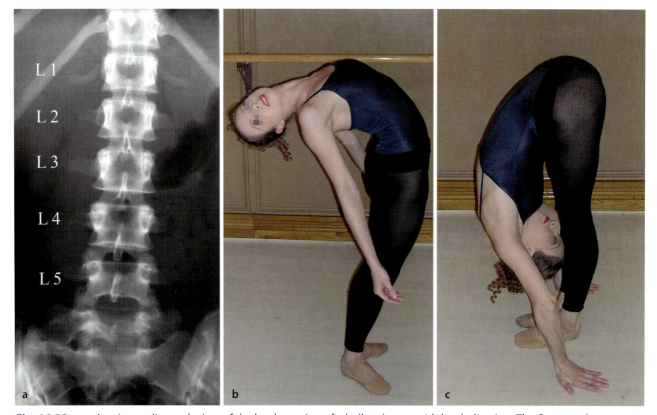

Fig. 14.22 a–c Ap view radiograph view of the lumbar spine of a ballet-dancer with lumbalization. The first sacral segment resembles the sixth lumbar vertebra with broad transverse processes. Spina bifida of the L5 and S1 segments can also be observed (**a**). The excellent range of motion of her dorsolumbar spine is demonstrated on the photos taken of her doing warming-up exercises (**b, c**)

14.1.7 Sacral Agenesis, Symphysis Agenesis, Symphyseolysis

Sacral agenesis is the term commonly applied to a group of disorders characterized by the absence of a variable segment of the caudal portion of the spine. Sacral agenesis is an uncommon congenital deformity of the spine occurring in approximately 1 of 25,000 live births. Prevalence of sacral agenesis in children of mothers with insulin-dependent diabetes mellitus is 1%. The appearance/condition of the patient depends on the extent of the vertebral involvement and on the degree of neurological deficit. Patients with sacral agenesis lack motor function below the level of their normal structured spine, similar to those with myelomeningocele. However, sensory function is impaired below the level of the affected vertebrae. In more severe cases part or all of the lumbar spine and even the lower thoracic spine may be absent.

Renshaw classified patients according to the amount of sacrum remaining and according to characteristics of the articulation between the spine and the pelvis.

- Type 1 is either partial or total unilateral sacral agenesis; vertebropelvic articulation is usually stable. Sensory loss corresponds to the distribution of the involved sacral roots. Usually, non progressive scoliosis develops.
- Type 2 is partial sacral agenesis with a bilaterally symmetrical defect, normal or hypoplastic sacral vertebrae, and a stable articulation between the iliac and the first sacral vertebra.
- Type 3 is variable lumbar and total sacral agenesis, when the iliac bone is articulating with the sides of the lowest vertebra present.
- Type 4 is variable lumbar and total sacral agenesis, with the caudal endplate of the lowest vertebra resting above the either fused iliac bone or an iliac amphiarthrosis (Figs. 14.23–14.28).

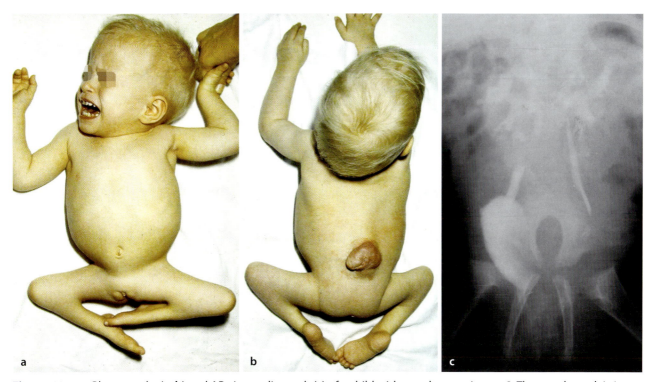

Fig. 14.23 a–c Photographs (**a**, **b**) and AP view radiograph (**c**) of a child with sacral agenesis type 3. The vertebropelvic junction is stable unless associated myelomeningocele is present. Hemivertebrae, may cause progressive congenital scoliosis. Note the serious contracture of the hip, knee and ankle joints

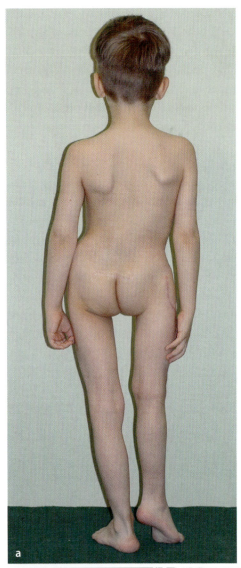

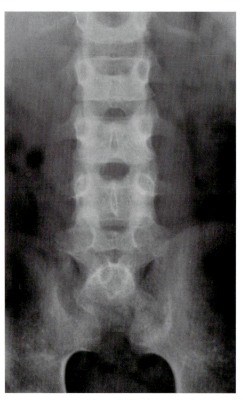

Fig. 14.25 AP radiograph of a complete sacral agenesis without scoliosis

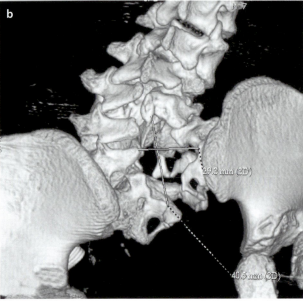

Fig. 14.24 a, b Posterior view (**a**) and 3D reconstruction CT of the lumbar–pelvic region of a 9-year-old boy, with complete sacral agenesis. Note the virtual shortening of the *right lower* extremity due to the fixed lumbar scoliosis

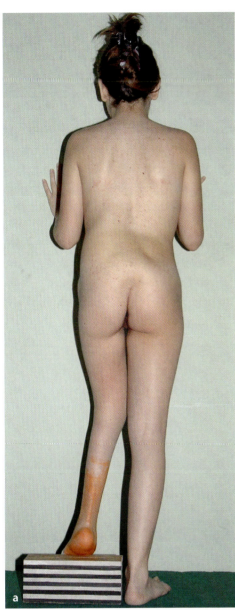

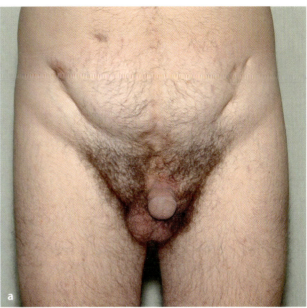

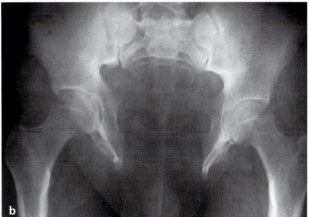

Fig. 14.27 a, b Photograph taken from a patient with symphysis agenesis (**a**). Despite the bilateral absence of the pubic bone (**b**), the patient has an almost normal gait and function

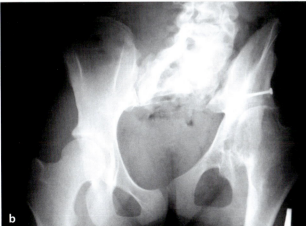

Fig. 14.26 a, b Photograph (**a**) and anteroposterior radiograph (**b**) of a 15 year-old girl with partial sacral agenesis

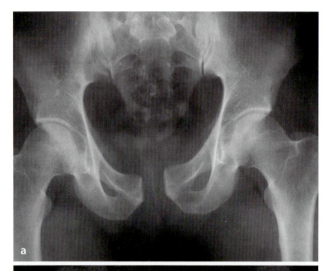

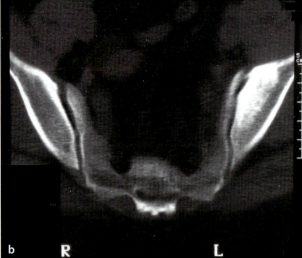

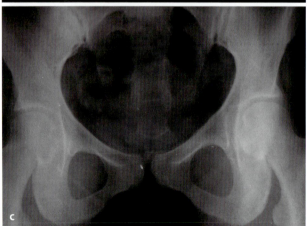

Fig. 14.28 a–c Symphysiolysis with 5 cm widening of the symphyseal joint (**a**). This can be associated with trauma, and more often with pregnancy. There is also a widening in the sacroiliacal joint as shown on the CT picture (**b**). This condition is very painful, sometimes the patient is not able to ambulate. Months later a spontaneous regression of the process results in closure of the symphyseal joint (**c**)

14.1.8 Spina Bifida Occulta

In case of spina bifida occulta, a bony defect is present at the arch of the vertebral body, but the lesion is covered by skin, and there is no meningeal herniation through the bony defect.

Spina bifida occulta is in most cases symptomless and an accidental finding on radiograph. It may result from a genetic mutation or may be an acquired deformity. The lumbar and lumbosacral regions are the most common sites for this lesion. Abnormal gait and foot deformities can also be associated with this disorder. Neurological problems can present/occur as back pain, radiculopathy, loss of sensation, hyperreflexia, weakness or atrophy and asymmetry of legs and in severe forms, neurogen bladder incontinence can be presented (Figs. 14.29 and 14.30).

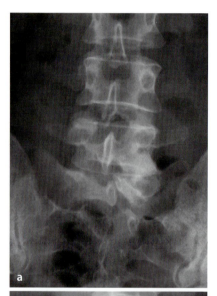

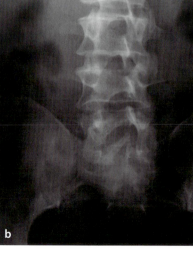

Fig. 14.29 a, b Anteroposterior view radiograph of spina bifida occulta at the transitional (**a**) and first sacral vertebras (**b**)

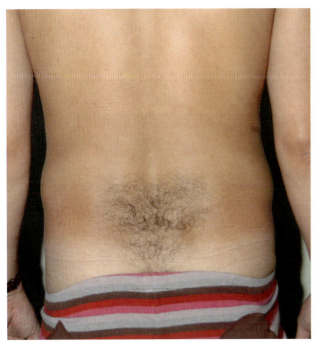

Fig. 14.30 Skin abnormalities can be observed at the level of the bony defect, as hypertrichosis, capillary hemangioma or dermal sinus that points to the presence of an occult spinal lesion

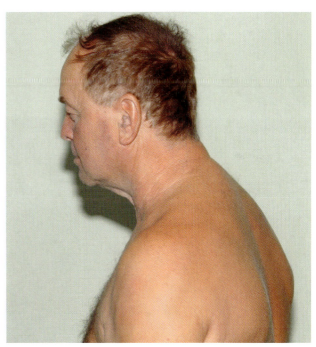

Fig. 14.31 Decreased cervical lordosis and spastic cervical muscles due to disc herniation result in antalgic posture of the patient

14.2 Degenerative Disorders

14.2.1 Cervical Intervertebral Disc Herniation

Deterioration of the intervertebral discs of the cervical spine can be brought on in many different ways; degeneration and trauma being the most frequent among them. Since the spinal cord and the discs are in close approximation at this level, mild disc disorders may just as well end up as severe symptoms. The most commonly affected levels are C5–6 and C6–7 causing generally sensory loss, muscle weakness, reflex abnormality and sometimes excruciating radiating pain in the upper limb. The severity of the disc disorder ranges from a disc bulge or a protrusion to a disc herniation, which – in most serious cases – can be sequestrated. The protruded disc can enter the foraminal space or narrow the spinal canal causing compression on the adjacent structures (Figs. 14.31–14.33).

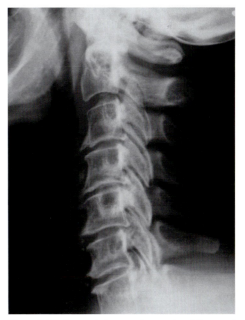

Fig. 14.32 Lateral view radiograph of the cervical spine of the same patient. Note the lowered intervertebral spaces between the affected (C 4–5 and C 5–6) vertebrae referring to disc disorder. Formation of osteophytes and foraminal narrowing can also be observed as the signs of cervical spondylosis

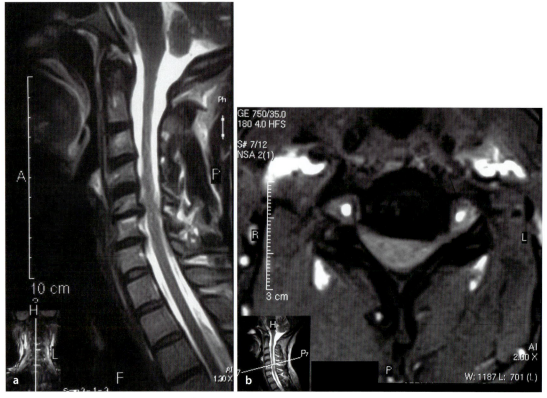

Fig. 14.33 a, b Sagittal MR picture of the cervical spine shows a herniated disc between the C 5/6 vertebras causing an impression on the chord (**a**). The horizontal section of the herniated C5/6 disc shown on the previous image (**b**)

14.2.2 Cervical Spondylosis

Degenerative changes affecting the cervical spine can be named as overall cervical spondylosis. It consists of the narrowing of the intervertebral space due to disc degeneration, osteophyte formation, hypertrophy of the ligamentum flavum, ossification of the posterior longitudinal ligament and osteoarthritic changes in the facet joints. Radiological signs of cervical spondylosis can be found in most of the aging population, only few of them having clinical syndromes, however. When the disorder is symptomatic, headache, neck or irradiating pain into the shoulder and arms (cervicalgia), stiffness, radiculopathy and cervical spondylotic myelopathy as the cause of paresis are the most common complaints (Figs. 14.34–14.37).

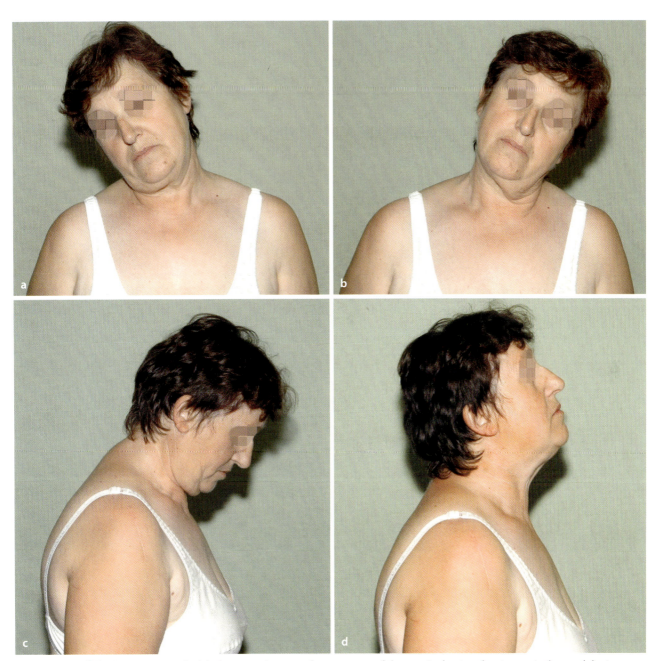

Fig. 14.34 a–d Patient presented with decreased range of movement of the cervical spine due to cervical spondylosis

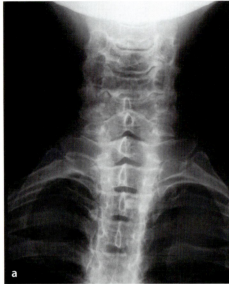

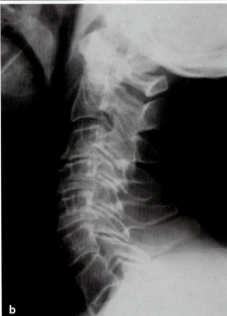

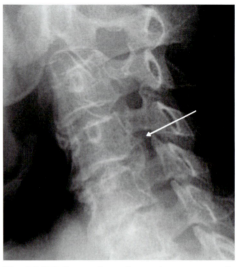

Fig. 14.36 Osteophyte formation narrows the intervertebral foramina between C4–5 level (*arrow*)

Fig. 14.35 a, b AP view radiograph of a spondylotic cervical spine with osteophyte formation and osteoarthritis of the facet joints. Slight degenerative scoliosis can also be observed (**a**). Cervical spondylosis with osteophyte formation at the anterior margin of the vertebrae. The sclerosis of the endplates are very apparent. Note the lowered intervertebral space between C 3/4, C 4/5 and C 5/6 that refers to disc degeneration (**b**)

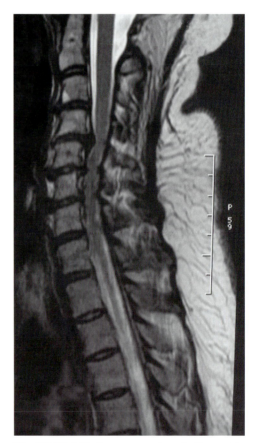

Fig. 14.37 MR picture reveals polydiscopathy: cervical intervertebral disc herniation at C4–5 level and disc protrusion between C5–6 and C6–7

14.2.3 Costochondritis (Tietze's Syndrome)

Tietze's syndrome is a benign inflammatory disorder of unknown origin, affecting the costochondral junction of the upper ribs. The syndrome occurs usually in the third decade, and is featured by chest pain and swelling. Males are twice as frequently affected as women (Figs. 14.38–14.41).

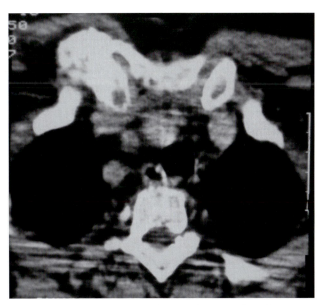

Fig. 14.40 Disorganization of the right costochondral articulation can be observed on the CT scan. Set against the left side the absence of the joint space and the deformed articulating bone ends is shown

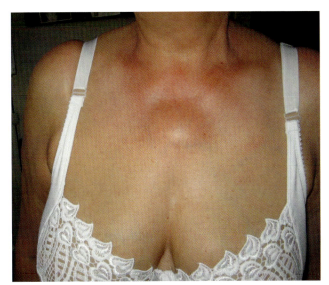

Fig. 14.38 Tietze's syndrome of the right side causing swelling of the costosternal junction

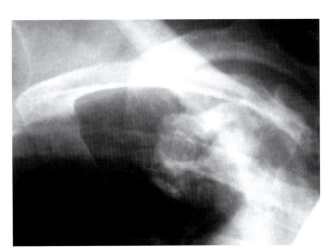

Fig. 14.39 Radiograph of the right costochondral junction showing excessive osteophyte formation causing deformation of the joint

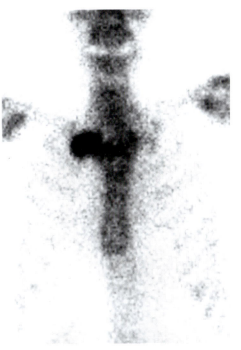

Fig. 14.41 Bone scan reveals an elevated technetium[99] isotope uptake in the right upper costosternal region corresponding inflammation due to costochondritis

14.2.4 Hyperostotic Spondylosis (Forestier's Disease)

Forestier's disease, also known as diffuse idiopathic skeletal hyperostosis (DISH), is described by ossification of the anterior longitudinal ligament and capsule insertions of the spine. Bony spurs can also be observed at tendon insertions; for instance heel spur is typical in DISH. The background of the disorder is not clear. It is often associated with elevated blood glucose level (diabetes mellitus) and obesity, no unambiguous link has been discovered yet, though. The patients are generally free of complaints with reduction in range of spinal motion (Figs. 14.42 and 14.43).

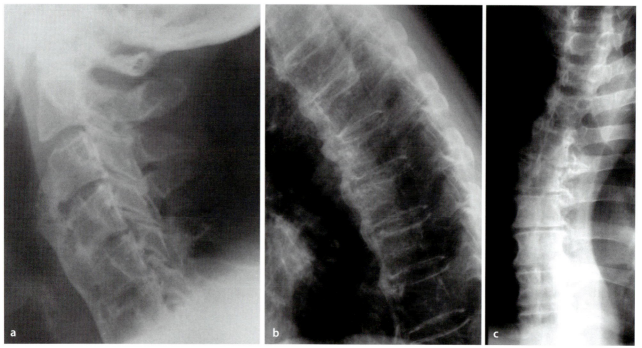

Fig. 14.42 a–c On radiological examination of DISH, characteristically the longitudinal ligaments, especially the anterior longitudinal ligament of the spine is calcified, while the intervertebral spaces, the facet joints and the sacroiliac joints are preserved. This typical ossification of the anterior longitudinal ligament of the cervical (**a**) and thoracic spine (**b**) is shown on the lateral view radiographs. Note, that the intervertebral disc spaces are preserved. Examining the AP view radiographs of the thoracic spine of the same patient the absence of ossification of the intervertebral ligaments at the sides of the vertebrae can be observed. Besides Forestier's disease this patient has scoliosis as well (**c**)

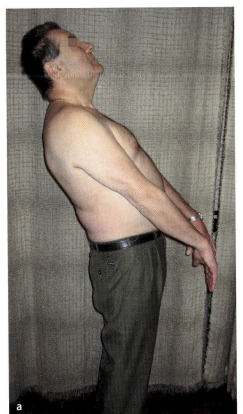

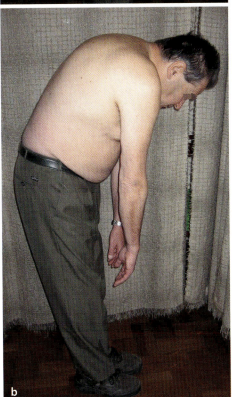

Fig. 14.43 a, b Decreased range of motion of the spine is shown at anteflexion (**a**) and retroflexion (**b**). Kyphosis of the dorsal spine can also be observed

14.2.5 Herniated Disc, Lumbar

Disc herniation as a part of the degenerative disorders affecting the spine occurs most commonly in the lumbar region, especially between L4–5 and L5-S1 levels. The severity may vary from protrusion to sequestration, causing local pain, muscle spasm, and various neurological symptoms such as muscle weakness, sensory loss, reflex changes and radiating pain (Figs. 14.44–14.47).

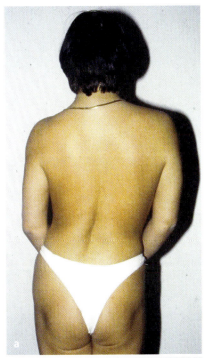

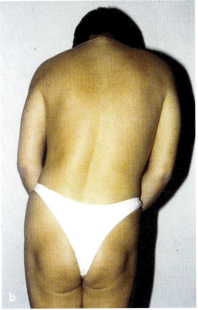

Fig. 14.44 a, b Patient having low back pain caused by herniated L5-S1 disc. Note the pathological posture

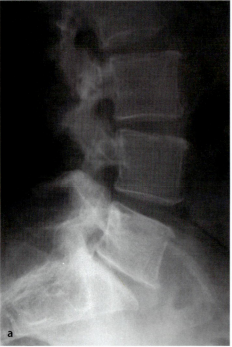

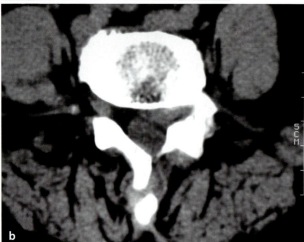

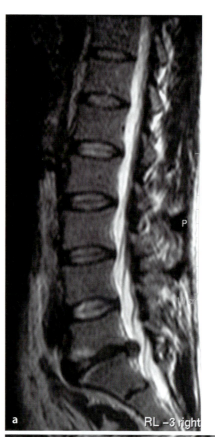

Fig. 14.45 a, b Lateral view radiograph of the lumbar spine of a patient having herniated L5-S1 disc. Note the narrow intervertebral space between L5 and S1. Osteophytes on the anterior rim of the vertebral bodies (**a**). CT picture reveals a marked paramedian disc herniation (**b**)

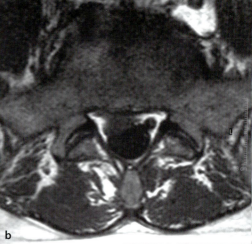

Fig. 14.46 a, b MRI of a herniated L5-S1 disc in the sagittal (**a**) and in the horizontal view (**b**). The herniated portion of the disc compresses the dura mater. Bone edema at the antero–inferior part of the L5 vertebra refers to instability (Modic's sign type I)

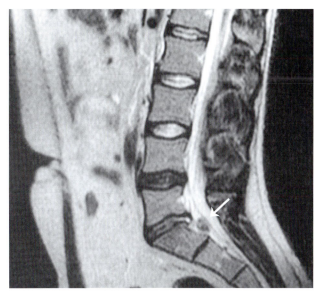

Fig. 14.47 Sequestrated L5-S1 intervertebral discus hernia-tion. The sequestrated piece is dislocated in the spinal canal. (*arrow*)

14.2.6 Deforming Spondylarthritis, Aging Spine

Like many other degenerative diseases, degenerative spine deformities can also be asymptomatic showing only radiological signs, such as intervertebral space narrow-ing, disc degeneration, osteophyte formation, ossification of the adjacent ligaments, facet joint osteoarthritis and/or instability. Osteophytes forming at the posterior border of the endplates, osteophytes of the facet joints or disc protrusion and herniation can narrow the spinal canal leading to spinal stenosis. Complaints usually consist of muscle spasm, pain, radiating pain, various neurological symptoms such as muscle weakness, sensory loss, bladder and bowel dysfunction or reflex changes. Pain associated with walking (neurogen claudication) refers to spinal ste-nosis. As degeneration makes its progress the osteophytes hypertrophize bringing on bony bars between the neigh-boring vertebrae. At the end stage of the process sponta-neous spinal fusion develops, abolishing the complaints contributed to instability, osteoarthritis or impingement (Figs. 14.48–14.52).

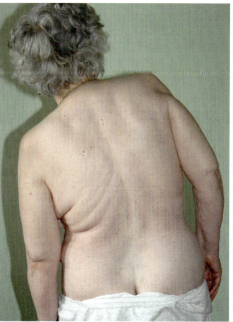

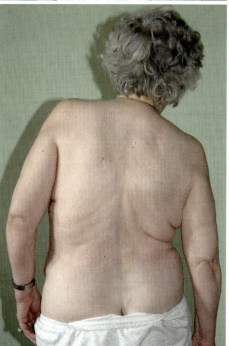

Fig. 14.48 a, b Patient presented with severe deforming spondylarthrosis of the spine shows the decreased range of movement while trying to bend to the side

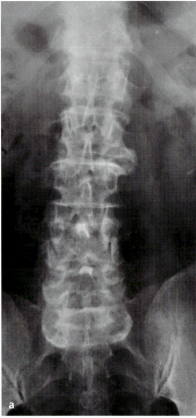

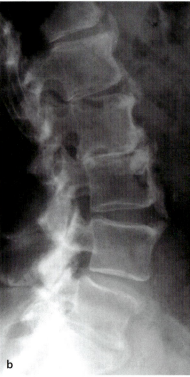

Fig. 14.49 a, b Lumbar spondylosis with bony bridge between L2–3. Degenerative retrolisthesis of L2 can also be seen. Note the narrowed L5-S1 intervertebral space referring to disc degeneration

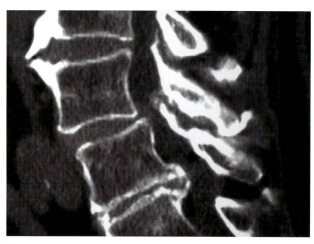

Fig. 14.50 Reconstructive CT scan of the same patient's lumbar spine. Bridging osteophyte formation can be seen both on the anterior and on the posterior side of the vertebral canal causing spinal stenosis. Almost complete fusion can be observed due to osteophytes

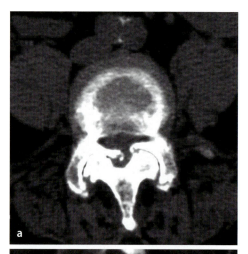

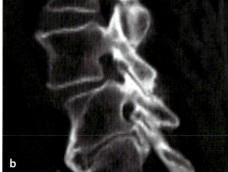

Fig. 14.51 a, b Severe narrowing of the lateral recess due to osteophyte formation on the edges of both facet joints on the left side ((a), CT scan). Stenosis of the intervertebral foramen can be observed at the same level on the right side ((b), reconstructive CT scan)

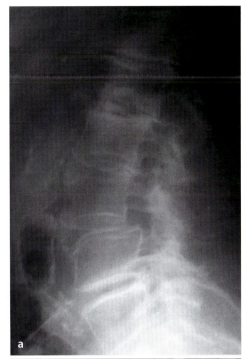

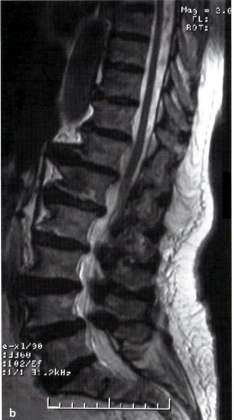

Fig. 14.52 a, b Radiograph reveals degenerative pseudo-spondylolisthesis at the L3/4 level (**a**). The *dark gray/grey* appearance of the lumbar discs and the protrusion at Th12-L1, L1-L2 and L4-L5 levels on the MRI sagittal plane refers to polysegmental intervertebral disc degeneration (**b**)

14.2.7 Morbus Baastrup, Arthritis of the Interspinous Neoarthros

Morbus Baastrup, also known as Baastrup's disease, Baastrup's sign, or kissing spine, is a pain syndrome of the spinous processes. As degenerative changes affect the spine, the intervertebral space narrows, bringing the adjacent vertebrae closer to each other. Besides, degeneration produces hypertrophied spinous processes, making it easier for the vertebrae to get into contact. Pain is caused by the compression developing between the enlarged spinous processes, especially when the spine is in extension. The syndrome is usually asymptomatic; however, stiffness and pain can occur (Figs. 14.53–14.55).

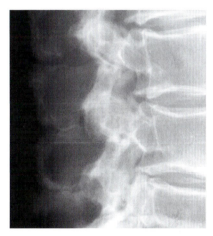

Fig. 14.53 Contacting hypertrophied spinous processes each other at L3–4 and L4–5 levels cause Baastrup's disease. Spondylosis and huge osteophytes can also be observed

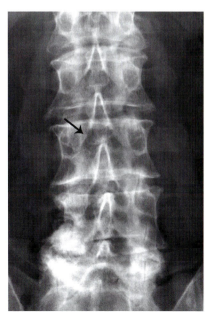

Fig. 14.54 Kissing spinous processes between L2–3–4 (arrow). The inferior pole of the L3 and L4 process deviate to the left due the proximity of L4 spinous process

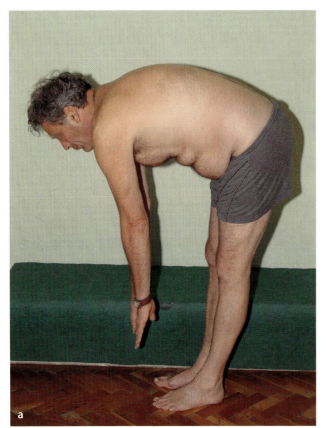

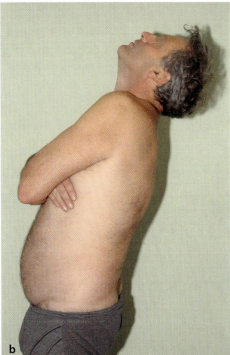

Fig. 14.55 a, b Decreased range of movement of the lumbar spine due to the degenerative changes seen on the radiograph of the same patient (**a**). Contacting spinous processes, restrain of lumbar lordosis even when the patient tries to bend backward (**b**)

14.3 Infection

14.3.1 Spondylodiscitis, Pyogenic Spondylitis

Spinal infections generally appear as vertebral osteomyelitis or spondylodiscitis. The most frequent source of spondylodiscitis is hematogenous spread, contiguous spread due to the infection of the adjacent structures, postoperative infection or direct open trauma. The site of the infection is most commonly the lumbar spine (60%), followed by the thoracic spine and the thoracolumbar junction (30%) and the cervical spine (10%). The most frequent infecting organism is Staphylococcus aureus (in app. 36%). Local back pain, fever, and fatigue are the most common complaints. Epidural abscess formation, neurological deficit and spinal instability can be the most serious complications, urging operative management of the usually conservatively treated disease (Figs. 14.56–14.59).

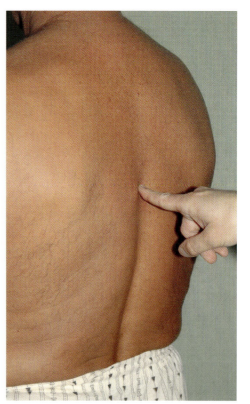

Fig. 14.56 Patient presented with spondylodiscitis of the Th6–8 levels. The examiner points to most tender segment of the thoracic spine. Despite of the severe inflammatory process, usually none of the typical signs of combustion (e.g., skin redness, swelling, etc.) can be observed

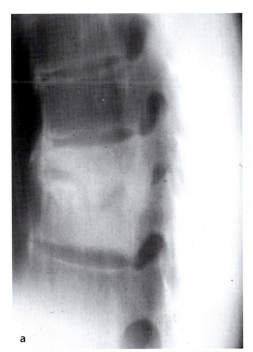

a

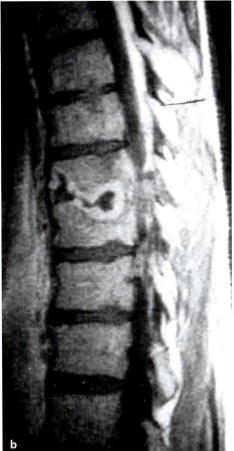

b

Fig. 14.57 a, b Conventional tomogram (**a**) and MRI image (**b**) of collapsing vertebrae due to spondylodiscitis at the Th6–8 level. Typically the inflammation process destroys usually the neighboring endplates of two adjacent vertebras

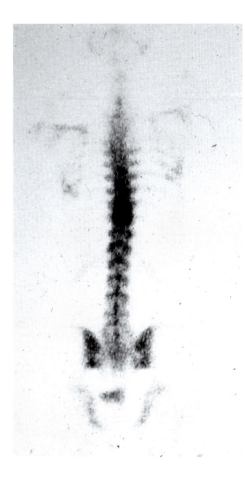

Fig. 14.58 Bone scan shows enhanced isotope uptake at the affected spine segments

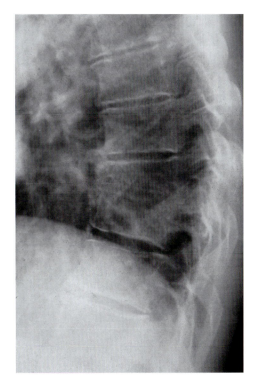

Fig. 14.59 Two years after ending the conservative therapy the infection healed by complete fusion of the affected vertebrae

Chapter 15

Shoulder, Upper Arm

Contents

Shoulder, Upper Arm

J. Kiss, G. Skaliczki

15.1 Congenital and Developmental Disorders

15.1.1 Phocomelia

Phocomelia (seal-limb) is a congenital developmental disorder, in which the terminal portion of the limb is attached directly to the trunk. Various types of phocomelia belong to the group of diseases, as the failure of formation (Swanson's classification) as an intercalated longitudinal arrest. Types are the following:

- Arm and forearm deficient type, when the hand attached directly to the shoulder
- Arm deficient type: when forearm attached directly to the shoulder
- Forearm deficient type: when the hand attached to the arm (Figs. 15.1 and 15.2)

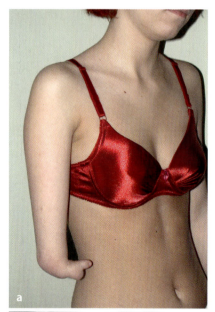

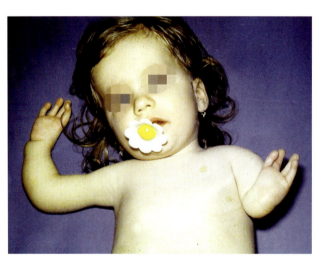

Fig. 15.1 Arm deficient type of phocomelia on the left side of a girl. The forearm attached directly to the shoulder

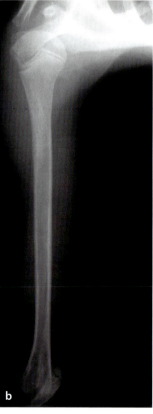

Fig. 15.2 a, b Forearm deficient type of phocomelia on the right side of an 11-year-old girl (**a**), radiograph of the same patient (**b**)

15.1.2 Congenital Radiohumeral Synostosis

Synostosis may exist between the humerus and one of the forearm bones, most frequently of the radius. Two third of the cases are unilateral. In this disease the proximal radial epiphysis and the distal humeral epiphysis is absent. This growth disturbance results in a considerable shortening of the upper extremity. Most cases are sporadic in occurrence, but though a genetic syndrome autosomal dominant inheritance is observed.

One third of the cases are associated with general skeletal abnormalities, such as hip dislocation; knee anomalies; clubfoot; polydactyly; syndactyly; Madelung deformity; ligamentous laxity; thumb hypoplasia; carpal coalition; and problems of the cardiac, renal, neurological, and gastrointestinal systems (Fig. 15.3).

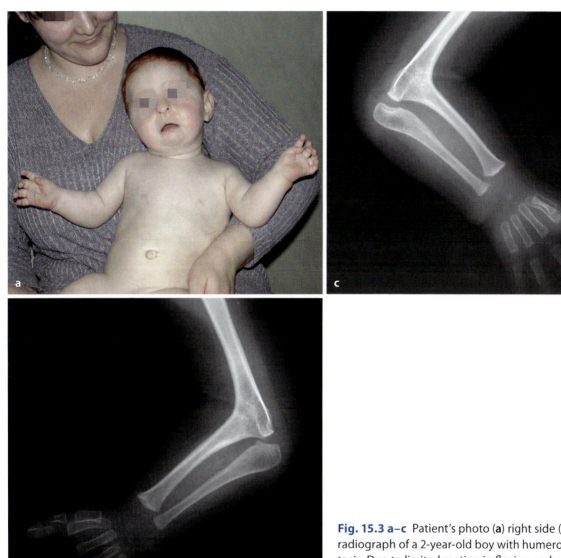

Fig. 15.3 a–c Patient's photo (**a**) right side (**b**) left side (**c**) radiograph of a 2-year-old boy with humeroradial synostosis. Due to limited motion in flexion and extension of elbow joint, the disorder is earlier diagnosed than radioulnar synostosis

15.2 Luxation, Subluxation, Instability

15.2.1 Chronic Acromioclavicular Dislocation

The chronic acromioclavicular (AC) joint dislocation is a late consequence of the acute displacement of the AC joint. The condition can be observed in case of untreated AC joint dislocations or in case of failed operative or conservative treatment. The severity of the disease depends on the extent of ligamentous injury and of clavicle displacement. The patients experience pain around the AC joint as a consequence of instability and secondary arthritis. The pain can be present at rest, but it is aggravated by overhead activities. If the displacement is severe the patients might have cosmetic problem as well (Fig. 15.4).

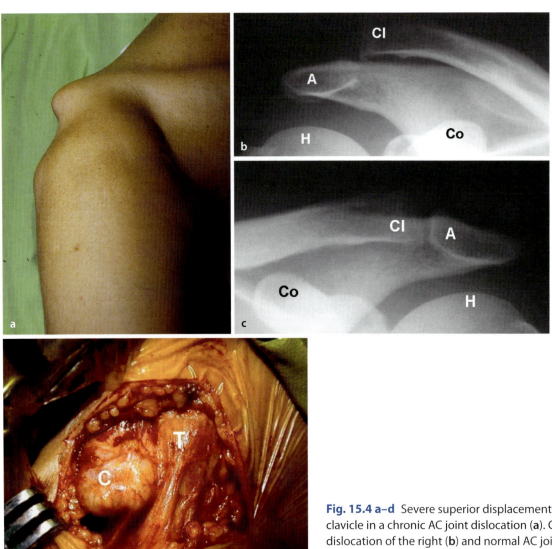

Fig. 15.4 a–d Severe superior displacement of the lateral clavicle in a chronic AC joint dislocation (**a**). Chronic AC joint dislocation of the right (**b**) and normal AC joint of the left (**c**) shoulder. (A = acromion, Cl = clavicle, H = humeral head, Co = coracoid process). Intraoperative picture of the same patient (**d**). The lateral end of the clavicle (C) is superiorly displaced and penetrated the trapezius fascia (T)

15.2.2 Multidirectional Shoulder Instability (MDI)

The abnormal amount of excursion of the humeral head on the glenoid without symptoms is called laxity. Instability is present if this laxity is associated with symptoms. Instability of the glenohumeral joint in more than one direction is considered as multidirectional instability. The condition is often bilateral but with different sever-

ity of instability of the two shoulders. The incidence of multidirectional shoulder instability is not known. The majority of patients are aged between 15 and 30 years. Bony and labrum abnormalities, ligamentous anomalies, impaired muscular control, and collagen abnormalities can lead to instability on their own or in combination. Some patients are able to dislocate the shoulder voluntarily (Figs. 15.5–15.10).

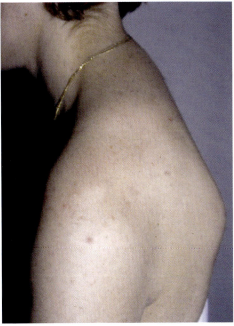

Fig. 15.5 Posteriorly displaced left shoulder of an MDI patient. Note the "pseudo-winging" of the scapula

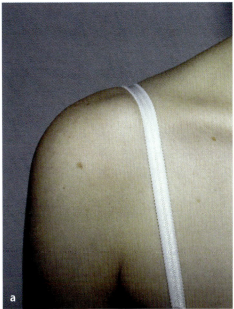

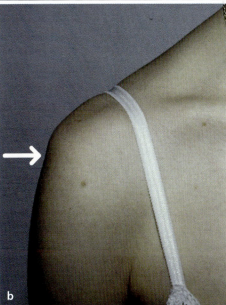

Fig. 15.7 a, b Positive sulcus sign of an MDI patient. An indentation can be seen (*white arrow*) on the lateral aspect of the shoulder due to the inferior displacement of the humerus on axial traction

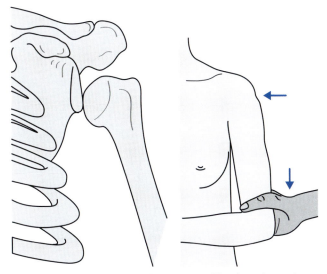

Fig. 15.6 The "sulcus sign," that is caused by the inferior displacement of the humeral head, is a typical finding in all cases

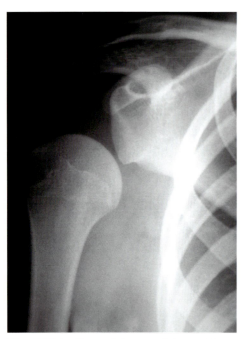

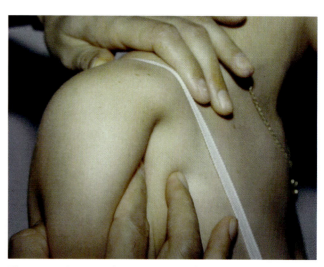

Fig. 15.10 Increased posterior translation (*posterior drawer sign*) of the humeral head of an MDI patient

Fig. 15.8 Radiograph image of the positive sulcus sign of an MDI patient. The humeral head is inferiorly displaced on axial traction

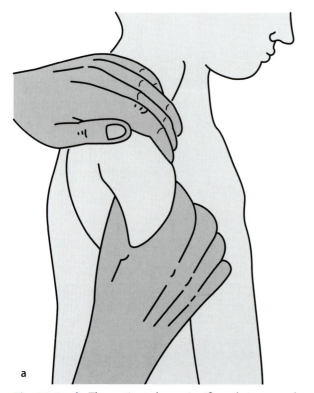

a

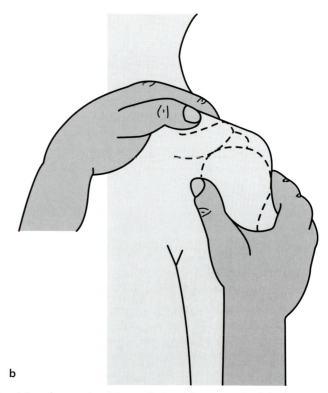

b

Fig. 15.9 a, b The patients have significantly increased anterior (**a**) and posterior (**b**) translation (*drawer sign*) of the humeral head

15.2.3 Recurrent Glenohumeral Dislocation

Instability is present if this laxity (abnormal amount of excursion of the humeral head on the glenoid) is associated with symptoms. Though recurrent shoulder dislocation can be present at any age group the typical patient is young. The instability can be classified according to etiology, direction, and position. Majority (some 96%) of shoulder dislocations are anterior traumatic dislocations, that are usually unilateral and commonly associated with the lesion of the anterior capsule–labrum complex (Bankart lesion). In older patients the recurrent shoulder dislocation is commonly associated with rotator cuff tear. Shoulder dislocation is often associated with the lesion of the axillar nerve or the brachial plexus. Anterior dislocation can occur when the arm is extended and externally rotated. Axial load on the arm in flexion and internal rotation can lead to posterior dislocation (Figs. 15.11–15.18).

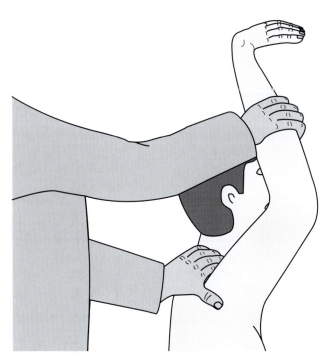

Fig. 15.13 Anterior apprehension sign for anterior shoulder instability. The patient is resisting extension and external rotation that is the typical position of the anterior instability

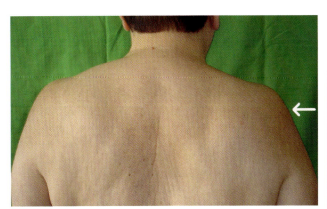

Fig. 15.11 Dislocated right shoulder. Note the abnormal right shoulder contour (*white arrow*)

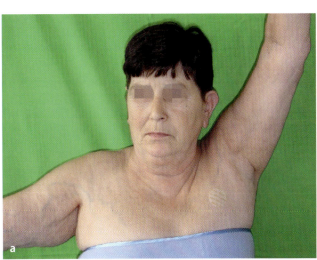

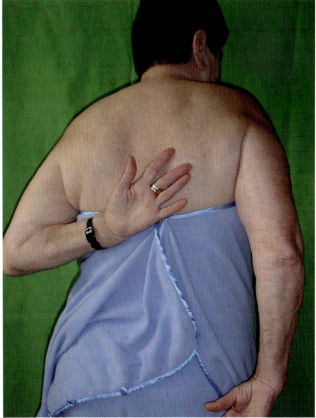

Fig. 15.12 a, b Elevation and rotation are limited due to right shoulder dislocation

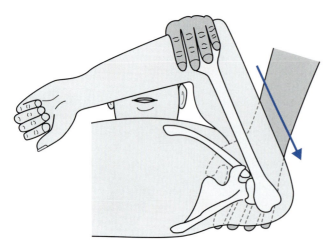

Fig. 15.14 Posterior apprehension sign for posterior shoulder instability. The patient is resisting flexion and internal rotation that is the typical position of the posterior instability

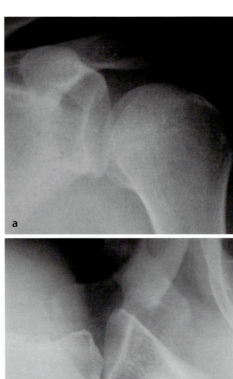

Fig. 15.16 a, b Posterior dislocation of the humerus. Note the overlap between the contour of the humeral head and of the posterior glenoid rim (a). Axillary lateral view of posterior dislocation. Note the impression fracture on the anterior aspect of the humeral head caused by the glenoid rim (reverse Hill–Sach's lesion) (b)

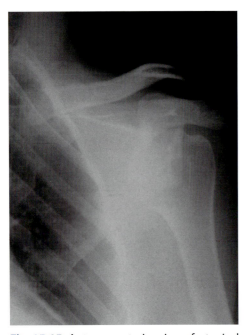

Fig. 15.15 Antero–posterior view of a typical anterior shoulder dislocation

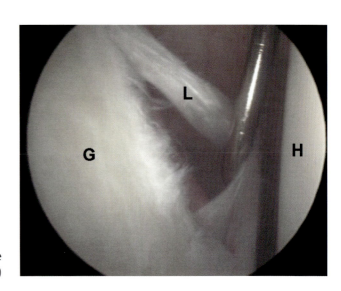

Fig. 15.17 Bankart lesion: torn anterior labrum and capsule (L = labrum, G = glenoid, H = humeral head)

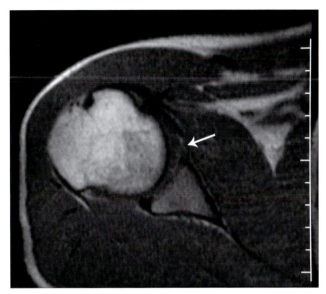

Fig. 15.18 MRI image of the torn anterior labrum and capsule. White arrow points to the rim of the glenoid where the labrum is absent. (Bankart lesion)

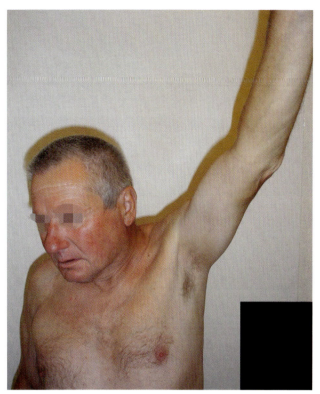

Fig. 15.19 Typical painful arc in case of subacromial impingement

15.3 Soft Tissue Disorders

15.3.1 Subacromial Impingement

Subacromial impingement is a painful condition typical of the middle aged and older patients (over 40 years of age). The patients experience pain on overhead activities but (typically) they have even more pain at night. Besides the pain there is a marked subacromial crepitation palpable on shoulder elevation. The greater tubercle and the anterior or posterior margin of the acromion are tender. There is no trauma in history. The pain arises from the inflammation of the subacromial bursa and from the tendinitis of the rotator cuff (Figs. 15.19–15.22).

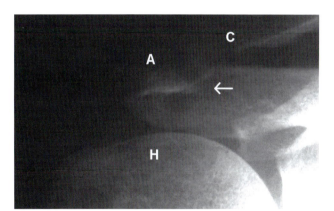

Fig. 15.20 "Eyebrow sign" – the undersurface of the acromion is sclerotic and there is a small spur at the medial side (*A* = acromion, *H* = humeral head, *C* = clavicle)

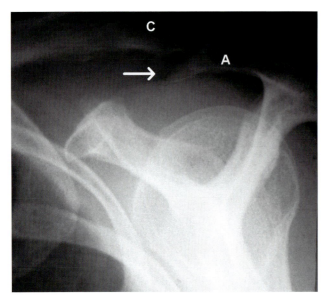

Fig. 15.21 Scapula–lateral (*Y* view) of the shoulder showing spur (*white arrow*) on the acromion (*C* = clavicle, *A* = acromion)

15.3.2 Rotator Cuff Lesion (Partial, Total)

Rotator cuff lesion is a painful condition typical of the middle aged and older patients (over 40 years). The symptoms are very similar to those of the symptoms of subacromial impingement. The patients experience pain on overhead activities but (typically) they have even more pain at night. Besides the pain and subacromial crepitation the patients complain to some extent, of weakness on elevation and external rotation. In most of the cases there is no trauma in their medical history especially in the elderly but younger patients have usually some kind of trauma in their medical history. The lesion can be classified as partial thickness tear (bursal or articular side tear) or by the size (small, large, massive). The more extensive the tear the most significant is the functional impairment but the severity of pain is not strictly related to the size of the lesion (Figs. 15.23–15.31).

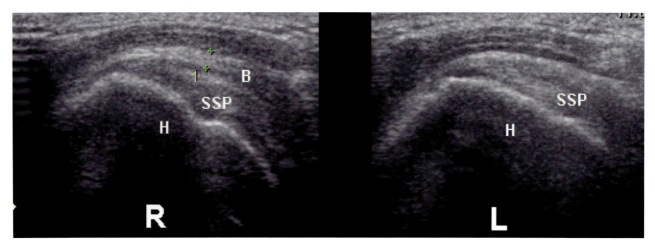

Fig. 15.22 Ultrasound examination in case of subacromial impingement. The subacromial bursa is enlarged on the right side (B = bursa, SSP = supraspinatus tendon, H = humeral head)

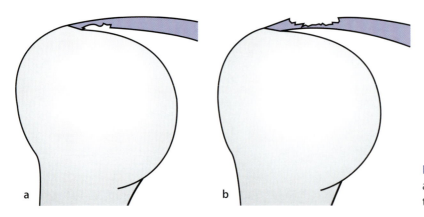

Fig. 15.23 a, b Articular side (*above*, (**a**)) and bursal side (*below*, (**b**)) partial thickness tear of the supraspinatus tendon

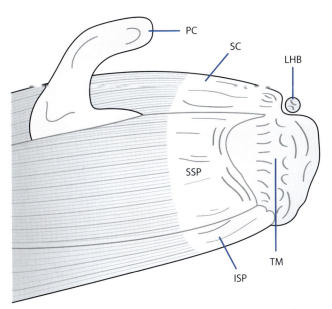

PC
SC
LHB
SSP
TM
ISP

Fig. 15.24 Full thickness tear of the supraspinatus tendon.
PC: Processus Coracoioleus, TM: Tuberculum Maius, SC:
Supraspinatus, ISP: Infraspinatus, LHB: Long head of biceps

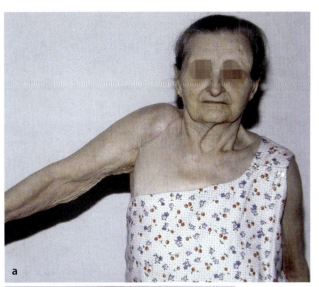

a

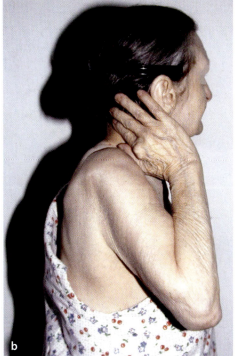

b

Fig. 15.26 a, b Loss of active elevation and external rotation due to massive rotator cuff tear

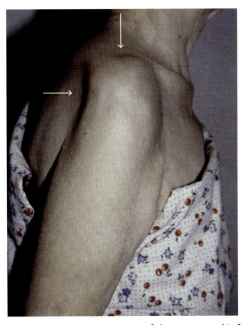

Fig. 15.25 Severe wasting of the supra and infraspinatus muscle belly (white arrows) in case of massive rotator cuff tear

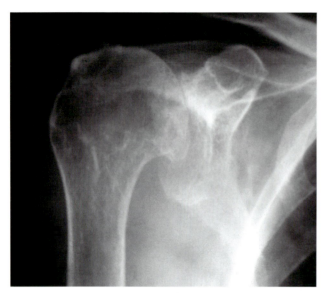

Fig. 15.27 Superior migration of the humeral head with rounding of the greater tuberosity in case of massive rotator cuff tear

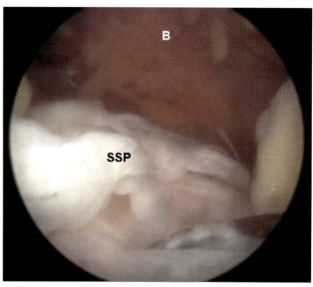

Fig. 15.29 Arthroscopic image of the complete tear of the supraspinatus tendon. The scope is introduced into the subacromial space (*SSP* = torn supraspinatus tendon, *B* = inflamed subacromial bursa)

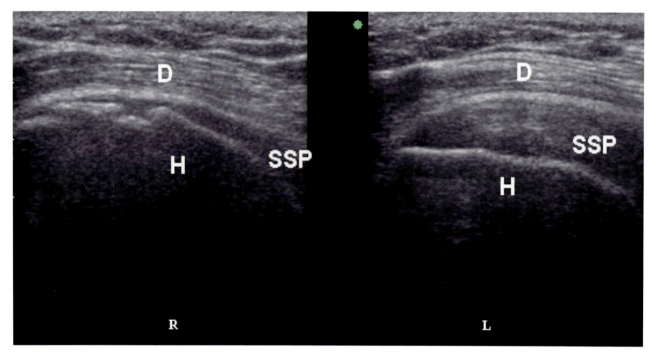

Fig. 15.28 Ultrasound image of the complete tear of the supraspinatus tendon of the right shoulder (*D* = deltoid, *H* = humeral head, *SSP* = supraspinatus tendon). The 'crescent' form is completely missing due to the retraction of the torn supraspinatus tendon

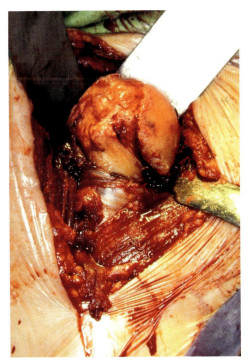

Fig. 15.30 Intraoperative picture of the same patient with massive rotator cuff tear. The humeral head is completely bold

15.3.3 Rupture of the Long Head of Biceps (Proximal)

There are two basic etiologies of the rupture of the proximal part of the long head of the biceps., One is caused by a sudden force during heavy physical activities in middle aged people. At this age there is already some moderate degeneration of the intraarticular part of the tendon that is a predisposing factor. The other is the spontaneous rupture without much force in elderly that is often associated with massive rotator cuff tear.

The patients feel a sudden painful snap around the upper arm or around the shoulder when the tendon ruptures. Later on a hematoma can appear on the arm. The patients mainly loose strength of supination and there is not much change of the strength of elbow flexion (Figs. 15.32 and 15.33).

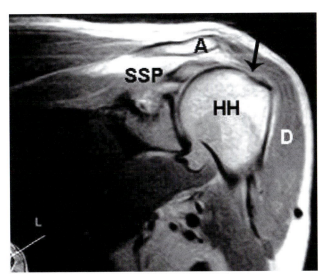

Fig. 15.31 MRI image of the complete tear of the supraspinatus tendon. Black arrow points to the complete absence of the retracted tendon: the humeral head is covered by the deltoid muscle only. (*A* = acromion, *D* = deltoid, *HH* = humeral head, *SSP* = torn and retracted supraspinatus tendon)

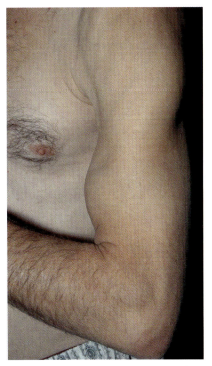

Fig. 15.32 Rupture of the proximal part of the long head of biceps. Note the bulging of the muscle belly on elbow flexion (Popey sign)

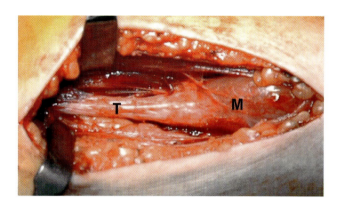

Fig. 15.33 Intraoperative view of partial biceps tendon rupture (*T* = thin partially ruptured tendon, *M* = muscle belly)

15.3.4 Frozen Shoulder (Idiopathic, Posttraumatic, Postoperative)

Frozen shoulder (adhesive capsulitis) is the severe restriction of shoulder movement in every direction without any significant radiological changes. This condition is usually painful at the beginning but the severe pain settles later on. The exact etiology is still unclear. The idiopathic form appears mainly in middle aged people without any history of trauma. It is more common among people who suffer from diabetes mellitus. The posttraumatic form can be present at any age group following soft tissue injuries around the shoulder. The same applies for the postoperative conditions (Figs. 15.34 and 15.35).

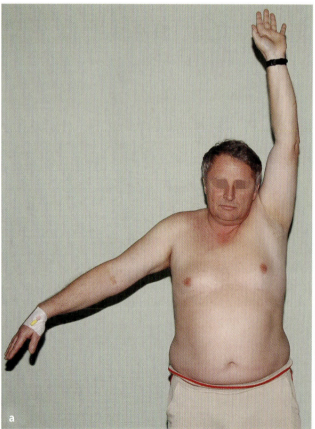

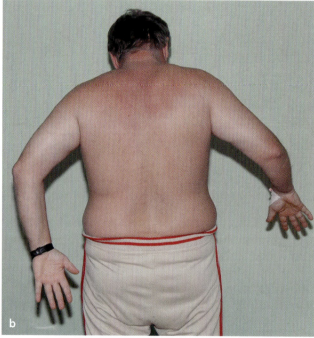

Fig. 15.34 a, b Limited elevation of the right shoulder due to frozen shoulder (**a**). The patient is unable to put his right hand behind his back (decreased internal rotation, (**b**))

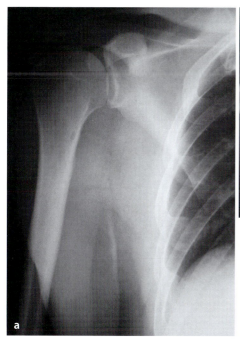

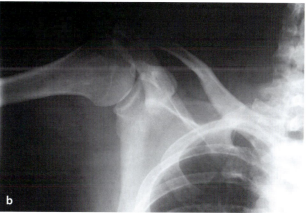

Fig. 15.35 a, b The radiograph clearly demonstrates the reason of the limited motions: from the normal position of the shoulder (**a**) a limited elevation (**b**) of the arm is possible by a compensatory elevation of the scapula. Note the unchanged position of the humeral head to the glenoideal fossa

15.3.5 Subacromial Bursitis

Subacromial bursa is a deep bursa located between the acromion and the rotator cuff. It helps the rotator cuff glide freely under the inferior surface of the acromion. Subacromial bursitis occurs most commonly due to re-petitive overhead activities or trauma. Less frequently inflammatory diseases can cause bursitis. Bursitis is often associated with supraspinatus tendinitis. The symptoms are swelling, tenderness, pain and limited range of movement (Figs. 15.36–15.40).

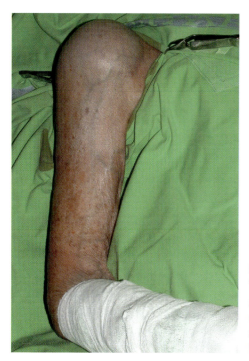

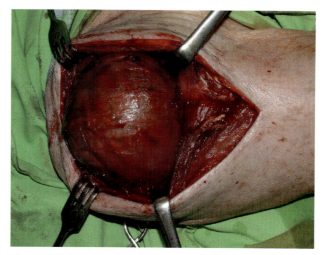

Fig. 15.36 The swollen shoulder refers to subacromial bursitis

Fig. 15.37 Splitting the deltoid muscle the enormous bursa is seen

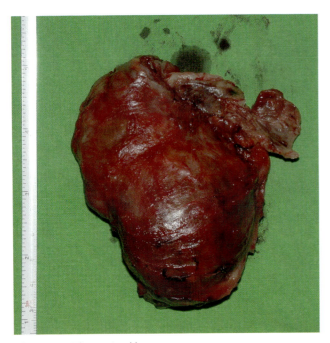

Fig. 15.38 The excised bursa

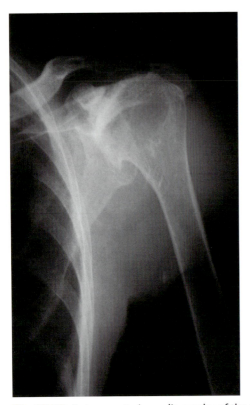

Fig. 15.39 Anteroposterior radiography of the patient. Cranial displacement of the humeral head along with signs of osteoarthritis refers to rotator cuff tear arthropathy. The subacromial bursitis may be a cause of the massive rotator cuff tear

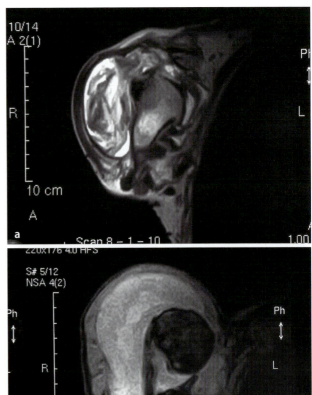

Fig. 15.40 a, b MRI image shows clearly separated areas with different signal intensity within the bursa. Note the thin deltoid muscle over the bursa (**a**). The enlarged bursa embraces the humeral head and neck (**b**)

15.3.6 Calcifying Tendinitis

This is a sudden onset of heavy pain around the shoulder without any history of trauma in middle aged patients. It is slightly more common in women. The exact etiology is still unclear. The pathology is that, different extent of calcium crystal deposits appear most commonly in the supraspinatus tendon (less commonly in the infraspinatus and subscapularis tendons) that is most likely to be some kind of an inflammatory disease. The calcium deposits can absorb by themselves (Figs. 15.41 and 15.42).

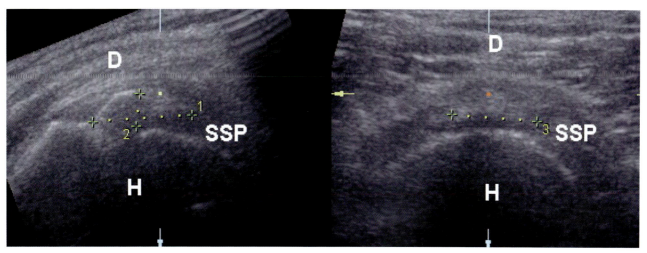

Fig. 15.41 Ultrasound image of calcifying tendinitis marked with the crosses and dotted lines (**D** = deltoid muscle, **SSP** = supraspinatus tendon, **H** = humeral head)

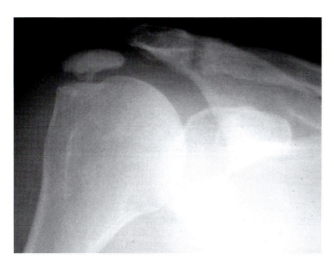

Fig. 15.42 Radiograph view of calcifying tendonitis: The cloud-like calcification refers to the degenerated area in the supraspinatus tendon near the attachment

15.4 Soft Tissue Lesions with Neurogen Etiology

15.4.1 Thoracic Outlet Syndrome

The thoracic outlet syndrome (TOS) is a combination of sensory, motor and vascular disturbance on the upper limb due to the various extent of compression of the brachial plexus and of the subclavian artery and vein. The compression can be caused by the cervical rib, by any kind of soft tissue anomaly around the neck and clavicle, and by any kind of anomaly of the clavicle (malunion of fracture, tumor etc.). Some of the symptoms may be present most of the time but some of them appear only on overhead activities. It is mostly the condition in middle aged people and it is more common in woman (Figs. 15.43 and 15.44).

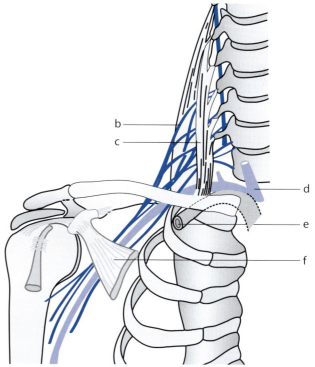

Fig. 15.43 Anatomy of the clavicular region (**a**) vertebral artery, (**b**) scalenus medius muscle, (**c**) scalenus anterior muscle, (**d**) subclavian artery, (**e**) subclavian vane, (**f**) pectoralis minor muscle

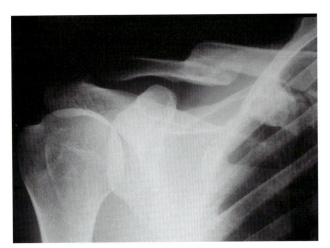

Fig. 15.44 Ap radiograph of a clavicle malunion causing thoracic outlet syndrome

15.4.2 Long Thoracic Nerve Lesion (Scapula Winging)

The winging of the scapula on active elevation is caused by the long thoracic nerve lesion that leads to the isolated paresis of the serratus anterior muscle. The nerve can get directly injured during thoracic surgery (first rib resection, introduction of chest drain etc.) or in case of direct trauma of the chest wall. Indirect injury can happen when the arm is overstretched in elevation. When there is no injury in the history, virus infection may be the reason of the nerve lesion (Fig. 15.45).

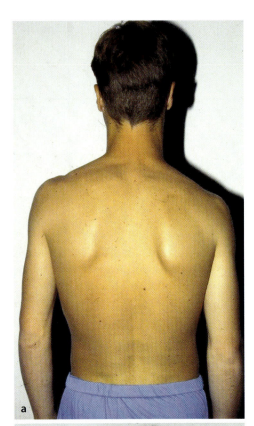

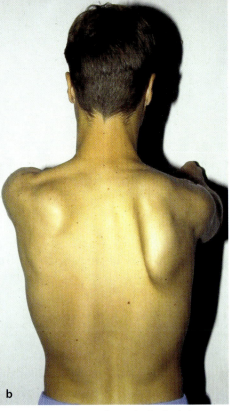

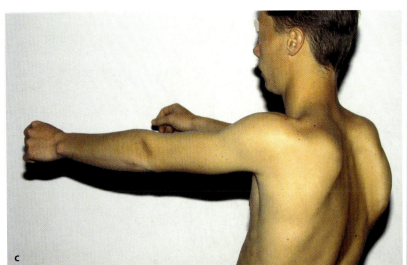

Fig. 15.45 a–c 17-year-old patient presented with the right long thoracic nerve lesion. His chest wall was kicked while playing football. There is no significant winging when the arm is at the side of the body (**a**). The right scapula is significantly winging when the arm is in forward elevation (**b**). The same patient in an oblique view (**c**)

15.5 Degenerative Disorders

15.5.1 Osteoarthritis of the Acromioclavicular Joint

Osteoarthrosis of the acromioclavicular (AC) joint is a painful degenerative condition of the AC joint. It can be present in the elderly like arthritis of any other joints. Some younger patients may develop arthritis especially if they do heavy physical activities or heavy sports (weight lifting, shot putting, etc.) (Figs. 15.46–15.49).

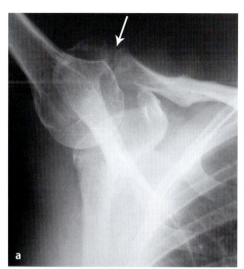

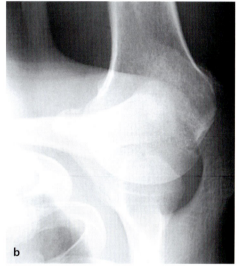

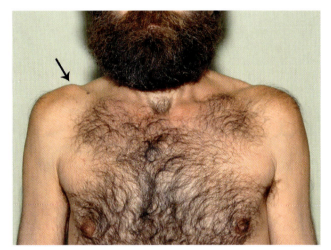

Fig. 15.46 Photograph shows the protuberant right (*arrow*) acromioclavicular joint of a heavy physical worker with osteoarthritis of the AC joint

Fig. 15.48 a, b Axillary lateral radiograph view of the right arthritic ((**a**), *arrow*) and normal (**b**) AC joints

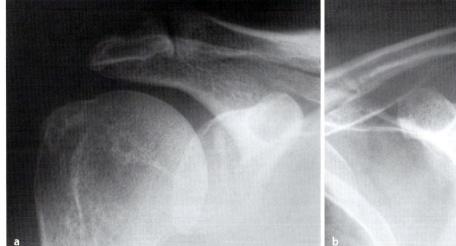

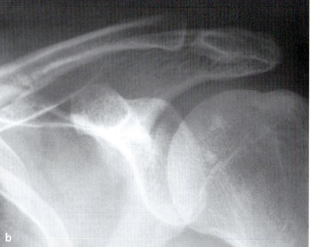

Fig. 15.47 a, b Antero–posterior radiograph view of the right arthritic (**a**) and normal (**b**) AC joints

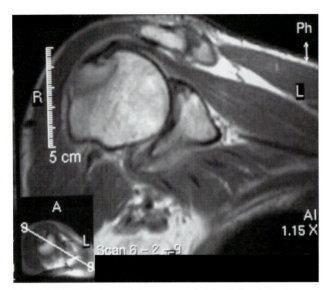

Fig. 15.49 MRI view of the osteoarthritis of the right AC joint

15.5.2 Primary Osteoarthritis of the Glenohumeral Joint

The pathology and etiology of primary osteoarthritis of the glenohumeral joint is similar to those of other articulations. It may be present less than 5% over the age of 65 years. Most of the patients have pain while performing activities and even at rest but the most significant problem is the limitation of function that may restrict everyday activities (combing hair, eating, perineal care, etc.) (Figs. 15.50 and 15.51).

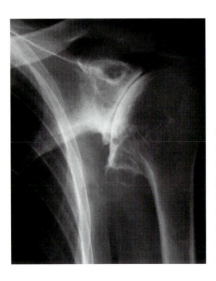

Fig. 15.50 Primary osteoarthritis of the glenohumeral joints. Note the irregular joint space and the big inferior osteophytes on the humeral head both side

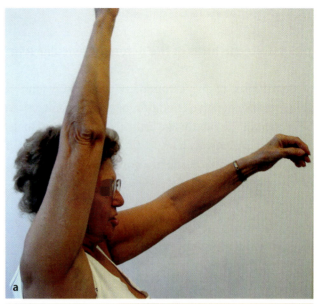

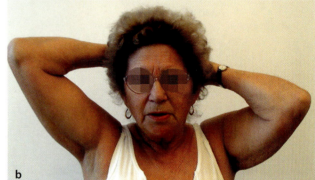

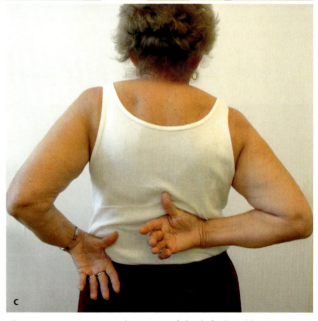

Fig. 15.51 a–c Active elevation of the left shoulder (**a**), external rotation in elevation of the left shoulder (**b**), and extension and internal rotation of left the shoulder is limited due to primary osteoarthritis of the glenohumeral joint (**c**)

15.5.3 Secondary Osteoarthritis of the Glenohumeral Joint

Secondary arthritis of the glenohumeral joint can develop due to inflammatory conditions (rheumatoid arthritis, infection), following trauma, following surgery of glenohumeral instability, avascular necrosis of the humeral head, massive tear of the rotator cuff. The patients have pain while performing activities and even at rest. The limitation of the function that may restrict everyday activities (combing hair, eating, perineal care, etc.) is even more severe than in case of primary arthritis (Figs. 15.52–15.57).

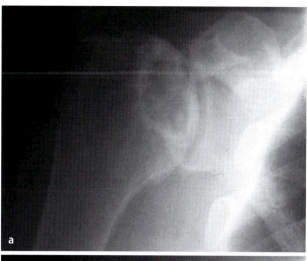

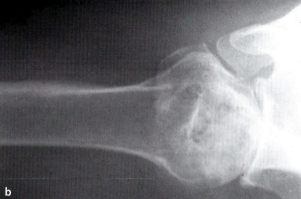

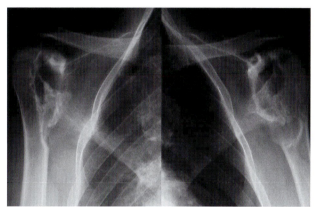

Fig. 15.52 Erosive form of glenohumeral destruction in rheumatoid arthritis

Fig. 15.53 a, b Avascular necrosis of the humeral head. Antero-posterior (**a**) and axillary lateral view (**b**)

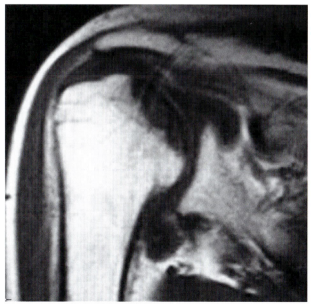

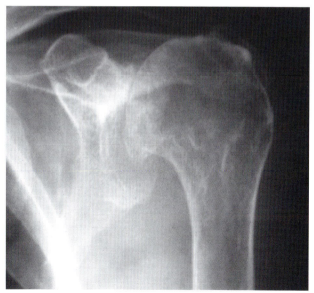

Fig. 15.54 MRI image of the avascular necrosis of the humeral head. Oblique coronal section

Fig. 15.55 Cuff tear arthropathy. The humeral head is superiorly migrated. The acromion is eroded and the greater tubercle is round

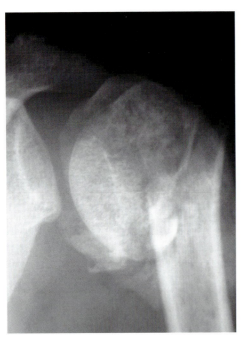

Fig. 15.56 Severe posttrauma condition of the left shoulder following a malunated four-part fracture dislocation

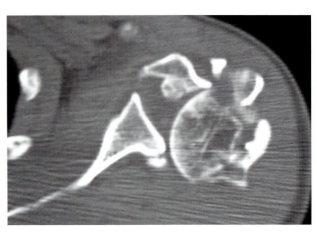

Fig. 15.57 CT scan of the same patient

Chapter 16

Elbow, Forearm

Contents

16.1 Congenital and Developmental Disorders

16.1.1 Congenital Radioulnar Synostosis

The rare condition of congenital radial-ulnar synostosis usually occurs between the proximal radius and the ulna. During the embryogenesis, for a short time, the radius and ulna share a common perichondrium. Abnormal events at this time can lead to failure of segmentation between them. Duration and severity of the insult can determine the degree of subsequent synostosis. Although the problem is present at birth, it usually is not discovered until early adolescence, when the patient presents with a lack of pronation and supination. A fibrous synostosis may allow limited motion. Regional soft tissue hypopla-

sia often is present in severe cases, including atrophy of the brachioradialis, pronator teres, pronator quadratus, and supinator muscles. The interosseous membrane also may be abnormal. With regard to frequency, there is no difference between the sexes, but more than half the cases are bilateral. One third of the cases is associated with general skeletal abnormalities, such as hip dislocation; knee anomalies; clubfoot; polydactyly; syndactyly; Madelung deformity; ligamentous laxity; thumb hypoplasia; carpal coalition; and problems of the cardiac, renal, neurologic, and gastrointestinal systems.

Posttraumatic radial-ulnar synostosis is an entity completely separate from the congenital synostosis and has different cause, treatment, and prognosis (Figs. 16.1 and 16.2).

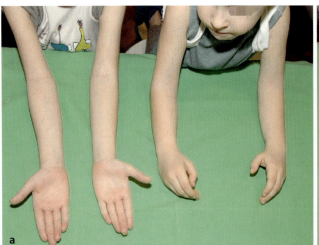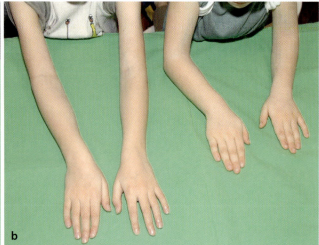

Fig. 16.1 a, b (**a**) Five-year-old boys with maximal supination in radioulnar joint, on the left normal and on the right with bilateral involvement of radioulnar synostosis. Severe fixed forearm pronation deformity is present, patients are partially able to compensate with glenohumeral motion.

Forearm usually lies in the pronated or hyperpronated position. Pain is usually not present. (**b**) 5-year-old boys with maximal pronation in radioulnar joint, on the left normal and on the right with bilateral involvement of radioulnar synostosis

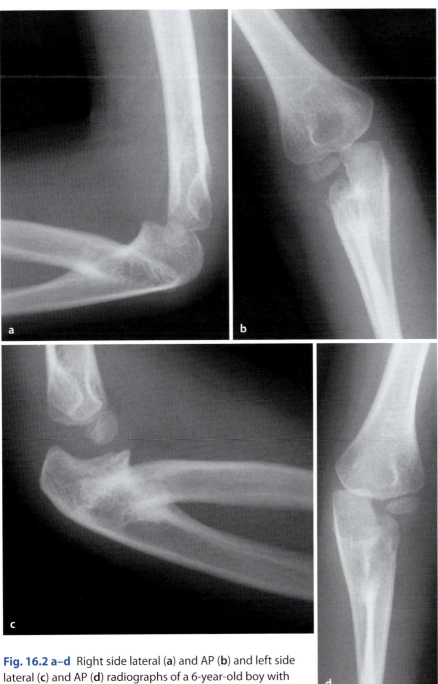

Fig. 16.2 a–d Right side lateral (**a**) and AP (**b**) and left side lateral (**c**) and AP (**d**) radiographs of a 6-year-old boy with radioulnar synostosis, bilateral involvement

16.1.2 Congenital Hypo-, Aplasia of Radius

Radial deficiencies, which characteristically affect only the structures on the radial border of the forearm and hand, are not clearly defined. Radial deficiency is described in a spectrum of osseous, musculotendinous, and neuromuscular dysplasias of the radial border of the upper limb.

Congenital longitudinal deficiency of the radius is characterized by radial deviation of the hand, significant shortening of the forearm, and subsequent bending of the ulna, presenting underdevelopment of the extremity. The thumb is usually absent or hypoplastic and the ulna is usually 60% of normal length. Isolated thumb hypoplasia represents radial deficiency in its mildest form, thumb hypoplasia and carpal anomalies represent an intermediate form, and absence or abnormality of all the radial structures (thumb, radial carpus, and radius) is at the extreme end of the spectrum. Although the etiology of radial deficiency is unknown, it is certainly multifactorial (Figs. 16.3 and 16.4).

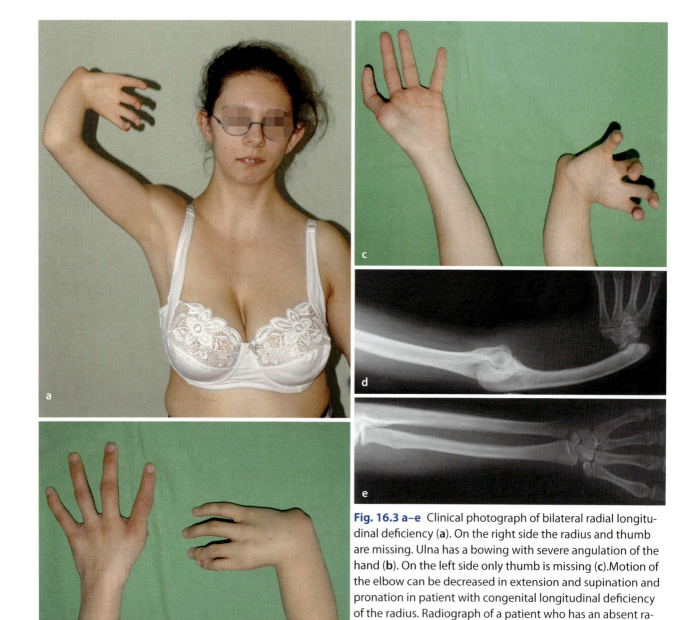

Fig. 16.3 a–e Clinical photograph of bilateral radial longitudinal deficiency (**a**). On the right side the radius and thumb are missing. Ulna has a bowing with severe angulation of the hand (**b**). On the left side only thumb is missing (**c**).Motion of the elbow can be decreased in extension and supination and pronation in patient with congenital longitudinal deficiency of the radius. Radiograph of a patient who has an absent radius. (**d**) Right carpal bones are angled and displaced radially with a secondary ulnar bowing. On the left side both ulna and radius are well matured; thumb is absent (**e**)

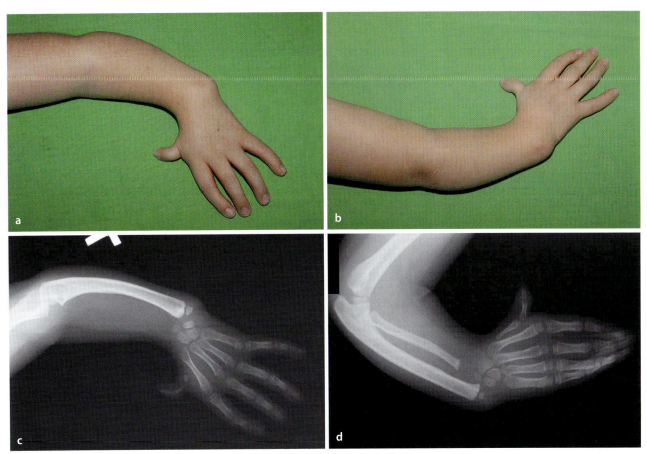

Fig. 16.4 a–d Patient photo and radiograph of a 9-year-old boy with radial aplasia on the left (**a, c**) and radial hypoplasia on the right side (**b, d**)

16.1.3 Madelung's Deformity

Madelung's deformity can be congenital and acquired. It is a deformity of the radius resulting in marked radial inclination, shorter forearm, dorsal dislocation of the ulnar head and a deformed carpal row. Posttraumatic Madelung's may follow partial growth arrest of the distal radius or technical failure of fracture management (Figs. 16.5–16.10).

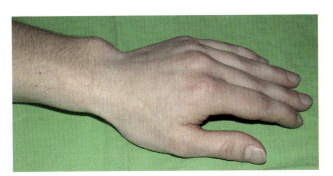

Fig. 16.5 Congenital Madelung may be due to an abnormal band tethering the radius proximally to the ulna

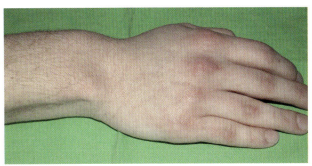

Fig. 16.6 Prominent distal radius and marked ulnar deviation

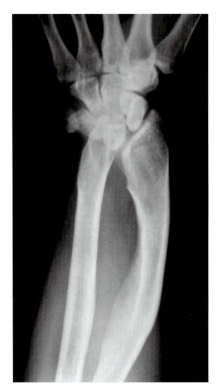

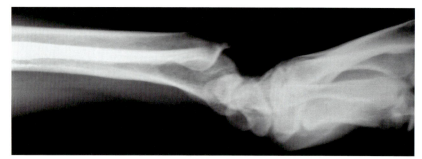

Fig. 16.8 Dorsal luxation of ulnar head and ulna "minus variant" in lateral view

Fig. 16.7 Radius diaphyseal curve with steep radial articular surface

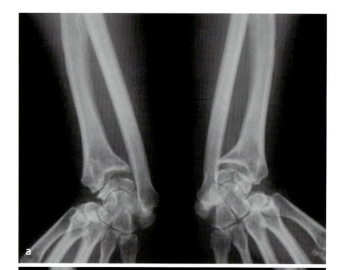

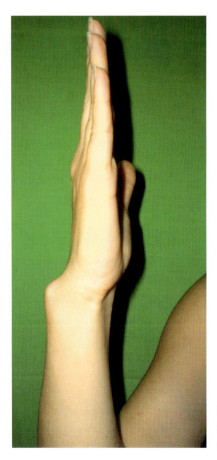

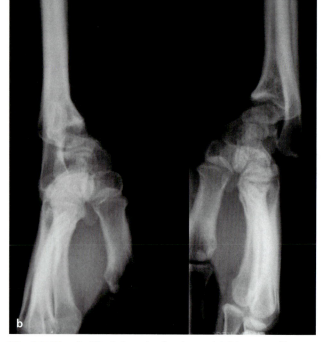

Fig. 16.9 Note the marked right ulnar displacement

Fig. 16.10 a, b The "ulna plus" variety with bizarre radiocarpal joint – AP view (**a**) and lateral view (**b**)

16.2 Primary and Secondary Osteoarthritis of the Elbow

Primary osteoarthritis of the elbow is a relatively uncommon disease compared to similar condition of the other major joints of the human body. It is more common in men than in women and in people who do heavy physical work. Secondary arthritis due to rheumatoid arthritis or trauma is more commonly seen. The main symptom is usually the limitation of flexion-extension and forearm rotation that can limit everyday activities. The pain can be disabling only in more severe cases (Figs. 16.11–16.14).

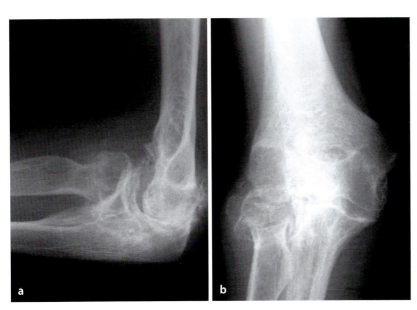

Fig. 16.11 a, b Severe primary osteoarthritis of right elbow. The joint space is narrow, subchondral bone is sclerotic and there is marked osteophyte formation

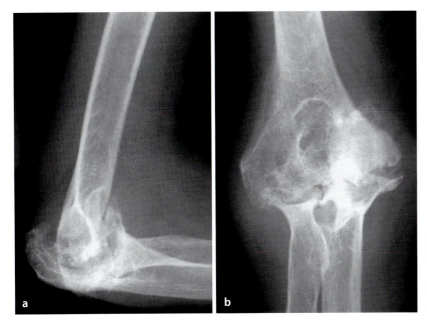

Fig. 16.12 a, b
Severe destruction of elbow due to rheumatoid arthritis. The subchondral bone is badly eroded. Surrounding bone is atrophic

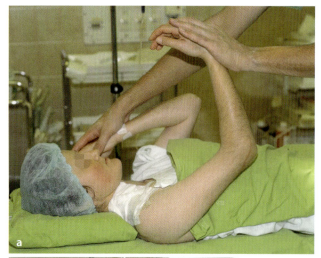

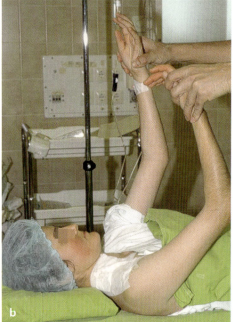

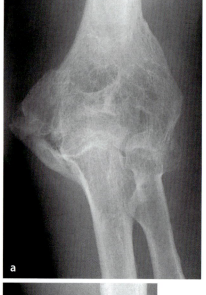

Fig. 16.13 a, b Elbow flexion (**a**) and extension (**b**) of right elbow of a patient presented with severe juvenile rheumatoid arthritis

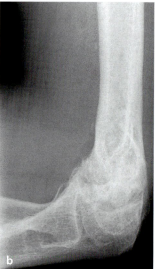

Fig. 16.14 a, b Secondary posttrauma arthritis of the left elbow of a 65-year-old patient

16.3 Elbow Instability

Stability of the elbow is provided mostly by the medial and lateral ligaments as static constraints. Of the three medial structures, the anterior medial collateral ligament is the most important, lateral stability is given mainly by the lateral ulnar collateral ligament. The head of the ra-dius is maintained by the annular ligament. Flexors and extensors, that transverse the joint are the dynamic stabi-lizers. Instability usually occurs as posterolateral rotatory instability or ulnar collateral ligament instability. Most common causes for instability are trauma, inflammatory disease (e.g., rheumatoid arthritis), dislocation, and pre-vious radial head resection (Figs. 16.15–16.17).

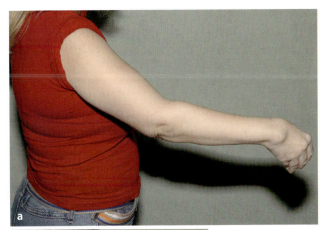

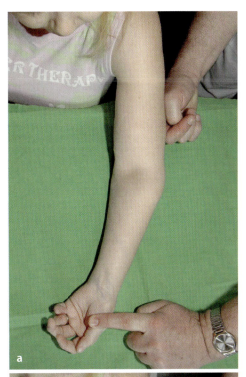

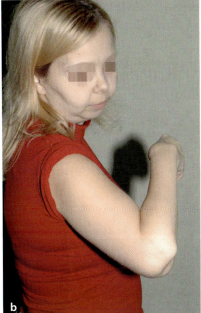

Fig. 16.15 a, b Patient with juvenile idiopathic arthritis (JIA). In extension, bones of the elbow are maintained in their original position. Note the swollen wrist and metacarpophallangeal joints due to JIA. Ulnar deviation of fingers also can be observed (**a**). Flexing the elbow, the ulna and the radius subluxate, humping the skin over the affected bones (**b**)

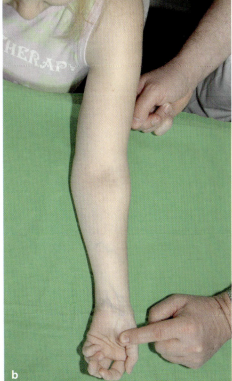

Fig. 16.16 a, b Applying varus (**a**) and valgus (**b**) stress on the forearm, instability of the elbow joint can be examined

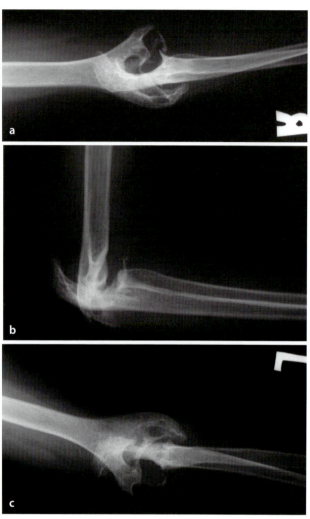

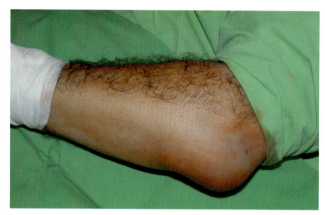

Fig. 16.18 Patient with olecranon bursitis: hump over the posterior aspect of the elbow refers to the swollen bursa

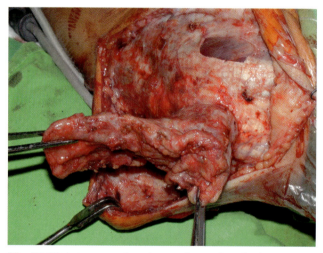

Fig. 16.17 a–c Right side lateral view radiograph of the patient with extended elbow. The articular surface is totally destroyed (**a**). Right side lateral view radiograph of patient with the elbow flexed showing the subluxated ulna. Note the marked instability of the joint (**b**). Anteroposterior radiograph shows that the articulating surfaces are seriously damaged due to JIA, resulting in instability of the joint (**c**)

Fig. 16.19 Intraoperative picture shows that the bursa is located superficially between the skin and the underlying muscles. It originates from the tip of the olecranon process

16.4 Olecranon Bursitis

Olecranon bursa helps the skin glide smoothly over the tip of the olecranon. Positioned superficially between the skin and the olecranon process, the bursa is disposed to inflammation. Olecranon bursitis (also known as elbow bursitis) can develop due to different mechanisms such as repetitive trauma, inflammatory disease or less frequently septic inflammation. Most common symptoms are swelling, redness and pain (Figs. 16.19–16.21).

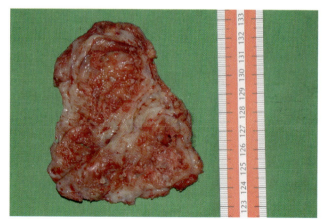

Fig. 16.20 Inflammated synovial tissue covers the inner surface of the excised bursa

Chapter 17

Wrist and Hand

Contents

Chapter 17

Wrist and Hand

Zs. Süth and J. Rupnik

17.1 Congenital and Developmental Disorders

17.1.1 Syndactylia

Congenital anomaly of the hand, marked by webbing between adjacent fingers. Syndactylies are classified as complete or incomplete according to the degree of joining. Syndactylies can also be simple or complex. Simple syndactyly indicates joining of only skin or soft tissue; complex syndactyly marks joining of bony elements (17.1–17.4).

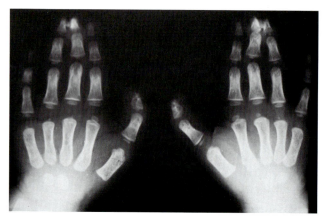

Fig. 17.2 Bony bridge present at the distal phalanges of 3–4 fingers

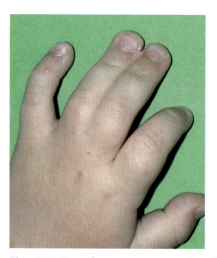

Fig. 17.1 Complete cutaneous syndactyly involving middle and ring fingers

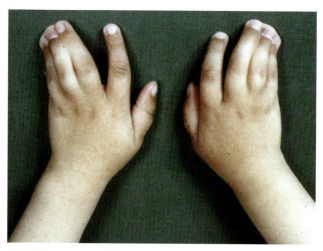

Fig. 17.3 Complex bilateral osteocutaneous syndactyly

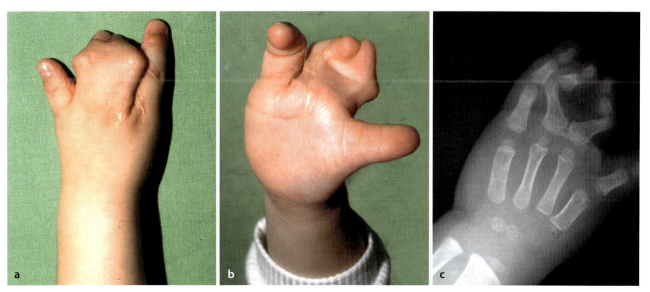

Fig. 17.4 a–c Complex syndactyly involving all long fingers, after a surgical release of the little finger (**a**). Palmar aspect of the same hand (**b**). Radiograph of the same patient: one ray is absent, and the two central fingers are in flexion and divergent position due to soft tissue abnormalities (**c**)

17.1.2 Pollex Duplex

Most common thumb duplication occurs at the metacarpophalangeal joint level. Four such types can be classified: hypoplastic, ulnar deviated, divergent and convergent (Figs. 17.5–17.9).

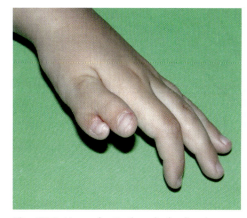

Fig. 17.6 Hypoplastic thumb duplication

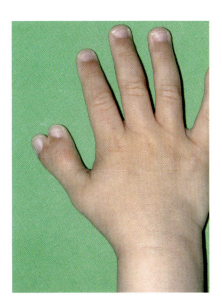

Fig. 17.5 Divergent type of pollex duplex

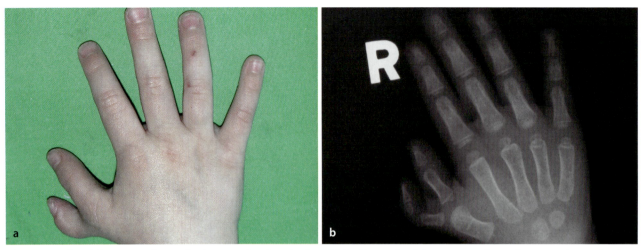

Fig. 17.7 a, b (**a**) Divergent–hypoplastic type of pollex duplex. (**b**) Radiograph of the same patient: divergent–hypoplastic type of pollex duplex with complete bony duplication of phalanges

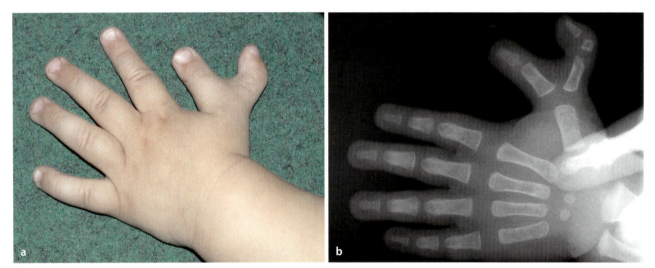

Fig. 17.8 a, b (**a**) Divergent type of pollex duplex. (**b**) Radiograph of the same patient shows divergent type of pollex duplex with complete bony duplication of the phalanges associated with delta phalanges

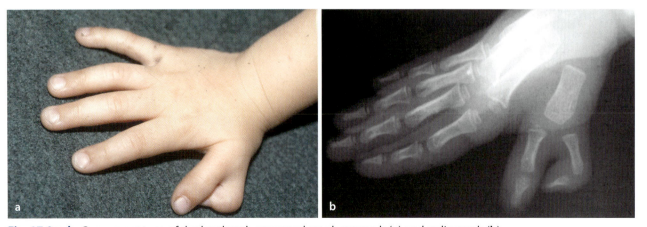

Fig. 17.9 a, b Convergent type of duplex thumb presented on photograph (**a**) and radiograph (**b**)

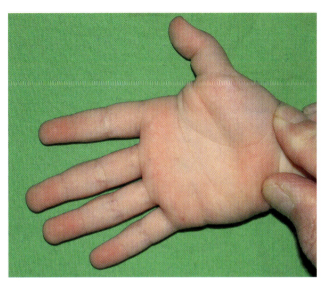

Fig. 17.10 A hard, palpable knot in the long flexor tendon of the thumb and flexion contracture in the interphalangeal joint

17.1.3 Pollex Flexus

The permanent flexion anomaly in the interphalangeal joint and a hard, palpable knot in the long flexor tendon of the thumb over the metacarpophalangeal joint are typical of this deformity. These changes are sometimes observed immediately after birth. The hypothesis that it is a hereditary, endogenous condition is supported by observations in twins, relatively frequent bilateral occurrence and a high familial incidence. Constriction of the synovial sheath over the basal joint of the thumb is a key pathogenetic factor (Fig. 17.10).

17.1.4 Congenital Hypoplasia of the Thumb (Floating Thumb)

Hypoplasia of the thumb is classified as follows: (1) Slight reduction in size but all structures normal. (2) Small thumb with abnormalities of the muscles and the tendons, instability (wobbliness) of the middle joint of the thumb and a tight restricted web space between the thumb and the index finger. (3) Small skeleton of the thumb, abnormalities of many of the muscles if not all, abnormalities of stiffness of the joints and a highly abnormal first web space. Position of the thumb may also be abnormal. (4) A floating thumb attached by only a thread. (5) Complete absence of the thumb (Fig. 17.11).

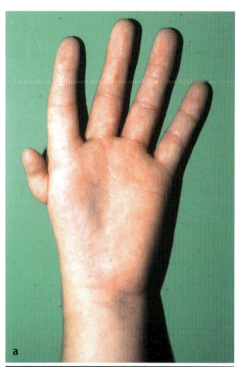

a

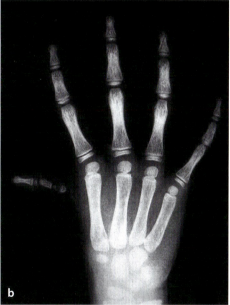

b

Fig. 17.11 a, b A floating thumb attached by only a thread. (type 4) (**a**), no bony connection can be recognized (type 4) on the radiograph (**b**)

17.1.5 Manus Fissa

Manus fissa (cleft hand or lobster-claw hand) is of two general types.

In the first type a deep palmar cleft separates the two central metacarpals. One or more rays are usually absent, and existing digits tend to be confluent and of unequal length.

In the second type of cleft hand the central rays are absent, and only short radial and ulnar digits remain. Oppositional pinch between these two digits may be impossible, the phalanges may be short or absent in one or both, one or more of their joints may be stiff, or the digits may be improperly aligned (Figs. 17.12 and 17.13).

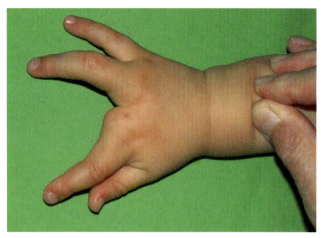

Fig. 17.12 Dorsal view of cleft hand Type I. One ray is absent

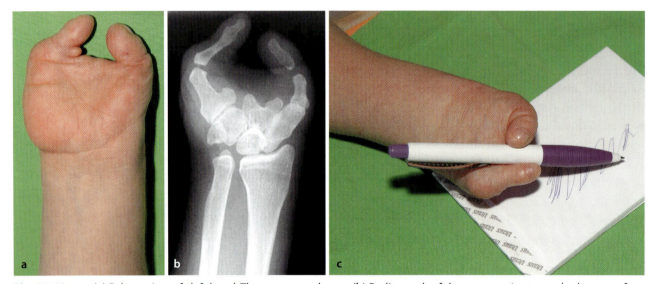

Fig. 17.13 a–c (**a**) Palmar view of cleft hand. Three rays are absent. (**b**) Radiograph of the same patient reveals absence of 2-3-4 metacarpal bones. (**c**) Function of cleft hand: patient is able to hold the pen but unable to write correctly

17.1.6 Macrodactylia

Macrodactylia (megalodactyly, macrodystrophia lipomatosa, dactylomegaly, local gigantism) can affect the fingers. The soft tissues ventral to the affected bones are diffusely enlarged and are predominantly of fat density, commonly mixed with bands of connective tissue. Usually multiple adjacent digits are affected on the lateral aspect of the hand or the medial aspect of the foot, although a single digit may also be involved. Histopathologic examination can distinguish fibrolipomatous macrodactyly or neural fibrolipoma with macrodactyly, from macrodactylia as a part of neurofibromatosis. Roentgenograms show bony enlargement, often with medial deviation in the hand. The cause of this rare condition is obscure but it may be related to fibrolipomatous tumors, often found at surgery, impinging on nerves supplying the enlarged digits (Fig. 17.14).

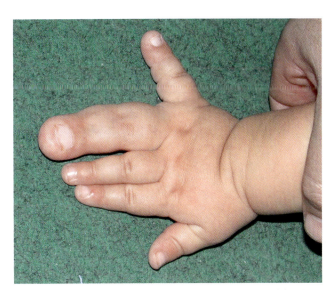

Fig. 17.14 Macrodactyly of ring finger in a 2-year-old girl

17.1.7 Metacarpal Hypoplasia

Relatively rare condition is the isolated congenital shortening of metacarpals resulting in shortening of the fingers. In most cases metacarpal hypoplasia is associated with other kinds of congenital maldevelopment. Often both metacarpal and metatarsal bones are bilaterally involved (See Chap. 20.1) (Fig. 17.15).

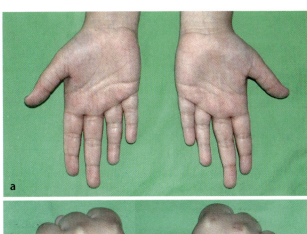

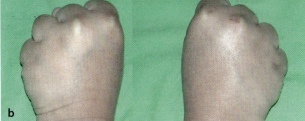

Fig. 17.15 a, b (**a**) Ring and little finger of both hands are shorter. (**b**) The heads of 4–5 metacarpal are sunk

17.2 Tenosynovitis

17.2.1 Digitus Saltans (Snapping or Spring Finger, Trigger Finger)

Flexion deformity of a finger(s) due to a tendon nodule which prevents tendon from sliding smoothly in its sheath. When the finger is flexed, this nodule may become trapped by the fibrotic zone at the base of the metacarpo–phalangeal joint. To straighten the finger, the patient has to extend it forcefully; this in turn results in triggering or snapping (Figs. 17.16–17.18).

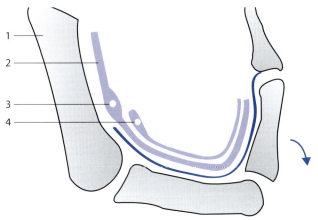

Fig. 17.16 Drawing presents pathomechanism of the trigger finger (1-metacarpal bone, 2- flexor tendon, 3- knot of the tendon, 4-concentric thickening of tendon sheath)

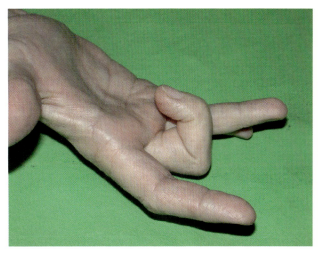

Fig. 17.17 The midfinger is in fixed flexion position, patient is unable to extend it

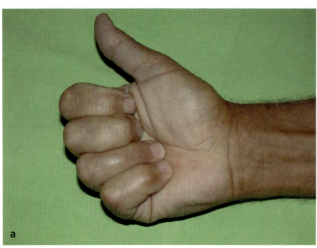

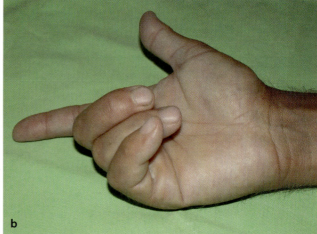

a

b

Fig. 17.18 a, b Unusual case: trigger phenomenon of middle, ring and little finger in a young male patient; he has full flexion (**a**) he is, however, unable to extend affected fingers without assistance (**b**)

17.2.2 Stenosing Tendovaginitis or De Quervain's Disease

Inflammation and thickening of tendon sheaths of extensor pollicis brevis and abductor pollicis longus. Usually presents in middle age. Pain noted over radial aspect of wrist. Often occurs after repetitive activity. Pain is often worsened by abduction of thumb against resistance. Symptoms can often be improved with conservative treatment. Persistent symptoms require surgery (Figs. 17.19 and 17.20).

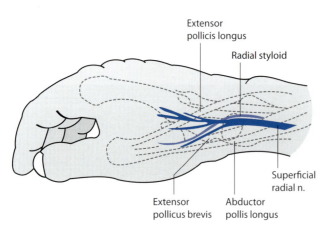

Fig. 17.19 Common sheath of the abductor pollicis longus and extensor pollicis brevis is demonstrated in this drawing

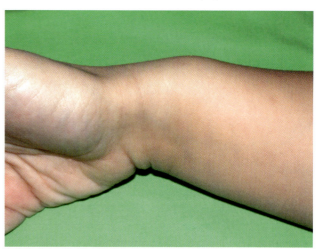

Fig. 17.20 Tendon sheath is thickened and tender over the radial styloid

17.2.3 Flexor Tenosynovitis

Tenosynovitis involves inflammation of the tendon and tendon sheath. Etiology of volar flexor tenosynovitis is often unknown. Flexor tenosynovitis often causes trigger finger phenomenon. Flexor tendons of the hand run in tight fibro-osseous tunnels. A series of ligaments, called pulleys loop around the tendons and their synovial sheaths. These pulleys hold the tendons close to the bones and joints. Inflamed pulley appears thick and fibrous. As the pulley thickens, it reduces the cross-sectional area of the tunnel (stenosis). When the tunnel becomes too narrow, the tendons no longer move freely through the tunnel and may develop a nodular deformity (Figs. 17.21–17.24).

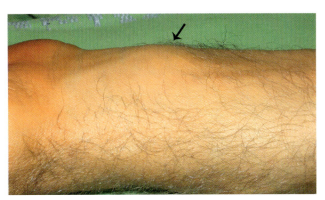

Fig. 17.21 Marked swelling due to inflammation (*arrow*)

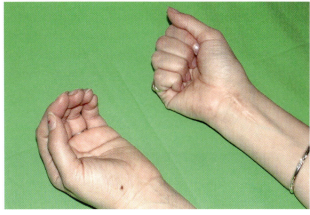

Fig. 17.23 Left palm is swollen; flexion of left fingers is restricted

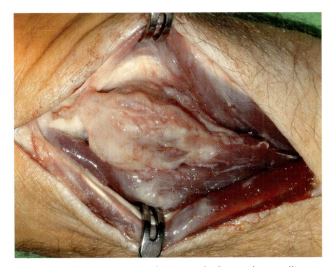

Fig. 17.22 Intraoperative photograph shows the swollen synovial tissue covering the flexor tendons

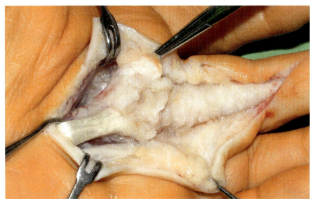

Fig. 17.24 Synovitis is present (synovial hypertrophy) around the middle finger's common flexor tendons in the palm

17.2.4 Extensor Tenosynovitis

Extensor tenosynovitis – inflammation of the tendons in the back of the hand and wrist. High risk occupation and activities associated with hand and wrist tendinitis include assembly line work, meat processing, manufacturing, knitting, typing, and piano playing. There is some evidence that workers exposed to risk factors such as high force and high repetition are at increased risk of hand and wrist tendinitis.

Clinical presentation of tendon disorders is characterized by the presence of pain at the site of injury. Specific physical findings on examination include tenderness when the area over the affected tendon is touched and may be associated with swelling, redness, and restriction of movement. Spontaneous tendon rupture may occur (Figs. 17.25 and 17.26).

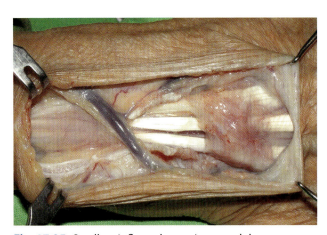

Fig. 17.25 Swollen, inflamed synovia around the extensor tendons on the dorsal part of the wrist

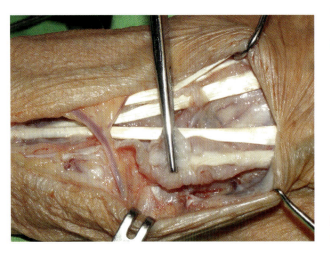

17.3 Disorders of the Carpal Bones

17.3.1 Post-Traumatic Necrosis of Scaphoid Bone

As a late complication of scaphoid fractures, avascular necrosis can develop. It serves as prearthrotic condition of wrist osteoarthritis (Fig. 17.27).

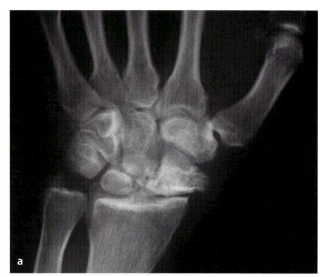

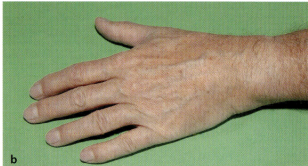

Fig. 17.27 a, b Radiograph shows typical appearance with marked necrosis of the proximal half of the bone (**a**), there are no apparent physical signs as demonstrated in the photograph (**b**)

Fig. 17.26 Extensor tendon rupture (instrument points to ruptured end of the tendon) caused by synovitis

17.3.2 Scaphoid Nonunion

A fall on the outstretched hand results typically in scaphoid fractures. These are the second most frequent fracture type of the hand. Ninety five per cent of the patients with acute scaphoid fractures are male, and the average age is approximately 25 years. Careful diagnostic and early therapy is especially important, because patients are mostly young. High numbers of nonunions develop on account of failure of first diagnosis and lack of proper treatment (Figs. 17.28 and 17.29).

17.3.3 Lunatum Malacia

Etiology of the aseptic necrosis of the lunate bone is not clear. Therapeutical problems result from late discovery of the disease. The goal attempted must be to keep the structures of the bone alive and prevent major pathological changes of the whole carpal bone system (Fig. 17.30).

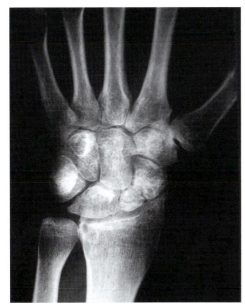

Fig. 17.28 Note the atrophic pseudoarthrosis line and loss of normal trabeculation, with narrowing of the radiocarpal joint space (arthrotic signs of the carpal joint)

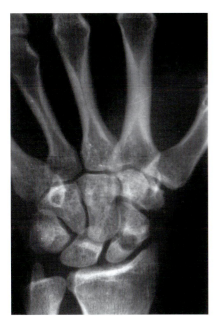

Fig. 17.29 Cystic–lytic changes in the scaphoid, dissociation of the scapho–lunar junction

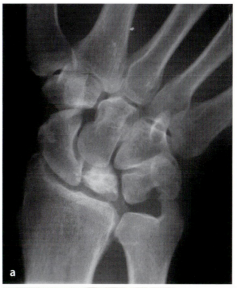

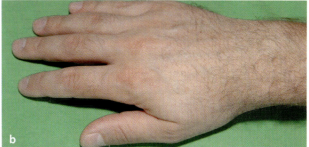

Fig. 17.30 a, b Radiograph reveals lunatum malacia. Note the condensity of the lunate (**a**). Photograph taken of the same patient: no apparent physical signs (**b**)

17.4 Osteoarthritis of Wrist and Small Joint of Hand

17.4.1 Wrist Osteoarthritis (OA)

OA of the wrist joint is uncommon except as the sequel to injury. Any fracture of the joint may predispose to degeneration, but the commonest is a fractured scaphoid, especially with nonunion or avascular necrosis. The patient may have forgotten the original injury; years later he/she complains of pain and stiffness.

Appearance is usually normal and there is no wasting. Movements of the wrist and radioulnar joints are limited and painful. Radiographs show irregular narrowing at the radiocarpal joint, with bone sclerosis, and the proximal portion of the scaphoid or the lunate may be irregular and dense (Figs. 17.31 and 17.32).

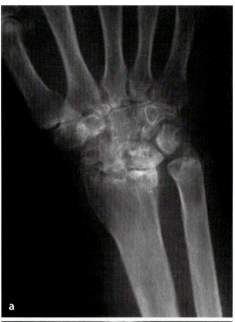

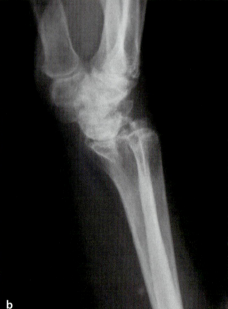

Fig. 17.32 a, b AP view of radiograph shows diminished radiocarpal joint space with sclerosis and degenerative cysts, and bony coalition of the scapho–lunar junction (**a**) lateral view (**b**) of the same case

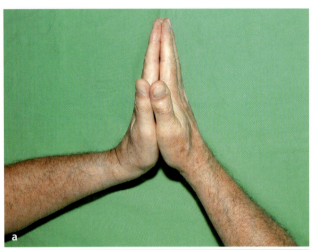

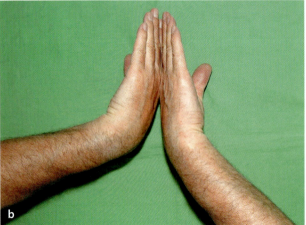

Fig. 17.31 a, b Both extension (**a**) and flexion (**b**) of the right wrist is restricted

17.4.2 First Carpometacarpal (CMC) Osteoarthritis

Painful function of the thumb is typical of osteoarthrosis of the first carpometacarpal joint ("rhizarthrosis"), which becomes particularly manifest when the patient opposes thumb and fingers for the purposes of apprehension.

Characteristic of rhizarthrosis is contracture of adductor pollicis muscles.

Clinical inspection as well as radiographs demonstrate that metacarpal bones of the thumb and the index finger are parallel, whereas here metacarpals otherwise spread out fanwise.

Restriction of movement in the carpometacarpal joint of the thumb, coupled with increasing compensatory hyperextensibility of the metacarpophalangeal joint, still enables the patient to grasp fairly large objects (Fig. 17.33).

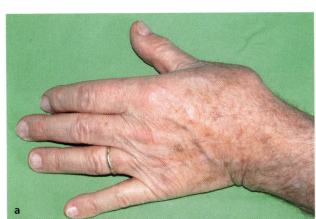

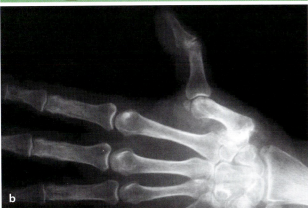

Fig. 17.33 a, b Photograph demonstrates characteristic "step formation" at the carpometacarpal joint and adduction contracture of the thumb, hyperextensibility of the metacarpophalangeal joint (**a**). Radiograph shows advanced osteoarthrosis of the carpometacarpal joint of the thumb with loss of joint space, subluxation and sclerosis between first metacarpal bone and trapezoid (**b**)

17.4.3 Osteoarthritis of the Lesser Hand Joints

Nodular osteoarthritis of the fingers: involvement of the proximal interphalangeal joints (Bouchard's nodes) and/or the distal interphalangeal joints (Heberden's nodes). This occurs more commonly in women. One or several of the joints may become periodically painful.

There is often a familiar element - the patient's mother, grandmother or a maternal aunt having had the same problem (Fig. 17.34).

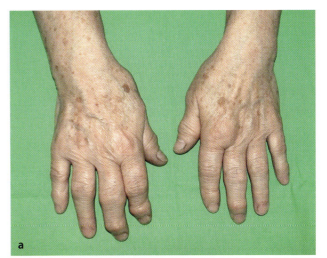

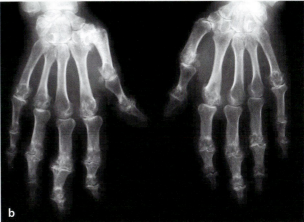

Fig. 17.34 a, b Typical Heberden's and Bouchard's nodes. Patient complains usually of swelling of distal or proximal interphalangeal joints and progressive development of unsightly nodes (**a**). The radiograph shows signs of osteoarthritis with narrow joint space, sclerosis and osteophyte formation, erosions (**b**)

17.5 Posttraumatic Axial Deformity

Fingers on the injured hand should line up the same way as fingers on uninjured hand. This means that if the fingers are straightened, they should come to the same length. Also while making a fist, fingers should not cross but should line up parallel to each other. Crossing of fingers is an indication that there may be a rotational deformity caused by malaligned fracture healing. This is a deformity that often needs correction and surgery may be necessary (Fig. 17.35).

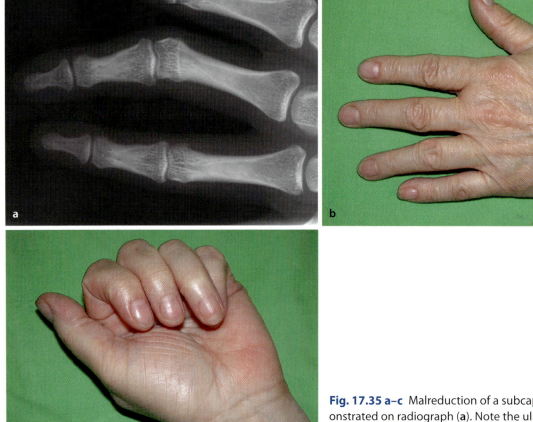

Fig. 17.35 a–c Malreduction of a subcapital fracture demonstrated on radiograph (**a**). Note the ulnar angulation in the PIP joint of ring finger (**b**) and the crossing sign of ring finger (**c**)

17.6 Contractures

17.6.1 Metacarpophalangeal (MCP) Joint Extension Contractures

If the hand is immobilized in inappropriate position, extension contractures of the metacarpophalangeal (MCP) joints can develop. MCP joint extension contractures can also result as a consequence of burn injuries or frostbite (Fig. 17.36).

17.6.2 Proximal Interphalangeal (PIP) Flexion Contracture

PIP flexion contracture may develop due to various etiologies. First some stiffness and slight swelling occur and antedate the onset of more severe joint symptoms. Chronic pain, deformity and function loss may follow. The joints involved most often are the proximal interphalangeal (Figs. 17.37–17.39).

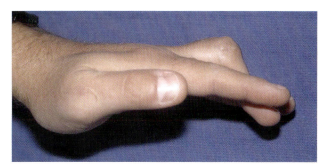

Fig. 17.37 Isolated flexion contracture in the PIP joint of third finger

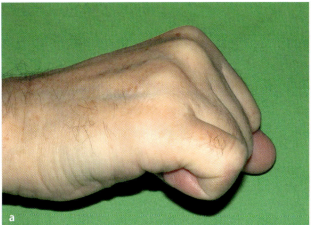

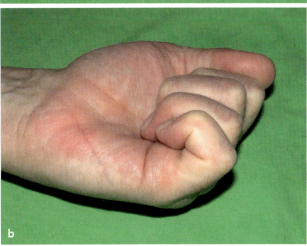

Fig. 17.36 a, b Flexion deficit of the fifth MP joint in dorsal view (**a**) and in palmar aspect (**b**)

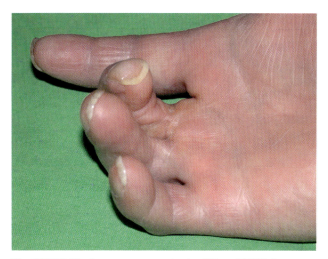

Fig. 17.38 Flexion contracture in the PIP and DIP joint because of burning injury

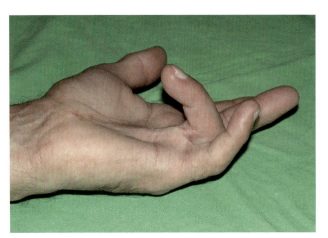

Fig. 17.39 Following palmar injury longitudinal deforming scar contracting fourth MP joint. Appearance of this disease can mimic Dupuytren's contracture

17.6.3 Volkmann's Ischemic Contracture

Volkmann's contracture occurs when there is ischemia of the forearm, usually caused by increased pressure that results from swelling (compartment syndrome). Trauma to the arm, including a crush injury or fracture, can decrease blood flow to the arm. A prolonged decrease in blood flow will injure the nerves and muscles, causing them to shorten and become stiff (scarred).

When the muscle shortens, it pulls on the joint at the end of the muscle just as it would if it were normally contracted, but because it is stiff the joint remains bent and cannot straighten. This condition is called a contracture (Fig. 17.40).

17.7 Entrapment and Compression Neuropathies

Peripheral nerves on the upper limb run through canals surrounded by bone and strong connective tissue. Discrepancy may develop between the extent of the canal and the size of its content, so the nerves can become compressed at various levels. Most common etiology are deformities following fractures, dislocations, scar formation after surgical interventions, tenosynovitis, hematoma, infection, and tumor which may all tighten the canal.

Consequences at the nerve supply area are: paresthesia – hypesthesia or partial or full paresis.

Most common compression neuropathies are the carpal, ulnar and supinator tunnel syndromes.

17.7.1 Carpal Tunnel Syndrome

Carpal tunnel syndrome (CTS) is caused by compression of median nerve in the carpal tunnel. Symptoms usually start gradually with pain, pins and needles, weakness, or numbness in the hand and wrist. As symptoms worsen, there may be feeling of tingling during the day, and decreased grip strength may make difficult to form a fist, grasp, or perform other manual tasks. In most of the cases no direct cause of the syndrome can be identified. (Figs. 17.41–17.45).

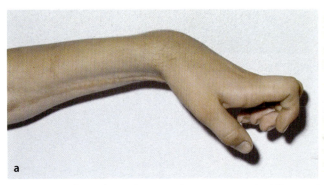
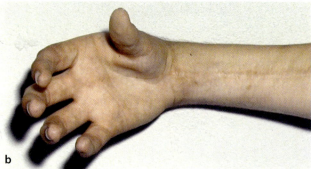

Fig. 17.40 a, b Archive photograph present a typical flexion deformity of the carpal and extension contracture of the MCP joints (**a**). Volar aspect of the hand (patient was already operated for its Volkmann's contracture) (**b**). (Courtesy of dr Wouters, Holland)

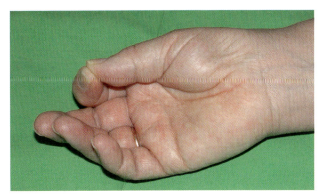

Fig. 17.41 Atrophy of the lateral part of the thenar eminence because of CTS

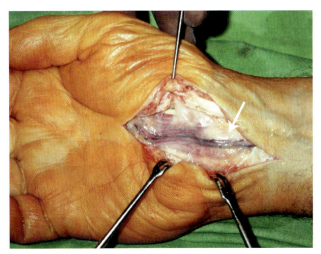

Fig. 17.42 Sand-glass like thickening in the median nerve caused by compression (*arrow*)

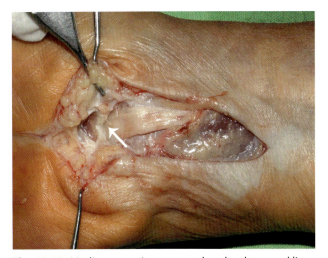

Fig. 17.43 Median nerve is entrapped under the carpal ligament (*arrow*). Synovitis of the flexor tendons is also due to carpal tunnel syndrome

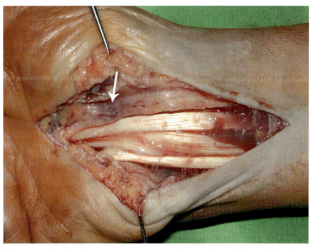

Fig. 17.44 Median nerve has now been freed. Note bluish entrapment zone on the nerve (*arrow*)

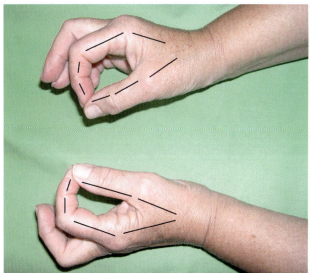

Fig. 17.45 Outline of opposition on the intact right side ("O"shaped); while on the abnormal left side, irregular opposition form an ellipsoid shape

17.7.2 Compression of the Ulnar Nerve

Ulnar tunnel syndrome: the ulnar nerve is compressed behind the medial epicondyle of the humerus. The nerve passes within the cubital tunnel posterior to the medial epicondyle. Compression is due to post–fracture valgus deformity, elbow osteoarthritis, chondromatosis, and tumors (Figs. 17.46–17.49).

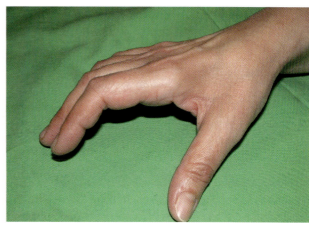

Fig. 17.47 Atrophy of adductor muscle of the thumb due to ulnar nerve entrapment

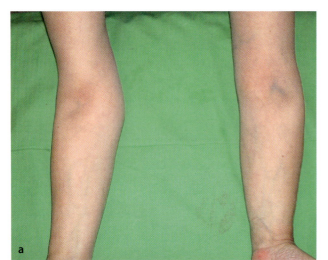

a

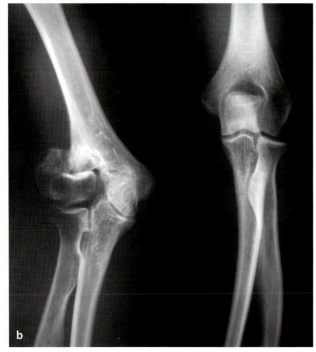

b

Fig. 17.46 a, b Valgus in right elbow as a consequence of a childhood supracondylar fracture (**a**), radiograph reveals severe valgus deformity of right elbow (**b**).Ulnar nerve is compressed at the former fracture level

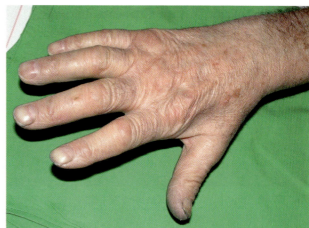

Fig. 17.48 Weakness of the intrinsic muscles, separation of fingers is weak due to ulnar nerve entrapment

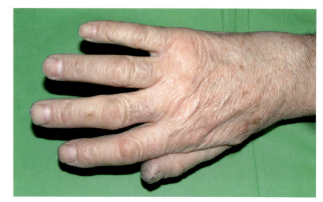

Fig. 17.49 Power of adductor muscle of the thumb is diminished due to ulnar nerve entrapment

17.7.3 Partial Palsy of Radial Nerve

Supinator tunnel syndrome: the motor branch of radial nerve which travels in the supinator tunnel and supplies the fingers long extensors is harmed. Innervation of the extensor carpi radialis muscle is intact. Usual causes are fracture of the radial head, operations, forced and extensive pro – supination, scar formation (Figs. 17.50).

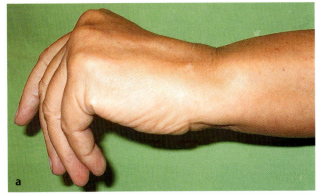

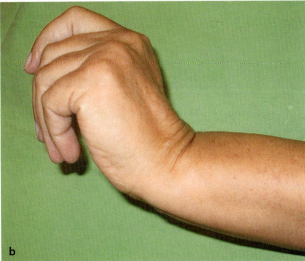

Fig. 17.50 a, b Active wrist extension is powered by the extensor carpi radialis muscle. Note loss of finger extension in the MCP joints due to partial radial nerve palsy (**a**). The PIP-s and DIP-s extension is powered by the interosseal muscles supplied by ulnar nerve

17.8 Tumors and Tumor like Lesions of the Wrist and Hand

The wrist and hand are rare locations for both primary and metastatic bone and soft tissue tumors. Less than 10% of the benign and 1% of the malignant bone tumors originate from the small tubular bones of the hand. There are, however, some tumor like lesions *ganglion, aneurysmal bone cysts*, benign tumors of the soft tissue *palmaris fibromatosis, localized giant cell tumor of tendon sheath, giant cell tumor of bone, enchondroma, enchondromatosis, chondroma of tendon sheath* and malignant tumors *chondrosarcoma* which often or mostly occurs in this region (See Table 17.1).

Table 17.1 Frequency of the most common bone and soft tissue tumors and tumor like lesions in the wrist and hand

(A) Tumor like lesions	
Ganglion	40–60%
Foreign body granuloma	40–60%
Aneurysmal bone cysts	3–4%
Myositis ossificans	1%
Osseous epidermoid cyst	90%
(B) Benign tumors	
Glomus tumor	20–30%
Palmaris fibromatosis	All
Giant-cell tumor of tendon sheath	80–85%
Chondroma of tendon sheaths	60–70%
Giant cell tumor of bone	12–15%
Enchondroma	25–50%
Osteoid osteoma	4–6%
Osteochondroma	1–3%
(C) Malignant tumors	
Chondrosarcoma	1–2%
Synovial sarcoma	7%
Metastatic tumors	1–2%

17.8.1 Palmar Fibromatosis (Dupuytren's Contracture)

Palmar fibromatosis (Dupuytren's contracture or disease) together with the plantar and penile fibromatosis belongs to the superficial fibromatoses. It arises from the palmar aponeurosis as a fibroblastic proliferation growing infiltratively. Adults are mostly affected with a rapid increase in incidence with advancing age. About 50% of the cases are bilateral. Its pathogenesis is multifactorial with genetic components (family history!) but other factors like trauma, diabetes, alcohol-induced liver disease also have a role in its etiology. It starts as an isolated firm palmar nodule, later shows a cordlike induration infiltrating the overlaying skin and extending most often toward the 4 and 5 fingers.

According to the progressivity of the lesion it can be classified:

- Nodules affected only palmar fascia without any contracture of the fingers
- One or more fingers are affected, the MP joints are in mild flexion contracture (0–45°)
- MP contractures are more severe (45–90°)
- Severe contractures of MP's (90–135°) (Figs. 17.51–17.57)

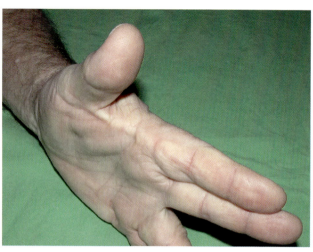

Fig. 17.52 Isolated cord involves the thumb; therefore it can not be fully extended

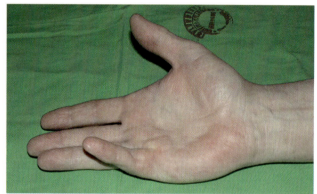

Fig. 17.53 Superficial pretendinous cord, which leads to contracture of the MCP joints and interphalangeal joints of the fingers. 30° flexion position in the MP joint of little finger

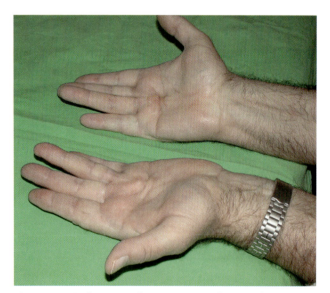

Fig. 17.51 Earliest manifestation is usually a tender nodule in the palm (most often at the third or fourth fingers). Bilateral nodules of the palm, mild flexion contractures of ring fingers' MP joint

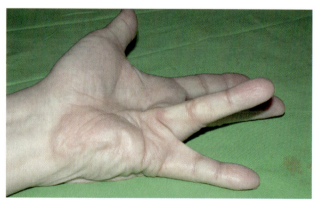

Fig. 17.54 Prominent cord overlying skin, isolated involvement of ring finger's ray

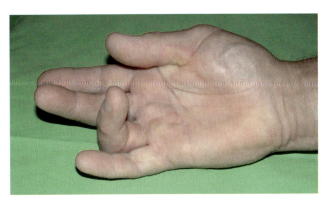

Fig. 17.55 Thumb in adduction contracture and PIP flexion contracture of the ring finger

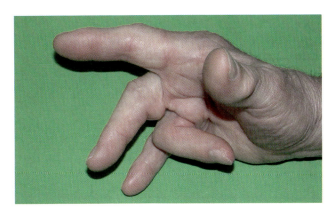

Fig. 17.56 Three rays are affected; the PIP joint of the ring finger is in flexion and can not be extended

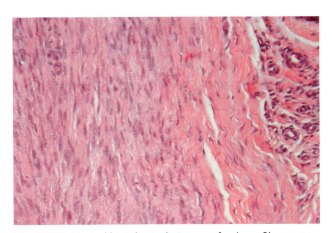

Fig. 17.57 Typical histological picture of palmar fibromatosis: early proliferative lesions showing bland fibroblastic cells in abundant dense collagen matrix

17.8.2 Ganglion

Common benign cystic lesion, develops from any synovial tissue (Figs. 17.58–17.61).

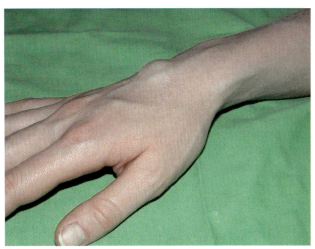

Fig. 17.58 Unilocular cystic lesion (1.5–2.5 cm in diameter) on the dorsal surface of the wrist of a young woman

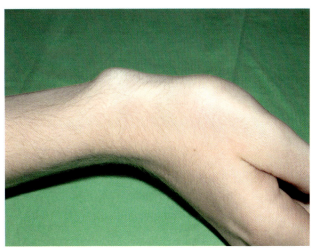

Fig. 17.59 Ganglions develop less frequently on volar surface of the wrist

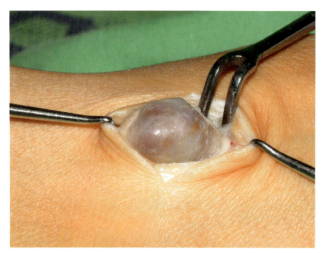

Fig. 17.60 At surgical exposure the ganglion appears as a thin walled cyst filled with transparent viscous myxoid fluid

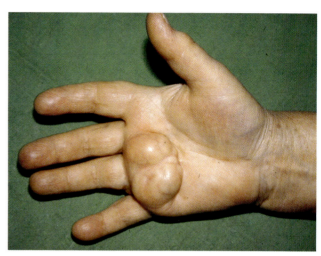

Fig. 17.62 Multilobular volar lipoma above the 4. and 5. metacarpal bone

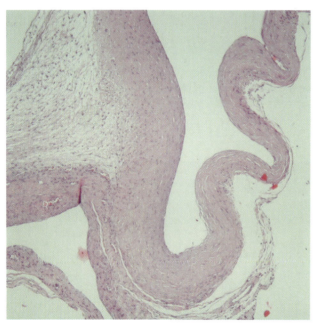

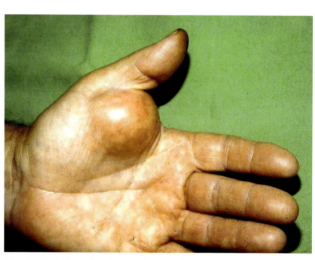

Fig. 17.63 Egg size lipoma in the thenar muscles

Fig. 17.61 Histologically wall of the ganglion consists of thin fibrous tissue rich in collagen fibers

17.8.3 Lipoma

Lipomas of the wrist and hand are usually deep-seated; they form irregular masses with multiple processes beneath the aponeurosis (Figs. 17.62–17.64).

Fig. 17.64 At surgical approach the well encapsulated tumor is seen with the second finger-nerve crossing the pedicle of the tumor

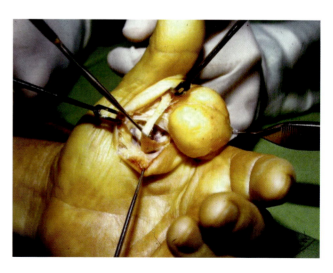

17.8.4 Giant Cell Tumor (GCT) of Tendon Sheath

This is a family of similar diseases arising from the synovium of bursae, joints and tendon sheaths. Its localized type (synonym: benign synovioma) is the most common soft tissue tumor of the hand. It occurs usually between 30 and 50 years, with a 2:1 female predominance (Figs. 17.65–17.68).

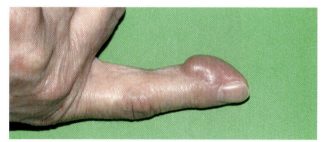

Fig. 17.65 Painless swelling, subcutaneous nodule in the distal phalanx of the forefinger –typical appearance of a GCT of tendon sheath

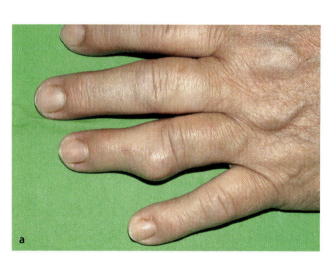

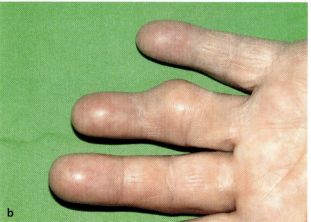

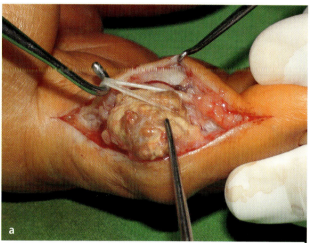

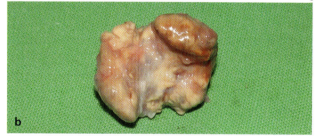

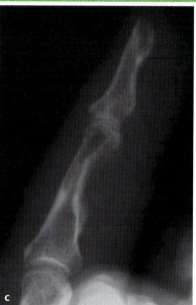

Fig. 17.67 a–c Digital nerves running on the capsule of the GCT of tendon sheath (**a**). Removed surgical specimen of the GCT of tendon sheath. Note the impression on the surface of the lobulated yellowish tumor due to the flexor tendons of the finger (**b**). Radiograph shows cortical erosion on the diaphyseal part of the phalanx due to pressure of GCT of the tendon sheath (**c**)

Fig. 17.66 a, b Swelling at the proximal interphalangeal joint of the ring finger – dorsal (**a**) and volar views (**b**)

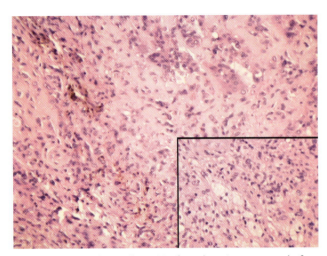

Fig. 17.68 Histologically, GCT of tendons is composed of variable amount of mononuclear cells, multinucleated giant cells, foamy macrophages, and siderophages containing haemosiderin pigments

17.8.5 Synovial Sarcoma

This is the most common soft-tissue sarcoma occurring in the hand. It is a highly malignant mesenchymal spindle cell tumor with variable epithelial differentiation (Also see Chap. 10, Soft tissue tumors) (Fig. 17.69).

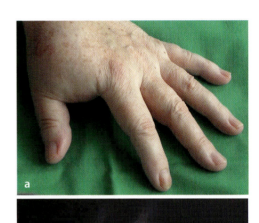

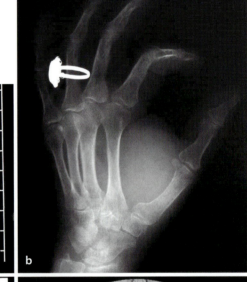

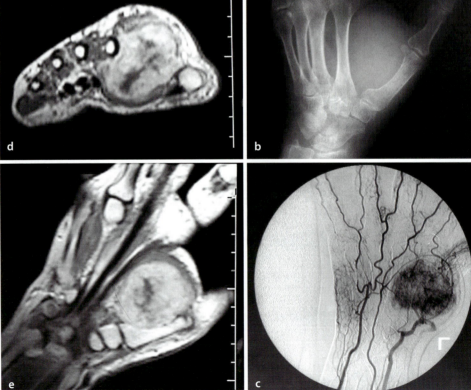

Fig. 17.69 a–e Photograph reveals a firm tumorous mass between the thumb and forefinger (**a**) Shadow of the soft tissue mass is also seen on the radiograph (**b**) Pathological vascularized tumor mass is shown in the angiography (**c**). MRI picture (transversal plane): the mass of the synovial sarcoma reaches both the ventral and dorsal superficial fascia pushing the bones from each other (**d**). MRI picture (frontal plane) shows extent of tumor mass between the metacarpals (**e**)

17.8.6 Glomus Tumor

A rare small benign tumor of mesenchymal origin which can occur anywhere, but typically affects young adults (women) characteristically in the subungual region of the hands (Figs. 17.70–17.72).

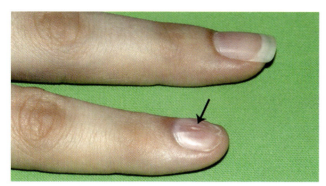

Fig. 17.70 Glomus tumor beneath the nail of the forefinger. Note the uneven surface of the brittle nail and the small bluish colored tumor underneath it (*arrow*)

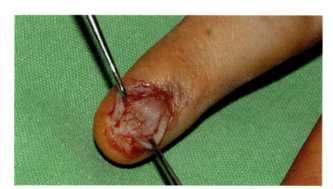

Fig. 17.71 Exposed nail bed with glomus tumor

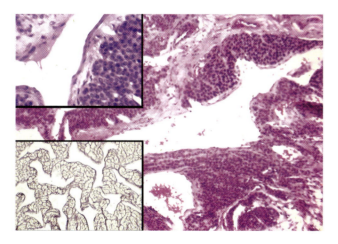

17.8.7 Traumatic Epithel Cyst of Fingers

Tumor like lesion which has a trauma caused implantation origin and can be found both in the soft tissue and in the bone (usually in the distal phalanx of the fingers) (Fig. 17.73).

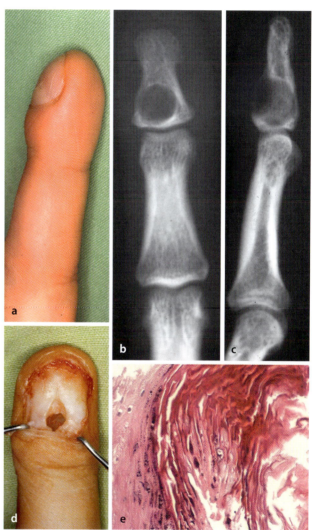

Fig. 17.73 a–e Swollen top of forefinger (**a**). Well defined lytic cystic lesion in the distal phalanx – ap view (**b**) and lateral view (**c**). Curetted defect intraoperatively (**d**). Histologically, the wall of the cyst-wall consists of normal epidermis; the defect is filled by detached squamous cells (**e**)

Fig. 17.72 Typical microscopic picture of the glomus tumor: solid areas of glomus cells surrounding vascular spaces. Insert: glomus cells presented by higher magnification (*above*) Cells are surrounded by reticulin fibers (Gömöri staining: *below*)

17.8.8 Foreign Body Granuloma

Splinters, fish-bones, glass-particles cause most often foreign body reaction in the hand, and fingers. The bone is rarely also involved (Fig. 17.74).

17.8.9 Aneurysmal Bone Cyst (ABC)

A rare benign cystic lesion of unknown etiology composed of blood-filled spaces separated by connective tissue septa (see also Chap. 11, Tumor like lesions of bone). It can affect the small tubular bones of hand and feet (Fig. 17.75).

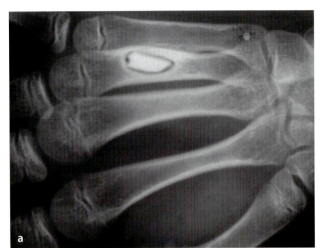

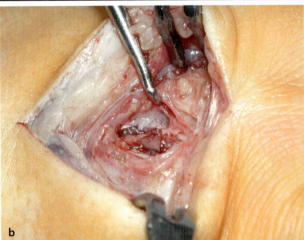

Fig. 17.74 a, b Radiograph reveals a lead-glass particle as a sequester in the fourth metacarpal bone (**a**). Intraoperative photograph taken from the glass particle in the bone (**b**)

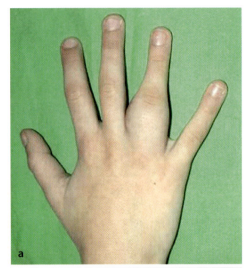

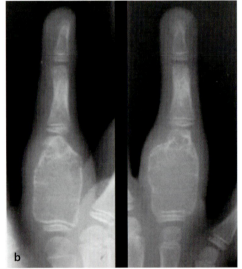

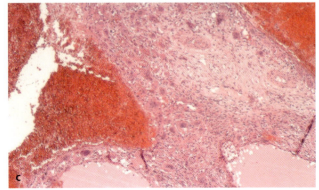

Fig. 17.75 a–c Thickened swollen ring finger of a young boy (**a**). Typical radiological appearance of an aneurysmal bone cyst: Proximal phalanx is expanded by radiolucent lytic lesion (**b**)Characteristic histological picture of the ABC. Irregular vascular spaces, connective tissue septae containing osteoclast giant cells (**c**)

17.8.10 Myositis Ossificans

Myositis ossificans is a localized, self-limiting reparative lesion that is composed of fibrous tissue and heterotopic bone. Trauma plays a role in its etiology. The
rapid growth, histological and radiological appearance
can mimic a true sarcomatous lesion. Myositis ossificans
rarely affects the hand (Fig. 17.76).

17.8.11 Chondroma of the Tendon Sheath

Chondroma of the soft tissues of hands and feet, synovial
chondroma can originate from the synovial membrane,
the fibrous tissue of the joint capsule, and the paraarticular tissues. Rather uncommon lesion (Fig. 17.77 and
17.78).

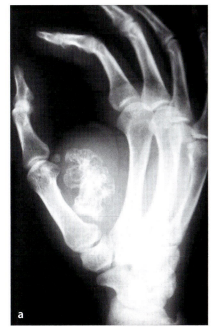
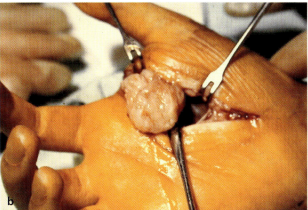

Fig. 17.76 a, b Radiograph presents large ossification area in the muscles of the thenar (**a**). Excised pseudotumor in operation (**b**)

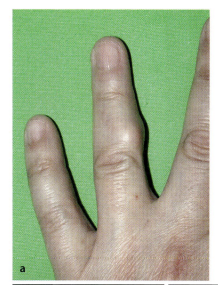
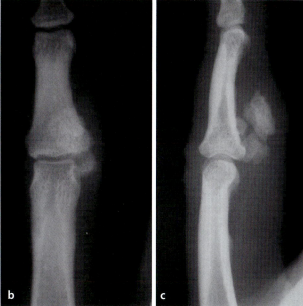

Fig. 17.77 a–c (**a**) Firm palpable tumor on radial site of the finger. Multiple calcified chondroma present around the capsule of the proximal interphalangeal joint on the ap (**b**) and lateral (**c**) radiographs

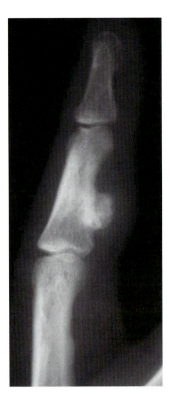

Fig. 17.78 Chondroma of the flexor tendon sheath as revealed by the radiograph

17.8.12 Osteochondroma of the Short Tubular Bones

Osteochondromas can also develop from the short tubular bones of the hand and feet (Fig. 17.79).

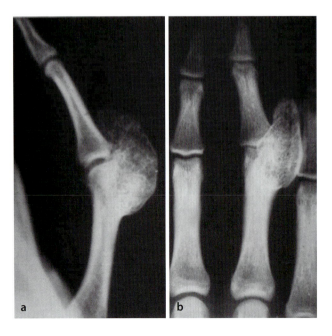

Fig. 17.79 a, b Osteochondroma deforms the proximal interphalangeal joints

17.8.13 Bizarre Parosteal Osteochondromatous Proliferation (Nora Tumor)

Bizarre paraosteal osteochondromatous proliferation mostly affects the small tubular bones of hands, but rarely the feet. The tumor has a cartilage cap but histologically it differs significantly from an osteochondroma (Fig. 17.80).

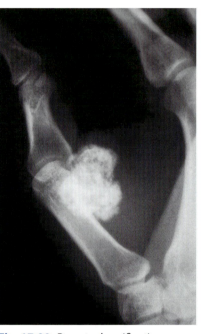

Fig. 17.80 Parosteal ossification seen on the radiograph in close relation with the cortex of the underlying bone

17.8.14 Osteoid Osteoma

This is a painful, small, benign bone forming tumor, with only 4–6% of them affecting the small bones of hands (Figs. 17.81 and 17.82).

17.8.15 Enchondroma, Periosteal Chondroma

These are benign hyaline cartilage forming tumors, appearing mostly singly but not infrequently in multiple form. The majority of the cases are asymptomatic and discovered incidentally after a pathologic fracture. Mild pain, deformation of the fingers, swelling are some symptoms which lead to recognition of the disease. Enchondromas are the most common bone tumors of the hand, half of them occur in the small tubular bone of the hand and feet. Radiographs show radiolucent lesion; the cortex is thinned, and characteristic spotty calcification in the cartilaginous matrix is present (Figs. 17.83–17.88).

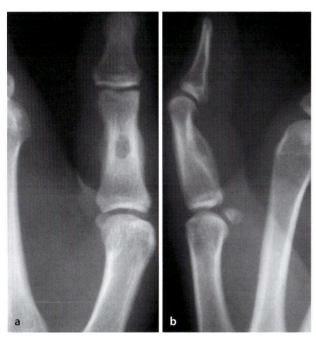

Fig. 17.81 a, b A typical nidus with sclerotic rim is present in the proximal phalanx of the thumb, anteroposterior (**a**) and lateral (**b**) view

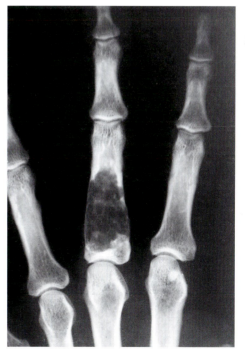

Fig. 17.83 Radiographs show radiolucent lesion, the cortex is thinned, characteristic spotty calcification in the cartilaginous matrix is present

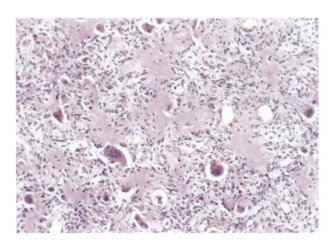

Fig. 17.82 Microscopic appearance of an osteoid osteoma

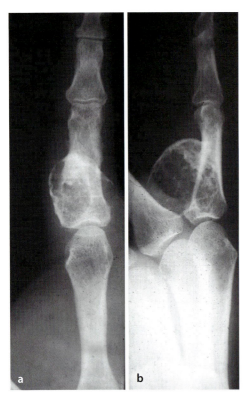

Fig. 17.84 a, b Enchondromas can grow eccentrically as *enchondroma protuberant* but a thin layer of cortical bone surrounds the lesion. a–p (**a**) and lateral (**b**) view

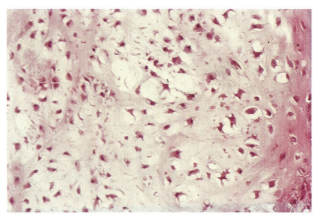

Fig. 17.86 Histology of enchondroma showing cartilage cells with small hyperchromatic nuclei of uniform size, in abundant hyaline cartilage matrix

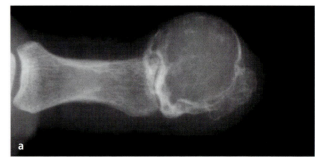

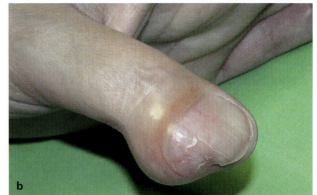

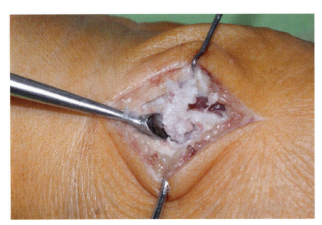

Fig. 17.85 At curettage, bluish–white cartilaginous material fills out the cavity

Fig. 17.87 a, b Enchondroma of terminal phalanx expanding the thinned cortex which is interrupted at one side (**a**). Deformed thumb of the patient (**b**)

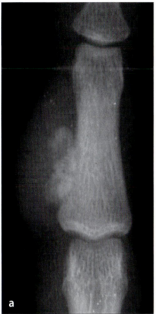

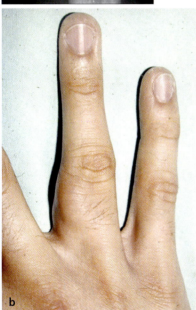

Fig. 17.88 a, b The periosteal chondroma *juxtacortical chondroma* is rather uncommon lesion, growing within or beneath the periosteal or parosteal connective tissue. It typically erodes the underlying cortex which is thickened and hollowed out (**a**) Palpable, painful mass on the finger caused by the periosteal chondroma (**b**)

17.8.16 Multiple Chondromas (Enchondromatosis, Ollier's Disease)

Multiple chondromas occur less frequently. They belong to developmental disorders *failure of normal enchondral ossification*. There is a predominant unilateral involvement, the most common site being the hand. Extent of the disease can be very different (Figs. 17.89–17.91).

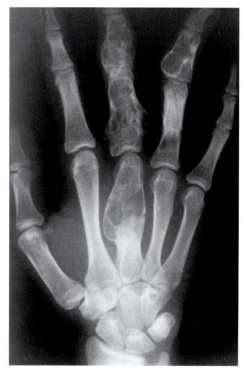

Fig. 17.89 Sometimes only a few small lesions are present

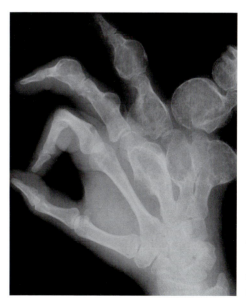

Fig. 17.90 In other cases the enchondromatosis affects many bones of the skeleton leading to crippling deformation

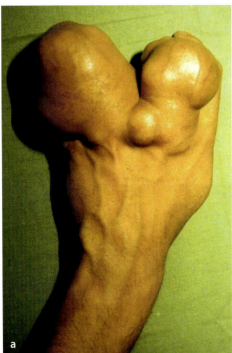

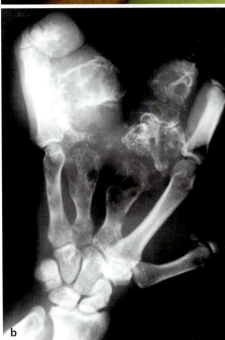

Fig. 17.91 a, b In advanced stage fingers are seriously deformed, the hand is useless. Sudden growth of one of the lesions refers to a malignant transformation (**a**). Radiograph of the same patient reveals huge tumor mass with spotty calcification (**b**). Histology reveals a secondary chondrosarcoma

17.8.17 Chondrosarcoma

Cartilage forming bone tumor of different grade of malignancy affect only very rarely the small bones of hand. They usually start de novo as sarcomas. Malignant transformation following curettage of an enchondroma has also been reported. Not more than 1 or 2% of all cartilage forming tumors of the hand are chondrosarcomas (Figs. 17.92–17.94).

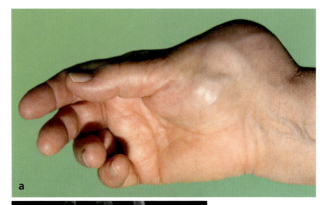

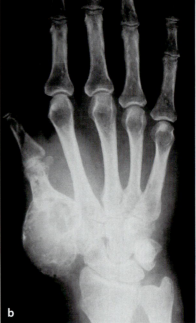

Fig. 17.92 a, b Leading clinical symptoms are swelling, palpable firm mass of the tumor (**a**) Affected bone is usually more expanded than in case of enchondroma as presented on radiograph (**b**)

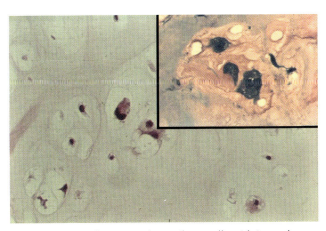

Fig. 17.93 Histology reveals cartilage cells with irregular plump nuclei. Differentiation of a low grade chondrosarcoma from an enchondroma can be extremely difficult

17.8.18 Metastatic Bone Tumors

Metastatic bone tumors affect the small bones of the hand and feet only in less than 2%. Clinical symptoms are unspecific: painful swelling, palpable tumor mass and decreased range of motion are usually present (Fig. 17.95).

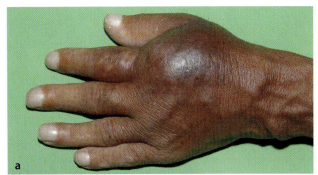

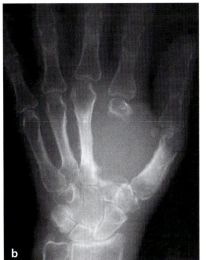

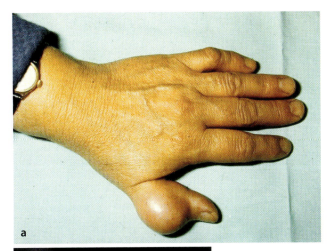

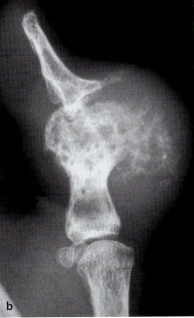

Fig. 17.94 a, b
A firm, palpable tumor of the thumb (**a**). The chondrosarcoma has destroyed the cortex of the phalanx and invaded the surrounding soft tissue (**b**)

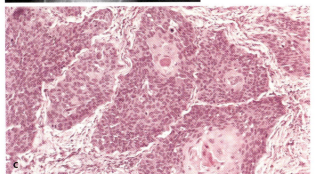

Fig. 17.95 a–c Painful swelling, palpable tumor mass of the hand is presented in this photograph (**a**). Radiological appearance of the metastasis is characteristic: destructive lytic lesion without periosteal reaction (**b**). Histology of the biopsy refers to the site of the primary tumor only in about half the cases. In this case it reveals a squamous cell carcinoma; the primary tumor was in the lung (**c**)

Chapter 18

Hip

Contents

Chapter 18

Hip

Z. Bejek, L. Sólyom and M. Szendrői

18.1 Congenital and Developmental Disorders

18.1.1 Proximal Femoral Focal Deficiency (PFFD)

The most frequent partial aplasia of the femur is the proximal femoral focal deficiency (PFFD), when the femur is shortened, flexed, abducted, and externally rotated. Flexion contractures of the hip and knee are present. The overall frequency of PFFD is 1/100,000. Bilateral involvement is seen in 15% of the cases. The etiology of PFFD is not known exactly, but may be due to a defect in maturation and proliferation of chondrocytes in the proximal growth plate (such injuries include anoxia, ischemia, irradiation, infections and toxins, etc). No evidence indicates a genetic etiology. Approximately 50% of patients with PFFD have other limb anomalies as fibular deficiency and valgus feet, cleft palate, clubfoot, congenital heart defects, and spinal anomalies.

Aitken's classification for PFFD:

- Class A, a shortened femur is present proximally, ending at or slightly above the level of the acetabulum. The femoral head is often absent but later ossifies; the acetabulum is well-developed. After ossification, there is subtrochanteric varus deformity.

- Class B has a more severe defect or absence of the proximal femur. At skeletal maturity, there is no connection between the femoral head and proximal femur; the proximal femur is above the acetabulum.

- Class C has an absent femoral head that does not ossify and has a markedly dysplastic acetabulum. The class C femoral shaft is shorter than in a person with class B. The entire proximal femur, including the trochanters, does not develop.

- In Class D, there is a severely shortened shaft, with an irregularly ossified tuft of bone proximal to the distal femoral epiphysis. No acetabulum is present because the lateral pelvic wall is flat (Figs. 18.1–18.4).

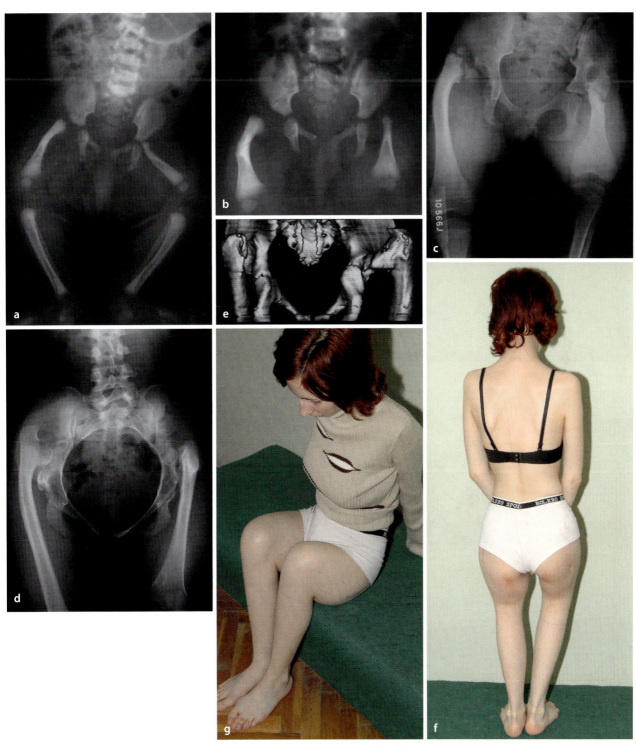

Fig. 18.1 a–g PFFD, Aitken class B on the right and class C on the left side of a 1-year-old girl. See the curved and shortened femoral shafts with virtual dislocation of the right femoral head (**a**). The same patient at the age of four: see the expressed curvature of the femoral shaft on the right and the sound dislocation of the left hip (**b**). At the age of 12 the femoral head is developing, and nonunion between head and neck is to be observed beside the coxa vara and curved femoral shaft on the right. The left side shows up a considerable shortening and aplasia of the proximal femur (**c**). Radiograph of the same patient at age of 17. Both hips are dislocated, there is a marked shortening of the left femur (**d**). 3D CT of the patient (**e**). Posterior view of the patient with visible limb length discrepancy due to severe shortening of the left femur (**f**). The patient in sitting position. Note that the shortening of the lower extremity is just at the femur. The tibia and fibula are normal in both sides (**g**)

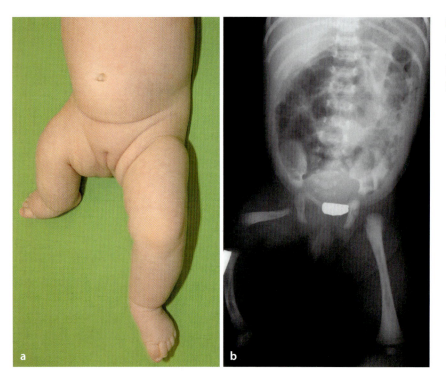

Fig. 18.2 a, b Unilateral PFFD of a girl at the age of one (a).The Radiograph of the previous patient at the age of four. Marked shortening of the right femur is present (b)

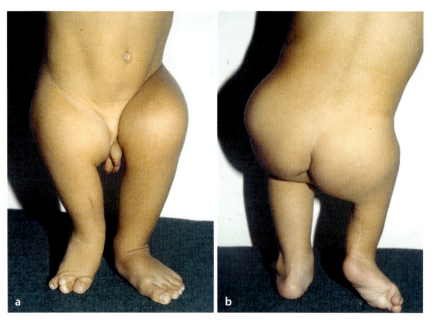

Fig. 18.3 a, b Bilateral PFFD (*more severe on right side*), with additional involvement of the rays of the foot

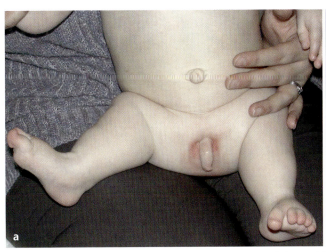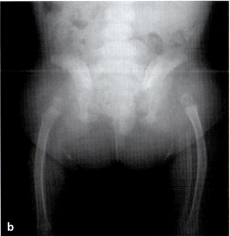

Fig. 18.4 a, b The most serious stage of the disease: bilateral femoral aplasia of an infant. Photograph presents the absence of the knees (**a**). Radiograph shows the abnormal hip joints: both proximal tibia are located beside the acetabulae (**b**)

18.1.2 Congenital Coxa Vara

Congenital coxa vara is a relatively rare developmental disorder with possible autosomal dominant inheritance. The incidence is about 6/100,000, and 50% of the cases are bilateral. This disease is characterized by the decreased femoral neck shaft angle less than 120° which presents/is seen at birth or presenting/seen clinically during early childhood and the deformation progresses with growth. In patients with congenital coxa vara a painless but progressive gait abnormality develops (Trendelenburg's limping) and in case of unilateral involvement it is frequently associated with a significant limb length discrepancy due to segmental shortening of the femur. Some authors refer to a close relationship of congenital coxa vara and the PFFD. The exact etiology is not known. Physiologic shearing stresses weight bearing cause pseudoarthrosis in the femoral neck or fatigue fracture of the local dystrophic bone (Fig. 18.5).

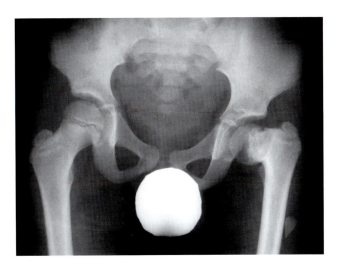

Fig. 18.5 Congenital coxa vara on the left hip. Note the 85° collodiaphyseal angle on the left, and the normal angle on the right side

18.2 Avascular Femoral Head Necrosis

This is a painful condition of the hip joint in the adult, mostly of an unknown origin. The anterolateral area or even the entire femoral head becomes necrotic and deformed. The supposed factors leading to the often bilateral disease are toxicity, as alcohol abuse or steroid medication and deterioration of vascular supply caused by trauma, caisson-disease, sickle cell anemia. Males are affected more commonly than females. The process itself leads to severe secondary osteoarthritis of the hip through different stages of progression (Ficat's stage 0–4).

Clinical symptoms: pain, restricted motion, limping.

Diagnosis of the illness is based on the history of the patient, clinical symptoms, in early cases MRI or isotope scan and later on radiographs.

- Ficat's stage 0: no alteration by any imaging techniques. This is the so called preclinical stage "silent hip".
- Ficat's stage 1: preradiographic stage, no radiological alteration on the a-p and frog position (Lauenstein's) radiographs are seen. On MRI pictures edema is present in the femoral head with a triangular shape.
- Ficat's stage 2: triangular sclerosis of the anterolateral quadrant in the femoral head appears on the radiographs showing the necrotic area.
- Ficat's stage 3: depression of the subchondral plate above the necrotic zone.
- Ficat's stage 4: severe secondary osteoarthritis develops with narrowing of the joint space, subchondral cysts and sclerosis, osteophytes at the margin of joint surfaces (Figs. 18.6–18.10).

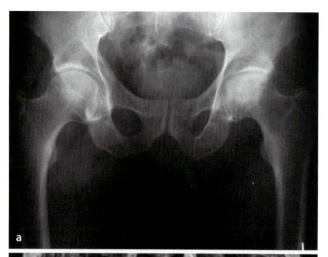

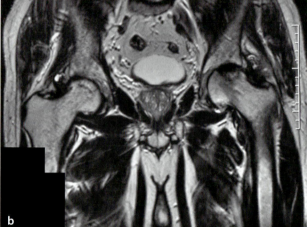

Fig. 18.6 a, b 61-year-old male with a stage 1 osteonecrosis of the right, and stage 3 one of the left femoral head (**a**). MRI picture of the same patient showing a demarcated area in the right and a severely necrotic area in the left hip with step building and depression (**b**)

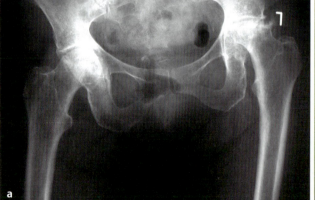

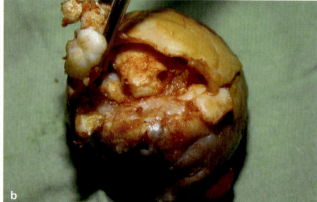

Fig. 18.7 a, b 53-year-old male patient with a stage 3 necrosis of the right and a stage 4 in the left hip. Note the progressed osteoarthritic changes of the femoral head (**a**). The resected femoral head of the patient with desquamation of the subchondral bone (**b**)

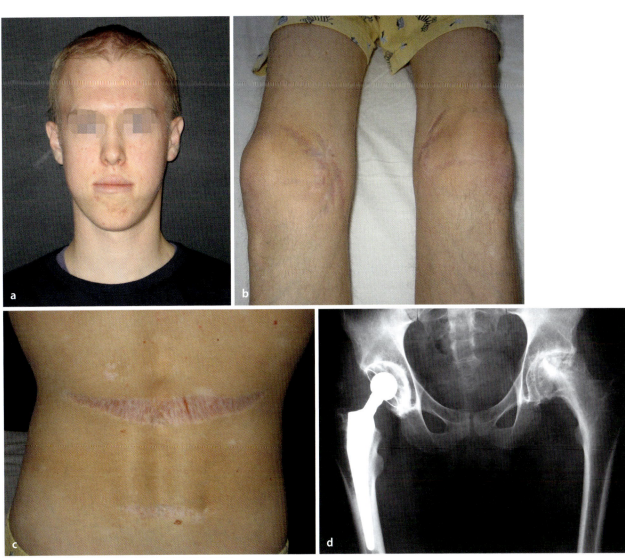

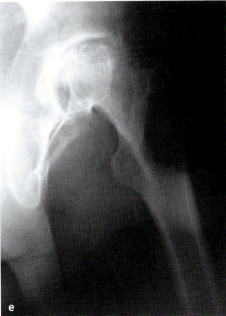

Fig. 18.8 a–e 18-year-old male has received steroid therapy because of acute myeloid leukemia. Note the steroid-altered face (a). Skin alterations (striae) on the knees and back are apparent as side effects of steroid treatment (b, c). Bilateral femoral head necrosis developed, the right hip treated already by total hip arthroplasty, on the left a stage 3–4 femoral head necrosis is present (d). The size of the necrotic area is best evaluated on the frog position radiograph (e)

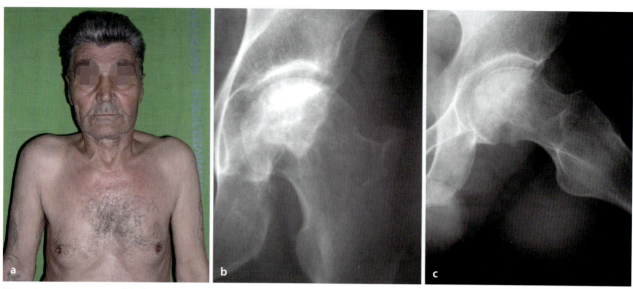

Fig. 18.9 a–c 60-year-old chronic alcohol abuser male patient (**a**). Ficat's stage 2 osteonecrosis of the femoral head with typical triangular sclerosis in the antero–lateral quadrant. A–P view (**b**) and frog position (**c**) radiographs of the left hip

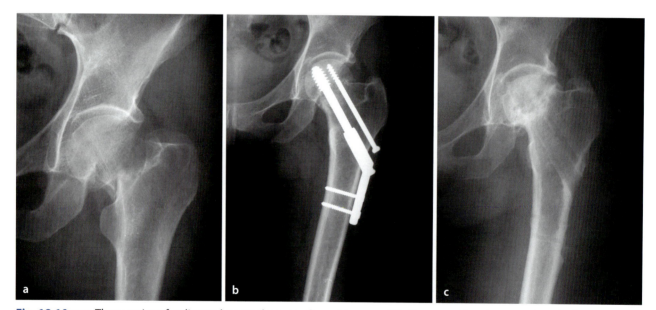

Fig. 18.10 a–c These series of radiographs reveal a secondary femoral head necrosis due to previous trauma. Radiograph of patient with femoral neck fracture (**a**). This was treated by reposition and osteosynthesis using dynamic hip screw (**b**). One year after the operation the femoral neck is shortened, and a secondary femoral head necrosis and osteoarthritis of the hip can be observed (**c**)

18.3 Contractures Around the Hip Joint

Causes leading to contractures: acute and chronic inflammations, septic and specific infections, diseases influencing the development of the hip joint as developmental hip dysplasia, Perthes, slipped capital femoral epiphysis, etc. Deformities following surgery can also lead to complex contractures.

18.3.1 Hip Contracture in Flexion

Hip contracture in flexion combined with extension contraction of the knee:
Isolated shortening of the rectus femoris muscle can develop after improper use of intramuscular injections or result in a partial rupture of the rectus femoris muscle (Figs. 18.11 and 18.12).

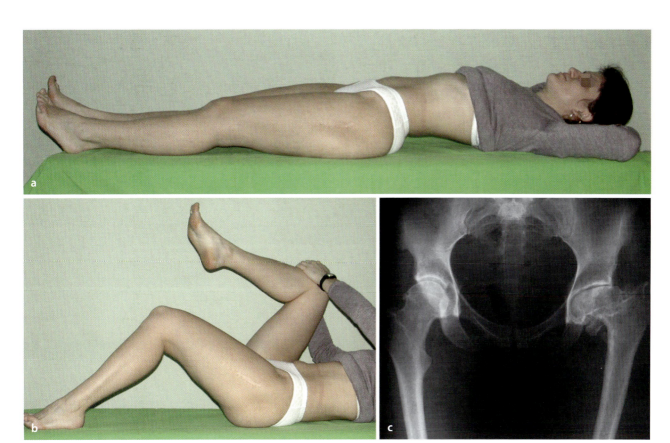

Fig. 18.11 a–c Flexion contracture of the left hip. The virtually full extension of the hip is produced by the patient's hyperlordosis (**a**). Maximal flexion of the opposite hip leads to the flattening of lumbar lordosis and presence of the flexion contraction becomes apparent (Thomas test) (**b**). Radiograph of the same patient: intertrochanteric osteotomy on the left side was performed in her childhood for congenital dislocation of the left hip. Note the marked coxa vara and severe secondary osteoarthritis with femoral head deformity which led to the contracture in flexion of the hip (**c**)

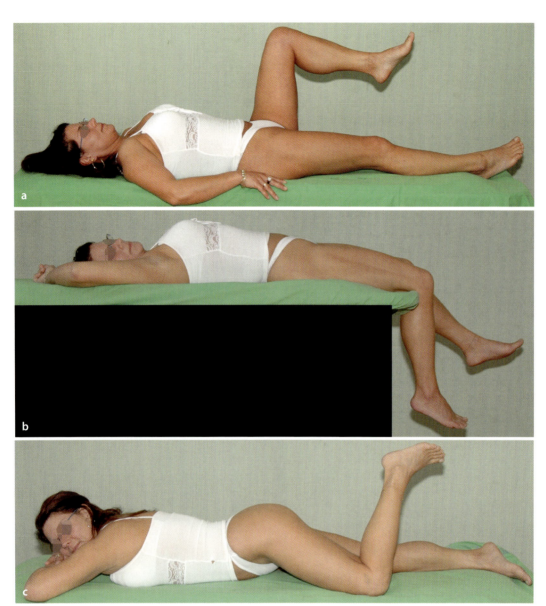

Fig. 18.12 a–c This patient was given repeatedly intramuscular antibiotic injections in her left thigh in childhood. Because the rectus femoris muscle overbridges both the hip and knee joints, the patient is able to flex the hip and knee in supine position (**a**).To flex the knee with extended hip is, however impossible on the affected side (**b**). To flex the knee in prone position is only possible when the patient simultaneously also flexes her hip (**c**)

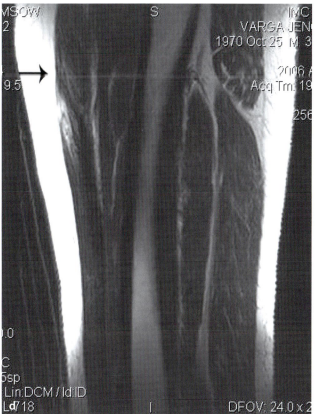

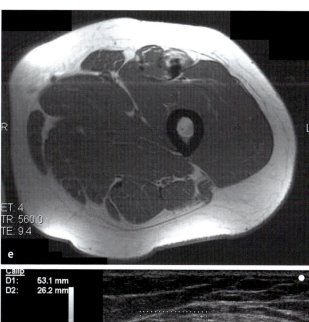

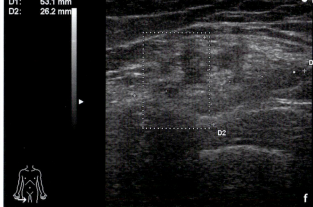

Fig. 18.12 d–f MRI imaging of contracted fibrotic rectus muscle of the left thigh (**d**, *arrow*). MRI horizontal picture of the left thigh. Note the scar formation in the rectus muscle (**e**). Color Doppler ultrasonography of the thigh: in the rectus femoris muscle an area of 5.3 × 2.6 cm with mixed echodensity is detected, with irregular structure, the muscle is hypovascularized – it refers to scar formation

Hip contracture in adduction

Congenital abnormalities, inflammatory conditions, neuromuscular diseases (infantile cerebral palsy, etc.) and osteoarthritis of the hip can lead to contracture of the adductor muscles. The patient is unable to carry out his duties, the leg becomes later fixed in an adducted position. This results in virtual shortening of the leg (Fig. 18.13).

18.3.2 Rupture of the Rectus Femoris Muscle

Causes leading to the lesion of the rectus muscle are: intensive sport activity at high level athletics, inadequate sport or heavy physical activity in untrained senior persons (Fig. 18.14).

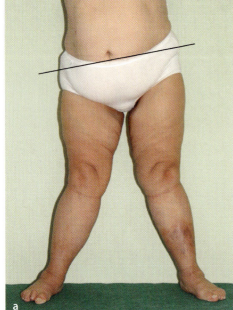

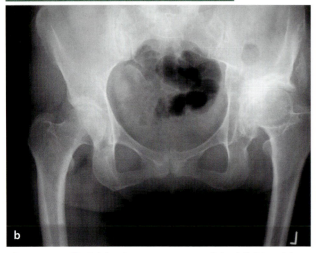

Fig. 18.13 a, b Adduction contracture of the left hip with consecutive genu valgum is evident when the patient stands feet wide apart. This can only be achieved by tilting the hip to the right because of left adduction contracture (**a**). The reason for the adduction contracture in this patient is a severe osteoarthritis of the left hip (**b**)

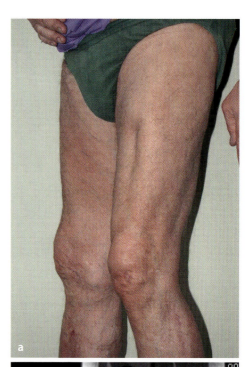

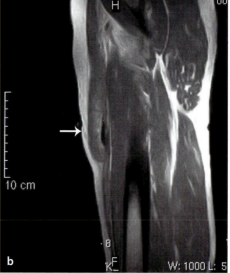

Fig. 18.14 a, b 63-year-old male patient: rupture of the rectus muscle during heavy physical work (**a**). On MRI picture the muscle belly is retracted (*arrow*) and migrated proximally leaving an excavation on the anterior thigh (**b**)

18.4 Deformities of the Collodiaphyseal Angle

Coxa vara

Diminishing of the collodiaphyseal angle under 120° is considered as coxa vara. It is associated with the high position of the major trochanter and insufficiency of the abductor muscles around the hip. It can be idiopathic, congenital (PFFD) or can arise from various causes and is a source of consecutive symptoms.

Coxa vara symptomatic

Secondary coxa vara can develop due to bone metabolic disturbances (Paget's disease, osteomalacia, rickets), slipped capital femoral epiphysis, fibrous dysplasia, or consequent deformities following treatment of congenital hip dysplasia (Figs. 18.15 and 18.16).

Coxa valga

Coxa valga is a developmental deformity of the proximal femur. A characteristic feature of this is the enhanced collodiaphyseal angle (over 135°) associated in some cases with shallow, dysplastic acetabulum and subluxation of the femoral head. It can be a source of pain following development of secondary osteoarthritis in the hip joint, Coxa valga is also often observed in spastic patients in association with muscle imbalance around the hip joint. The condition is more often detectable in female than male patients (Figs. 18.17 and 18.18).

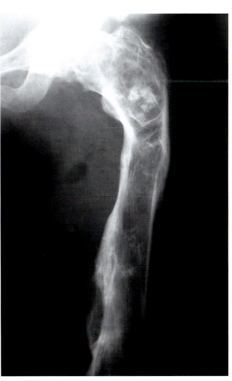

Fig. 18.16 Secondary coxa vara of an 81-year-old lady due to fibrous dysplasia of the left femur

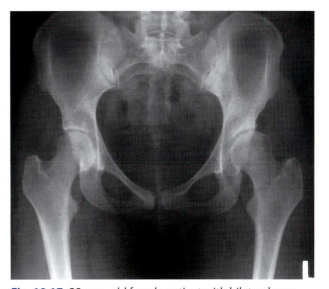

Fig. 18.17 28-year-old female patient with bilateral coxa valga. The collodiaphyseal angles are 150° on both sides. Shallow acetabulum, subluxation and early osteoarthritic signs (acetabular subchondral sclerosis, femoral head deformity) represent the late consequences of a developmental hip dysplasia in the left hip

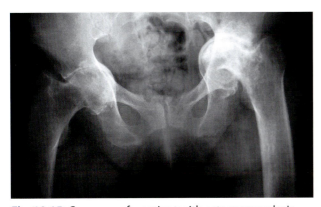

Fig. 18.15 Coxa vara of a patient with osteoporomalacia. The condition leads to secondary acetabular protrusion and osteoarthritis

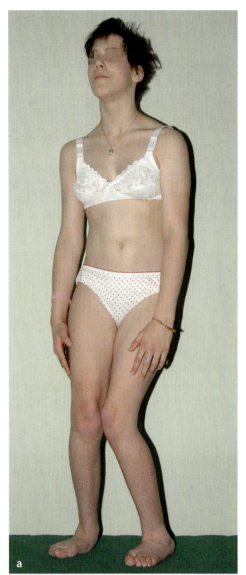

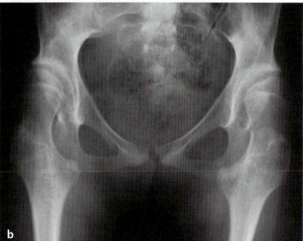

Fig. 18.18 a, b 18-year-old spastic female patient with characteristic posture (**a**). Radiograph taken from the pelvis of the same patient. Coxa valga is present on both sides (**b**)

18.5 Osteoarthritis of the Hip

18.5.1 Primary Osteoarthritis of the Hip

Degenerative process of the hip joint, which is characterized by wear up of the cartilage surface, osteophyte formation, synovitis, capsular and muscular contractures, muscle atrophy, leading to severe deterioration in life quality of the patient. Five to ten percent of population over 60 years of age can be affected with the number varying in different geographic areas.

Clinically it is characterized by pain around the hip and the lower limb, at the start of motion in the beginning and growing pain at activity later, even experiencing pain at rest finally. The range of motion becomes restricted in abduction, internal rotation, and finally concentrically as well. Limping arises because of pain, joint stiffness, shortening and muscle insufficiency.

Radiologically narrowing of the joint space, bony spurs, deformity, subchondral sclerosis and cysts are observed.

Osteoarthritis (OA) can arise without any proven cause, as a primary one. Heavy physical labor, excessive sport activity can play a pathogenetic role as it is supposed to. (Figs. 18.19–18.21).

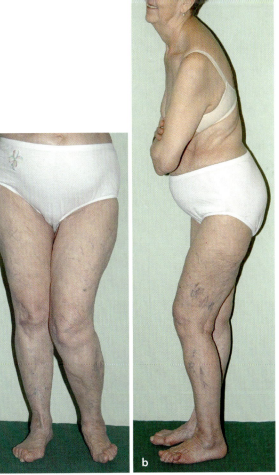
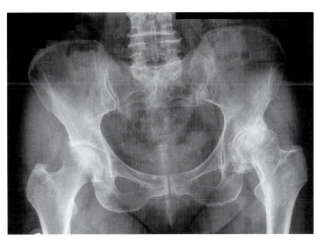

Fig. 18.20 Primary osteoarthritis of the left hip is presented on the radiograph. Note the narrowing of the joint space, the lateral dislocation of the femoral head on the left site due to the central acetabular osteophyte formation

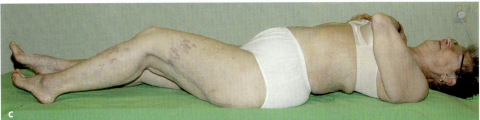
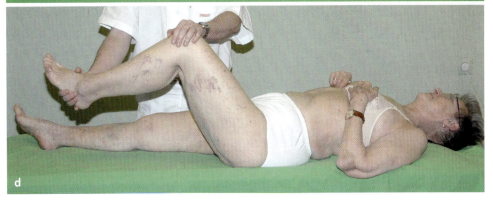

Fig. 18.19 a–d 69-year-old female patient with primary osteoarthritis of the hips (**a**). Note the antalgic posture and adduction and flexion contracture of the left hip (**b**, **c**). Even flexion of the left hip is restricted to 70° (**d**)

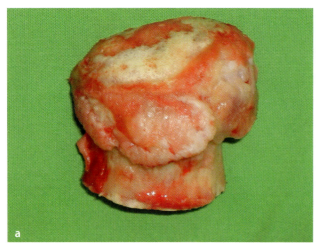

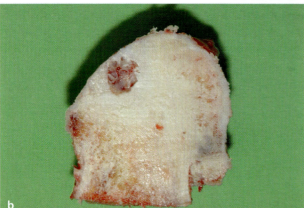

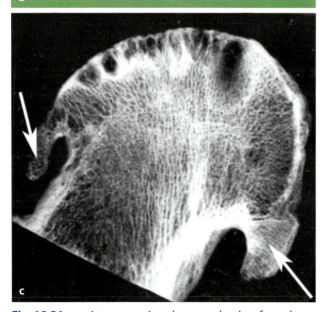

Fig. 18.21 a–c Intraoperative photograph taken from the resected femoral head. Note the eburneated surface and the remnants of cartilage (**a**). On the surface of the specimen subchondral sclerosis and degenerative cysts can be observed (**b**).Radiograph of the surgical specimen. Note the osteophytes around the neck (*arrows*), and the subchondral degenerative cysts (**c**)

18.5.2 Secondary Osteoarthritis of the Hip

Secondary osteoarthritis is caused by previous illnesses and congenital conditions, as congenital hip dysplasia, coxa vara, systemic bone disorders, dysplasias, metabolic diseases, as gout and pseudogout, hematological diseases, as hemophilia, that can lead to deterioration in joint shape, function and cartilage quality as well.

Acquired conditions as M. Perthes, slipped upper femoral epiphysis, inflammation, trauma, tumor, osteonecrosis can also lead to secondary OA of the hip.

Inflammations which can cause OA later on can be of septic, specific and aseptic origin, latter as RA, Bechterew's, SLE or PVS.

Several classifications are described according the dislocation of the femoral head in secondary OA (Figs. 18.22–18.31).

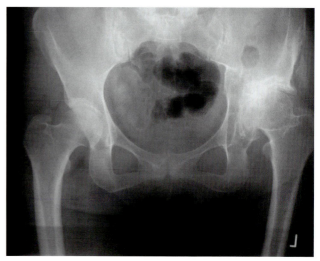

Fig. 18.22 The radiograph reveals a stage 1 dysplastic hip regarding the dislocation of the femur according to Eftekhar's. The femoral head is located in the true acetabulum

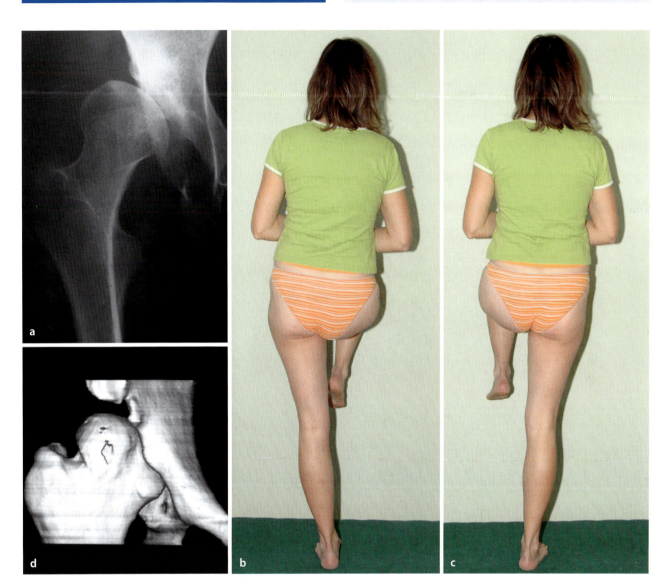

Fig. 18.23 a–d Radiograph of a 30-year-old female patient with Eftekhar's stage 2 dislocation. The centre of the head of the femur is at the level of the acetabular roof. It forms a secondary acetabulum deforming the upper edge of the primary one (**a**). When the patient is standing on her affected side, the left hip sinks because of the insufficient medial gluteal muscles (positive Trendelenburg's test) (**b**). Standing on the healthy limb the opposite pelvic region is moderately elevated by the gluteus medius muscle (negative Trendelenburg's test) (**c**). Eftekhar's stage 2 dislocation is presented on the 3D CT picture (**d**)

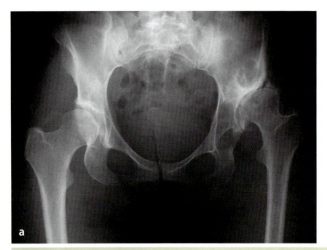

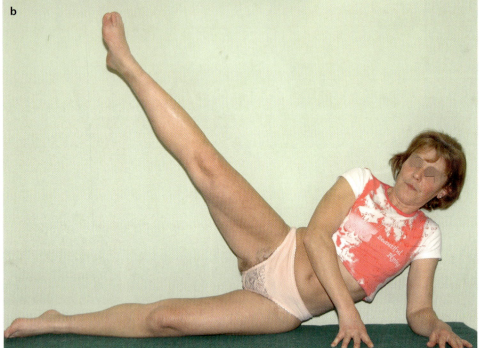

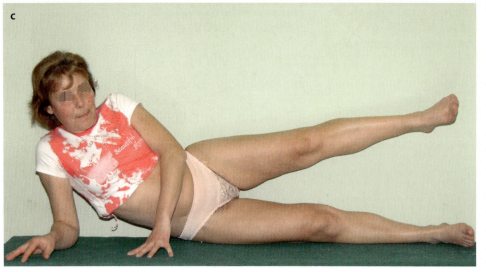

Fig. 18.24 a–c Eftekhar's stage 3 dislocation on the left side. Radiograph shows (**a**) that the deformed femoral head is placed above the level of the primary acetabulum and it formed a secondary acetabulum, on the iliac bone photograph taken from the patient demonstrates that she can normally elevate her right leg (**b**) against the gravitation but not her left one (**c**) due to the weakened abductor muscles and contracture of the adductors

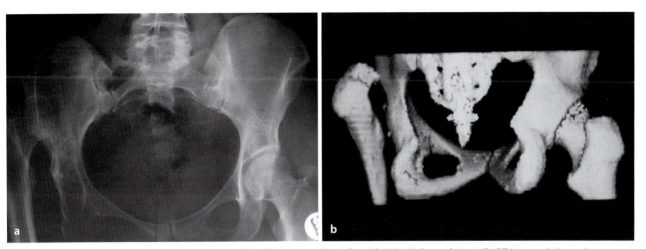

Fig. 18.25 a, b Eftekhar's stage 4 dislocation of the femur on the right side (**a**). With applying 3D CT image, it is easier to understand the localization of the femoral head (**b**)

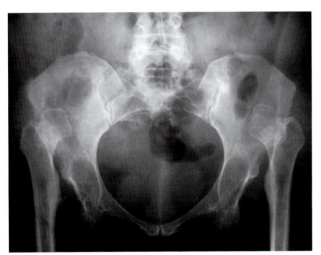

Fig. 18.26 Eftekhar's stage 4 dislocation on both sides. The upwards and posteriorly dislocated femoral heads are supported by the elongated joint capsule and the gluteal muscles

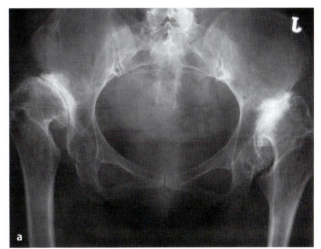

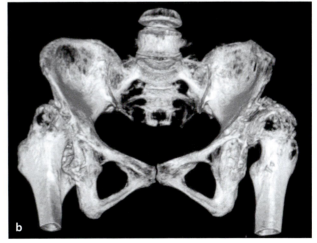

Fig. 18.27 a, b 46-year-old female with secondary osteoarthritis of both hips due to bilateral hip dysplasia (**a**). 3D reconstruction CT picture of the same patient (**b**)

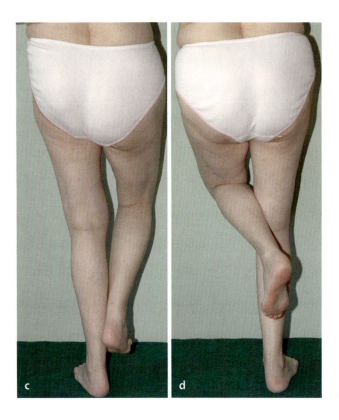

Fig. 18.27 c, d The Trendelenburg's test is positive on both side (**c**, **d**)

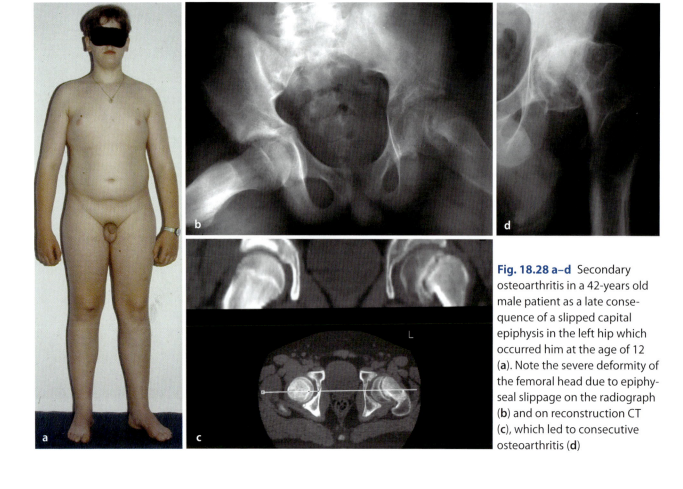

Fig. 18.28 a–d Secondary osteoarthritis in a 42-years old male patient as a late consequence of a slipped capital epiphysis in the left hip which occurred him at the age of 12 (**a**). Note the severe deformity of the femoral head due to epiphyseal slippage on the radiograph (**b**) and on reconstruction CT (**c**), which led to consecutive osteoarthritis (**d**)

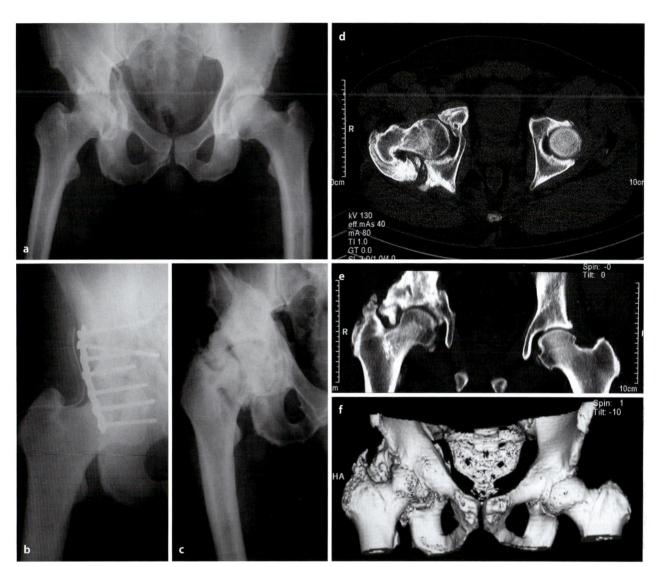

Fig. 18.29 a–f Trauma, as femoral neck fracture, fracture of the acetabulum, central dislocation of the femoral head, damaging the integrity of the joint, lead frequently to secondary osteoarthritis of the hip joint. This 50-year-old female patient had a car accident with an acetabular fracture 16 years ago (**a**), fixed by plate and screws (**b**). The radiograph shows protrusion of the medial wall of the acetabulum and secondary osteoarthritis of the hip joint (**c**). Horizontal (**d**) and vertical (**e**) CT images and 3D CT (**f**) reconstruction of the affected hip joint of the same patient

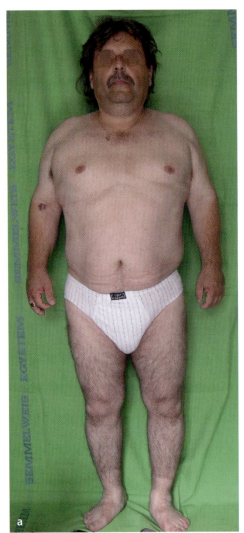

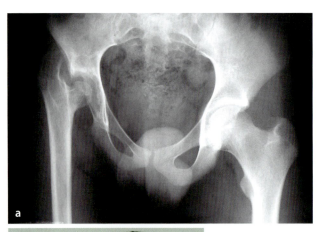

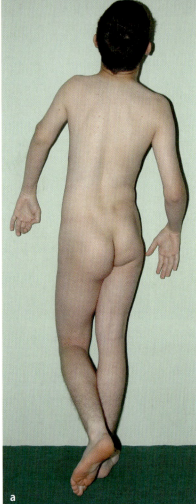

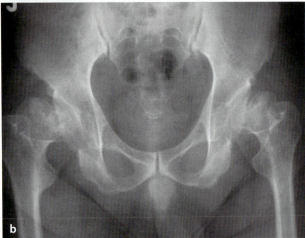

Fig. 18.30 a, b 44-year-old male patient with spondyloepiphyseal dysplasia. Disproportion of the body and shortened extremities are typical (**a**). Maldeveloped hip joint with dislocation of the femora is characteristic for the spondyloepiphyseal dysplasia which caused the secondary osteoarthritis (**b**)

Fig. 18.31 a, b The radiograph of an 18-year-old male who had septic arthritis of the right hip in his childhood. Note the adduction contracture, the small and deformed femoral head, shortened femoral neck and overgrowing of the greater trochanter as a consequence of the septic arthritis (**a**). He has a significant leg length difference and decreased range of motion in the right hip. Note the positive Trendelenburg's test on the right (**b**)

Chapter 19

Knee

Contents

Knee

M. Szendrői, G. Skaliczki and L. Bartha

19.1 Developmental Disorders

19.1.1 Congenital Dislocation of the Knee

Congenital dislocation of the knee is a rare congenital abnormality, due to shortening and fibrosis of the quadriceps muscle, causing muscular imbalance during the prenatal period. Hyperextension of the knee joint evidently manifests itself at birth. In simple cases the hyperextension of the knee with moderate elongation of the cruciate ligaments is observed. In severe cases subluxation or complete dislocation of the tibia is present in relation to the femur with anteriorly displaced hamstring tendons, and elongated cruciate ligaments. Almost half of the cases are with bilateral involvement. Dislocation of the knee can appear as a part of complex orthopedic defects, as club foot, vertical talus, developmental dysplasia of the hip or congenital dislocation of the patella. In Larsen's syndrome the knee dislocation is combined with facial abnormalities.

Congenital dislocation of the knee can also appear in a more variable form, in a part of complex congenital abnormality of the lower extremity. In these cases not the muscular imbalance, but the shortening of the long tubular bones and the ligamentar deficiencies determines the deformation (Figs. 19.1–19.3).

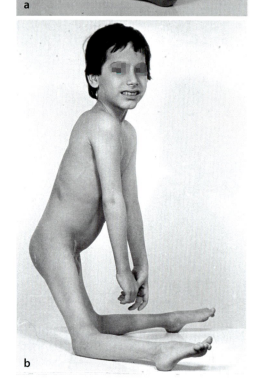

Fig. 19.1 a, b Severe and untreated case of congenital luxation of the knee of a 9-year-old boy. While he was present at our department, he was able to walk on his dislocated knees. (photos from our archives)

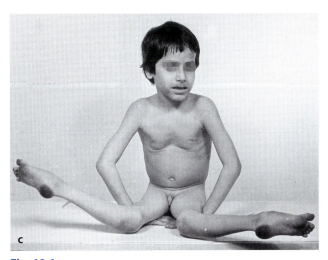

Fig. 19.1 c

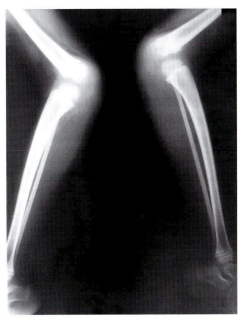

Fig. 19.2 Lateral radiograph of the same patient. The bilateral knee dislocation is well visible, the angle of anterior dislocation is about 90°

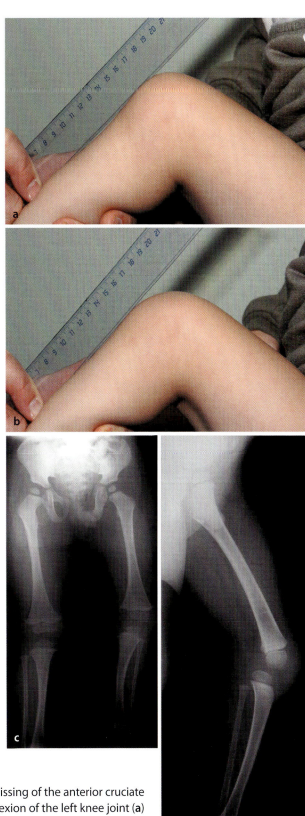

Fig. 19.3 a–d 3-year-old boy with missing of the anterior cruciate ligament (ACL). Photos in 90° of flexion of the left knee joint (**a**) and the possible anteposition of the tibia due to ACL defect. Anteroposterior (**c**) and lateral (**d**) radiographs of the same patient. Note, that the femur and the tibia are also shortened on the left side, and in relaxed position the knee is dislocated posteriorly

19.1.2 Congenital Disorders of the Patella (patella aplasia, bi-, tripartita)

The patellar aplasia or hypoplasia is a very rare disorder. Hypoplastic patella is observed in association with congenital syndrome, for example patella-nail syndrome (See Chap. 1) In case of patella bi- or tripartita, the patella has got multiple (two or three) ossification centers which persist as separate bones even after the end of the growth. The separated and smaller ossification center is generally at the lateral and proximal part of the patella. The congruency of patellar articular surface is intact, the patients are complaint free. It is recognized usually as accidental finding on radiographs taken after knee trauma and it can cause problems in differentiating between a developmental innocent disorder and fracture of patella which latter needs to be operated on (Figs. 19.4 and 19.5).

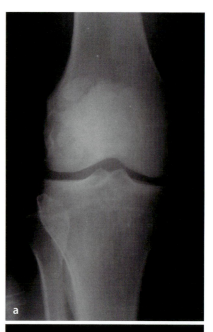
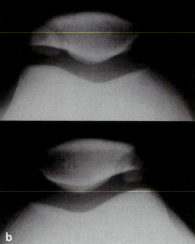

Fig. 19.5 a, b Bilateral patella tripartita presented on a-p (**a**) and sunrise radiographs (**b**)

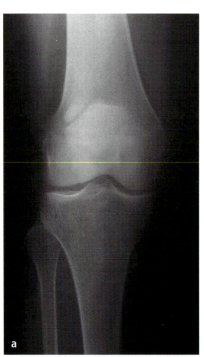

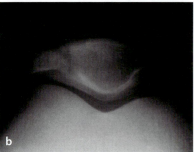

Fig. 19.4 a, b
Patella bipartita
on the right side.
Anteroposterior (**a**)
and sunrise view (**b**)

19.1.3 Congenital Disorders of Fibula (hypoplasia, aplasia)

Fibular hemimelia is the most frequent congenital deficiency of the long bones. Initially it was described as being related to aplasia or hypoplasia of the fibula. Fibular hypoplasia has a variable penetrance, ranging from a minimal shortening of the fibula with an absence of the fifth toe to immediately apparent complete absence of the fibula. Males are affected twice more than females, the disorder being more often unilateral. Fibular hemimelia means rather a total limb involvement, and not just a simple absence of a bone, it is classified as a postaxial hypoplasia of the lower extremity.

Associated abnormalities may include the following: Proximal femoral focal deficiency (PFFD), coxa vara, femoral hypoplasia with external rotation, lateral patella subluxation, hypoplastic lateral femoral condyle, genu valgum with lateral mechanical axis displacement (Figs. 19.6–19.8).

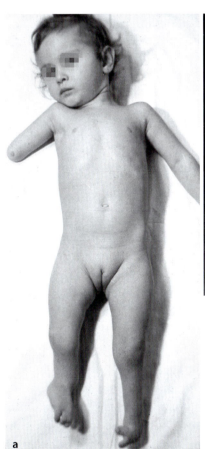
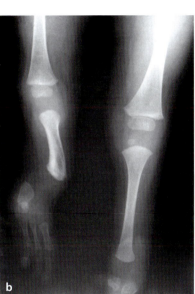

Fig. 19.6 a, b Clinical view (**a**) and radiograph (**b**) of a 4-year-old girl with multiple limb congenital abnormalities from our archives. Bilateral fibular aplasia is well demonstrable on the radiograph. Shortened femur and short and bowed tibia with absence of the fourth and fifth ray is present on the right side. During the fetal period, the fibular field of the limb bud controls the development of the proximal femur, explaining the frequent association of femoral abnormalities

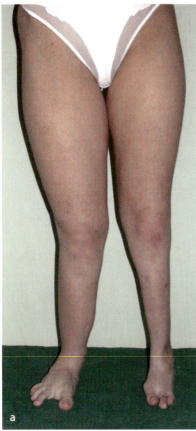

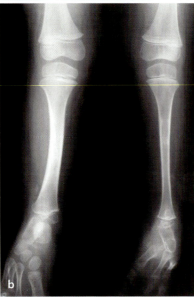

Fig. 19.8 a, b Clinical view (**a**) and radiograph (**b**) of bilateral aplasia of the fibula with shortened tibia and missing of the second ray on the right and the fourth and fifth rays of foot on the left side

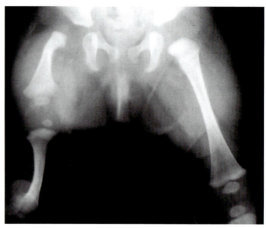

Fig. 19.7 Fibular aplasia associated with PFFD. Typical anteromedial tibial bowing is shown due to abnormal distal tibial epiphysis. Proximal femoral focal deficiency with external rotation and hip dislocation is present on the right, hypoplastic femur on the left side

19.1.4 Congenital Disorders of Tibia (crura vara, tibia aplasia, pseudoarthrosis)

Congenital disorders of tibia are less common than fibular disorders. In most of the cases the etiologic causes are unknown. Variable kinds of deformities are crura vara, tibia hypo- or aplasia with partial- or total absence of the tibia so it is rather a total limb involvement and not just a simple absence of a bone. Pseudoarthrosis of the tibia can be present or incipient at birth. It is a rare malformation involving only 4 in 1,000,000 live births, and this disorder is frequently associated (50–90%) with neurofibromatosis. Classification of Boyd in congenital pseudoarthrosis includes: Anterior bowing and defect present at birth; hourglass constriction at birth; congenital cyst; sclerotic segment with medullar obliteration; dysplastic fibula; presence of neurofibroma or schwannoma. Associated abnormalities may include the following: Proximal femoral focal deficiency, coxa vara, femoral hypoplasia with external rotation, lateral patella subluxation, hypoplastic lateral femoral condyle, genu valgum with lateral mechanical axis displacement, flattened tibial eminence with absent cruciate, shortened and bowed tibia, ankle in valgus position, ball-and-socket ankle, absent tarsal bones, tarsal coalitions, absent foot rays (Figs. 19.9–19.12).

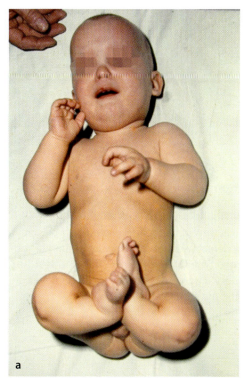

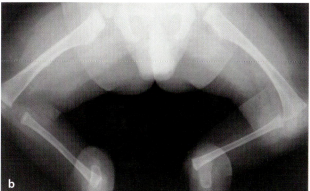

Fig. 19.9 a, b Clinical view (**a**) of a patient and radiograph (**b**) of bilateral tibia aplasia

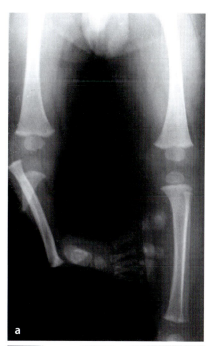

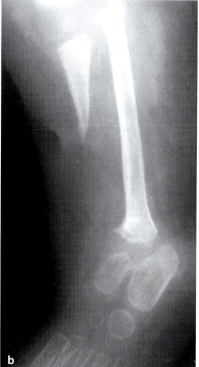

Fig. 19.10 a, b Anteroposterior (**a**) and lateral (**b**) radiographs of a boy with tibia hypoplasia (underdeveloped distal two-third of the long bone) on the right side. Fibular shortening is also present, and in consequence of it the fibula is extremely thickened

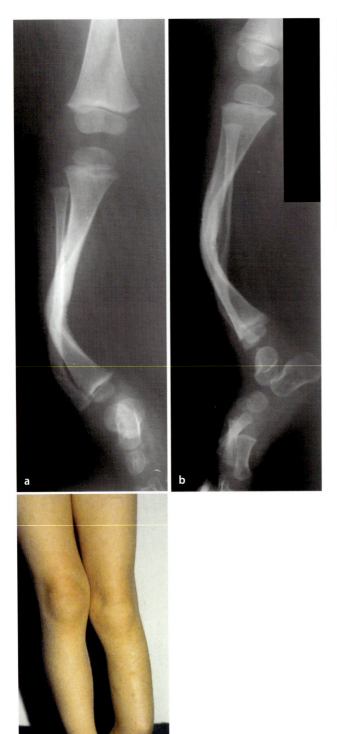

Fig. 19.11 Clinical view of congenital pseudoarthrosis: at birth presenting defect with anterior bowing of the tibia on the right side (Boyd type I.) of a newborn. The pseudoarthrosis may be manifest in adolescence as an incorrect development of one of the main bone articulations

Fig. 19.12 a–c Anteroposterior (**a**) and lateral (**b**) radiographs and clinical view (**c**) of a boy with crus varum on the left side

19.2 Deformities

19.2.1 Genu Varum

Genu varum –called also "bow leg"– is defined as a malalignment that doesn't reach the normal 7–10° femorotibial valgus angulation. It is a commonly occurring deformity in childhood which is gradually corrected spontaneously. Adolescent idiopathic genu varum may be familial, or it may occur sporadically. Secondary varus deformity can develop because of different reasons: injury or any other disease, as femoral or tibial condyle fractures, spontaneous osteonecrosis of the medial femoral condyle. Growth disorder of epiphyseal plate because of osteomyelitis or dyschondroplasia, osteitis deformans and osteomalacia can also cause varus knee deformity. In these cases anterior and medial knee pain is common.

Severe varus deformity can lead to early osteoarthritis of the knee due to the overload of the medial compartment.

Blount's disease (tibia vara epiphysarea) is caused by the abnormal ossification of the medial part of the proximal tibial physis. The deformity is progressive, causing varus angulation in the proximal metaphyseal region of the tibia, due to irreversible growth disturbances of the subjecent physis at the medial portion of the proximal tibial epiphysis. It is thought that the etiology of Blount's disease is a biomechanical overload of the proximal tibial physis due to static varus alignment and excessive compressive forces on the proximal medial metaphysis of the tibia inducing a disruption in the normal endochondral bone formation. This disease can occur in growing children aged 2–10 years. The occurrence is approximately 7 of 100,000 children, predominantly in males, but obese and black population have a greater risk (Figs. 19.13–19.16).

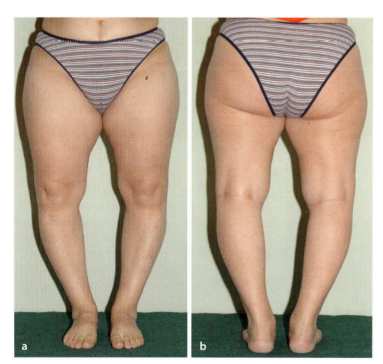

Fig. 19.13 a, b Anterior (**a**) and posterior (**b**) view of typical adolescent idiopathic genu varum

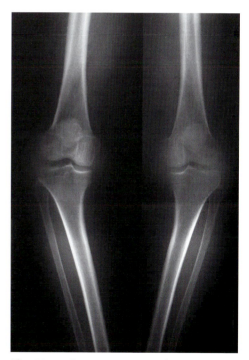

Fig. 19.14 Anteroposterior radiograph of genu varum deformity in the previous patient

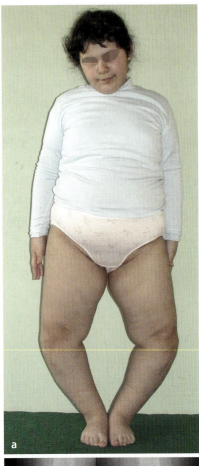

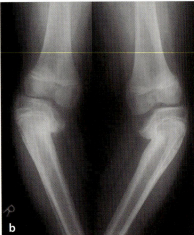

Fig. 19.15 a, b Blount's disease. Abnormal growth of the proximal medial physis, epiphysis, and metaphysis of the tibia results in a progressive varus deformity below the knee. Anterior clinical view (**a**) and radiograph (**b**) of an 8-year-old girl with Blount's disease. Note the closed growing plate on the medial sides

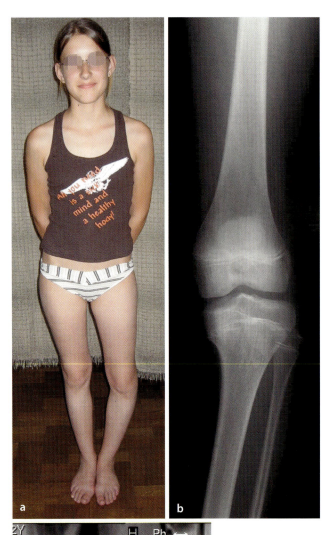

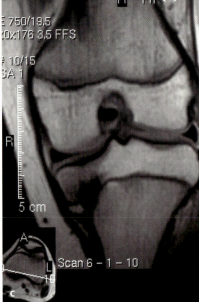

Fig. 19.16 a–c Secondary varus deformity of the left knee is presented (**a**) due to an injury of the growing plate in the childhood of this girl. The axial malalignment of the knee is well demonstrated on the radiograph (**b**) and also the partial closure of the medial physis is shown on the MR picture (**c**)

19.2.2 Genu Valgum

Genu valgum – called also "knock knee"– is defined as a malalignment that exceeds the normal 7–10° femorotibial valgus angulation. It's a commonly occurring deformity in childhood which is gradually corrected spontaneously. Adolescent idiopathic genu valgum may be familial, or it may occur sporadically. This deformity could be the result of a dysplastic lateral femoral condyle that contributes to over-loading of the lateral compartment of the knee and subsequent bone and cartilage destruction. Secondary genu valgum develops due to injury or any other disease, as femoral or tibial condyle fractures, spontaneous osteonecrosis of the femoral condyle, primary or secondary osteoarthritis. Damage and early closure of the lateral part of the epiphyseal plate because of osteomyelitis or dyschondroplasia, osteitis deformans and osteomalacia are rare causes of valgus knee deformity. In these cases anterior and medial knee pain is common. These symptoms reflect the pathologic strain on the knee and its patellofemoral extensor mechanism (Figs. 19.17–19.19).

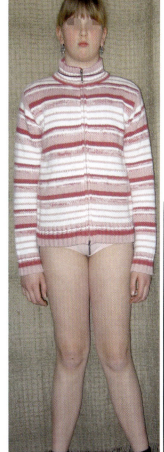
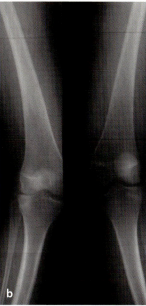

Fig. 19.17 a, b Anterior view of a valgus deformity of the knees of a 14-year-old girl (**a**) and her radiograph (**b**), in weight-bearing standing position

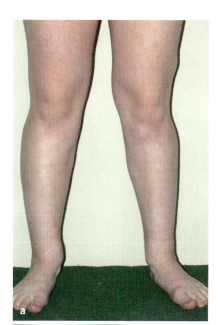
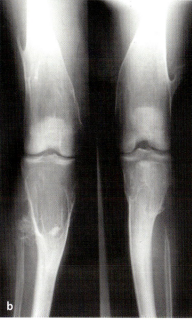

Fig. 19.18 a, b Anterior view (**a**) and anteroposterior radiograph (**b**) of a bilateral secondary genu valgum, due to multiple exostoses

19.2.3 Genu Recurvatum

In case of genu recurvatum the extensibility of the knee joint is more than 10°. In the congenital form of this deformity the tibial plateau inclines anteriorly. Idiopathic genu recurvatum may present due to irregular weight bearing and weakness of the dorsal joint capsule of the knee. This deformity could also be the result of trauma, when the ventral part of the tibial growth plate is destroyed. Genu recurvatum may occur compensatorically in neuromuscular diseases (e.g., Heine–Medin disease or secondary iatrogenic events) (Fig. 19.20).

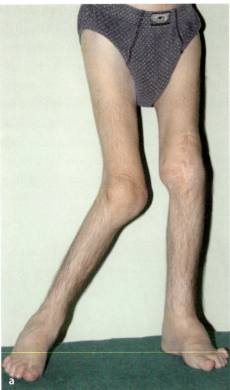

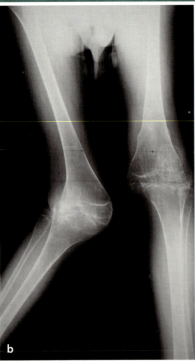

Fig. 19.19 a, b Anterior clinical view of a patient with juvenile chronic arthritis (**a**) and radiograph (**b**) of secondary genu valgum on the right site. The left knee is already fused. Often genu valgum is observed in association with outward torsion of the femur, tibia, or both. Look for retropatellar crepitus and tenderness and note a patellar tilt, tracking, and stability

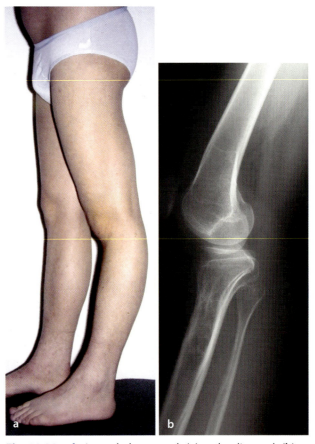

Fig. 19.20 a, b Lateral photograph (**a**) and radiograph (**b**) of an 18-year-old boy with genu recurvatum at the left side. Trauma by traffic accident caused an early closure of the ventral epiphyseal part in his childhood

19.3 Meniscal Lesions

19.3.1 Meniscal Cyst

Meniscal cysts arise spontaneously, due to degenerative changes in the intrameniscal mesenchymal cells, but also often there is a history of previous injury. The lateral meniscus is affected seven times more often then the medial one. Especially young adults (between age 20 and 40), complain of painful swelling at the level of lateral (or medial) knee joint gap usually anteriorly to the collateral ligament (Figs. 19.21–19.23).

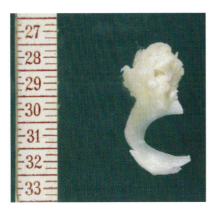

Fig. 19.21 Excised meniscus with meniscal cyst

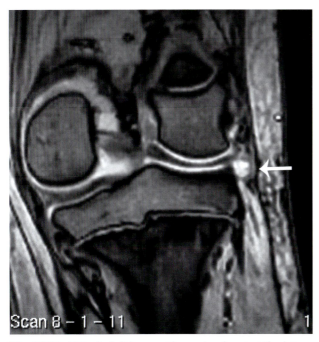

Fig. 19.22 MRI of a left knee with meniscal cyst at the lateral compartment (*arrow*)

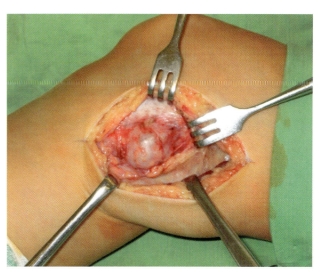

Fig. 19.23 Intraoperative picture of a meniscal cyst in a 25-year-old woman

19.3.2 Discoid Meniscus

Discoid meniscus is a developmental anomaly of the menisci that usually affects the lateral meniscus. Discoid lateral meniscus is presented in the normal population at a rate of 1.5–3%, the incidence is higher in the Asian population. Based on its coverage to the tibial plateau it can be classified as complete and incomplete types, also stable and unstable forms can be differentiated. The most common symptoms are pain, giving way, joint effusion or snapping phenomenon (Figs. 19.24–19.26).

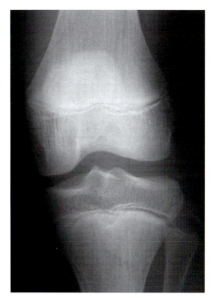

Fig. 19.24 The widened lateral tibiofemoral joint space refers to a lateral discoid meniscus

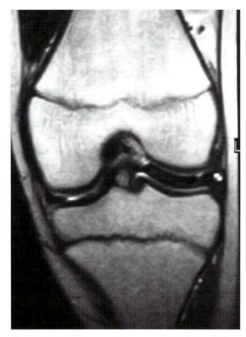

Fig. 19.25 MR reveals a complete lateral discoid meniscus covering the whole tibial plateau

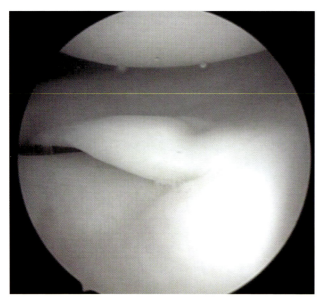

Fig. 19.26 Arthroscopic view of an incomplete lateral discoid meniscus, that leaves only a small portion of the tibial joint surface uncovered

19.3.3 Meniscal Tear

Being anchored to the capsule tighter, the medial meniscus has less mobility than the lateral one, provoking a greater risk for ruptures. Meniscal tears can occur as acute injuries with a history of an adequate trauma (most commonly twisting), or they can be presented as a degenerative rupture usually without any memorable violent event. Intermittent pain at the joint line and swelling are the most frequent symptoms; depending on the size and the pattern of the tear where the knee can become "locked" in a bent position (Figs. 19.27–19.32).

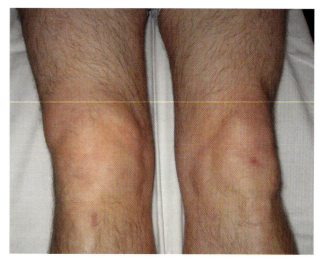

Fig. 19.27 Swollen knee joint after a previous twisting sport injury. At arthroscopy a medial meniscal tear was found

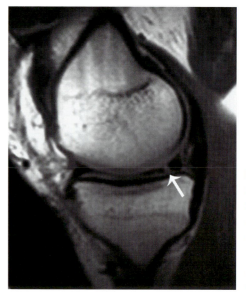

Fig. 19.28 Posterior horn tear of the medial meniscus. The *arrow* points to the tear

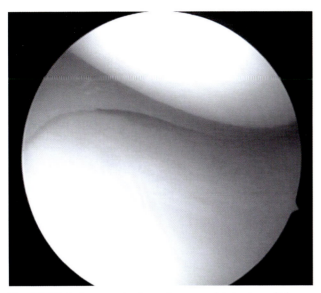

Fig. 19.29 Arthroscopic view of a normal, intact medial meniscus

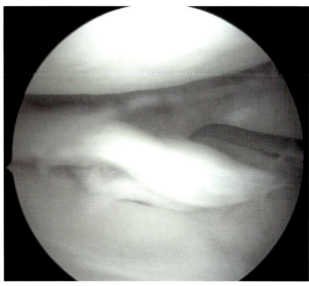

Fig. 19.31 Ruptured medial meniscus, showing a posterior tag, one of the most common varieties of meniscus rupture

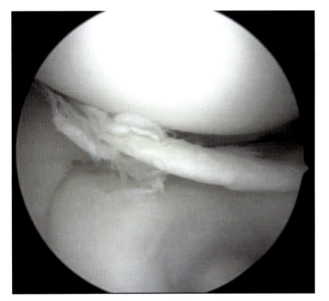

Fig. 19.30 Posterior horn tear of the medial meniscus

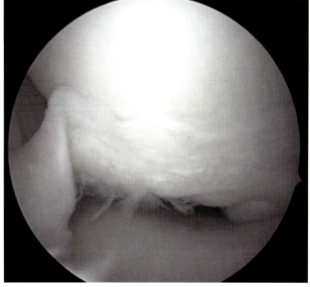

Fig. 19.32 "Bucket-handle" tear of the medial meniscus, the torn part is dislocated anteromedially locking the knee in flexion

19.4 Cysts Around the Knee

19.4.1 Baker Cyst

Baker cyst –also called "popliteal cyst"– is the most common synovial cyst in the popliteal fossa resulting from fluid distension of the gastrocnemio–semimembranosus bursa. It may serve as a protective mechanism for the knee. Intrinsic intraarticular disorders cause joint effusion. The knee effusion is displaced into the Baker cyst, thus reducing potentially destructive pressure in the joint space. Two types of Baker cysts may form:

A primary or idiopathic cyst has a valvular connection with the joint cavity. Idiopathic cysts usually are seen in young patients without symptoms. Cyst contents usually are viscous.

A secondary or symptomatic cyst communicates freely with the knee joint and contains synovial fluid of normal viscosity, and it reveals the underlying articular disorders, as osteoarthritis, rheumatoid or psoriatic arthritis, meniscal tears, and patella chondromalacia (Figs. 19.33 and 19.34).

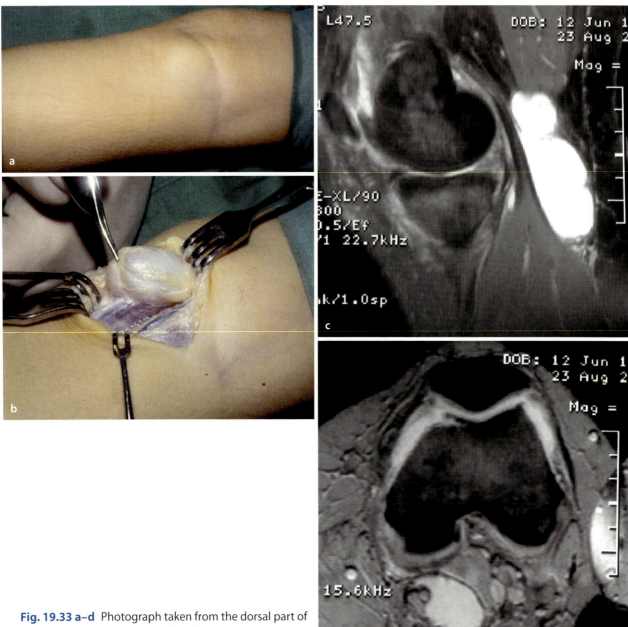

Fig. 19.33 a–d Photograph taken from the dorsal part of the knee (**a**) and intraoperative (**b**) pictures of a primary Baker-cyst exstirpation from the popliteal fossa of a 16-year-old girl. Lateral (**c**) and horizontal (**d**) MR picture of a Baker cyst

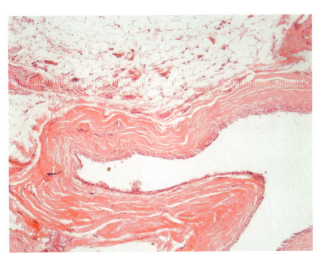

Fig. 19.34 Histologic picture of a Baker's cyst: thick septum consisting of connective tissue rich in collagen fibers lined by synovial cell layer

19.4.2 Ganglion

Ganglions consist of thin-walled sacs filled with glary viscous fluid, and the fibrous wall is usually connected with the tendons of the extensor muscles that originate from the fibular head. The knee joint is the fourth most common region for ganglion formation, after wrist, hand and foot. The diameter of this ganglion is up to 5 cm. Clinically it appears as a firm tense subcutaneous mass (Figs. 19.35–19.38).

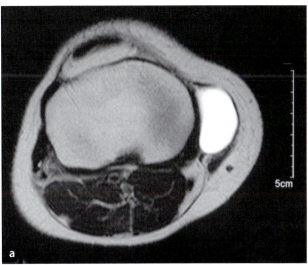

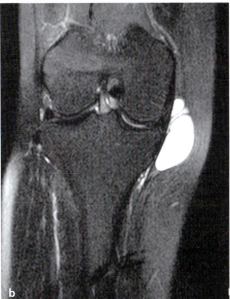

Fig. 19.36 a, b Horizontal (**a**) and frontal (**b**) MRI pictures of the right knee of the same patient, with a well remarkable sac filled with fluid

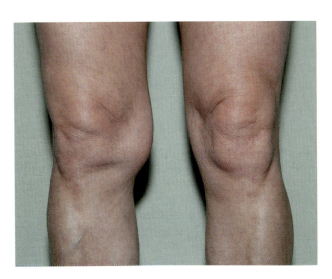

Fig. 19.35 Anterior view of the knees of a 41-year-old woman. Protruding, tense subcutaneous ganglion is present at the medial side of the right knee

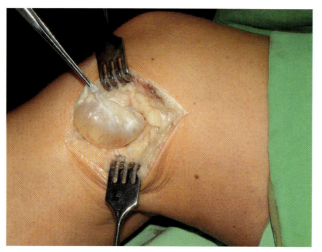

Fig. 19.37 Intraoperative picture at excision of the ganglion

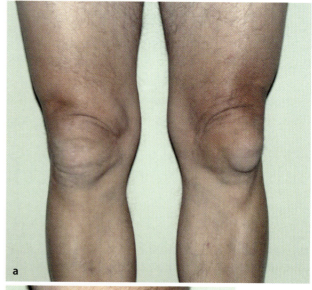

a

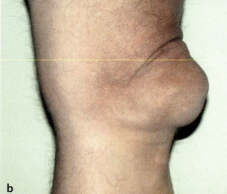

b

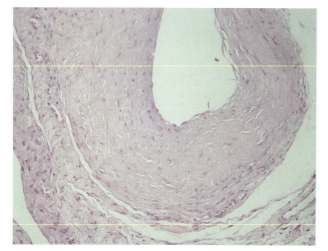

Fig. 19.38 Photomicrograph demonstrates the wall of a ganglion: mature mesenchymal cells and collagen fibers form the septum which is lined inside by flattened thin cells

19.4.3 Bursitis Prepatellaris

The prepatellar bursa is located in front of the proximal part of the patellar tendon and the distal half of the patella. Two types of prepatellar bursitis are known. The knee joint is unaffected in both forms. The most common is the irritative bursitis due to repeated friction. The demarcated softly fluctuant swelling in front of the distal part of patella is seen with the fibrous thickening of the wall of the serous fluid distended bursa.

The suppurative form of this bursa is caused by pyogenic infection. Behind the hot and reddened skin the bursa is distended by the pus (Fig. 19.39).

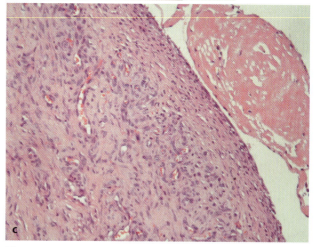

c

Fig. 19.39 a–c Anteroposterior (**a**) and lateral (**b**) view of an irritative prepatellar bursitis of the left knee of a 44-year-old man. Note that the prepatellar bursa is distended, but the knee joint is unaffected (**b**). Histological picture of the inflamed bursa: thick wall consisted of inflammatory and mesenchymal cells and connective tissue rich in small vessels. The cavity is lined by synovial cells. Eosinophil stained amorph mass of fibrin is attached to the wall (**c**)

19.5 Contractures of the Knee

The knee *contracture in extension* is defined as the limited motion in flexion, and the *contracture in flexion* is defined as the limited motion in extension. The origin of the contracture can be a muscular disease, or an innervation defect, or shrinkage of the joint capsule, ligaments and skin. Arthrofibrosis (fibrous ankylosis) can occur after surgical intervention. The origin of the congenital form of knee contracture in extension –where the quadriceps femoris muscle is partially or totally shortened– is not known, but is frequently accompanied by other developmental disorders. Intramuscular injections –especially antibiotics to the vastus lateralis and vastus intermedius muscles– in childhood, can cause shrinkage. In these cases patients walk with abducted and externally rotated hip, without knee flexion. In infantile cerebral paresis the flexion contractures of the knees are common, due to spasm of knee flexors (Figs. 19.40 and 19.41).

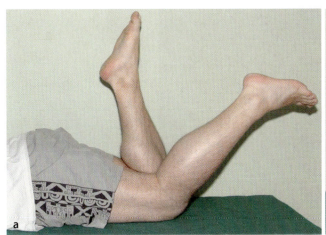
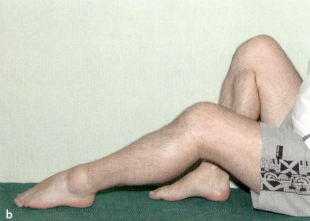

Fig. 19.40 a, b Contracture of the knee in extension: Clinical view of a patient in a lying position (**a**) and in sitting position (**b**) with knee contracture in extension in left side, due to shrinkage of joint capsule and ligaments

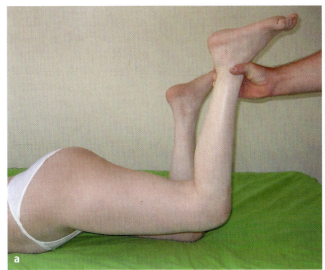
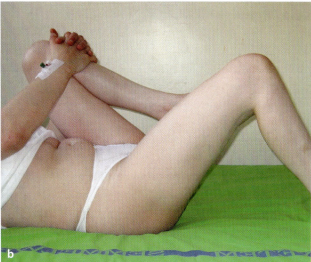

Fig. 19.41 a, b Contracture of the knee in flexion: 110° of flexion contracture of knees and 50° of flexion contractures of hip joints of a 46-year-old female. The alcoholic patient was using a wheel chair for a year, and during this period a progressive hip and knee contracture developed. The patient in supine (**a**) and prone (**b**) position: note, there is limited motion in knee joints (between 70 and 90°)

19.6 Dislocation of the Patella

19.6.1 Congenital Dislocation of Patella

The lateral dislocation of the kneecap is persistent and irreducible, representing a complex abnormality of the joint and quadriceps mechanism, often familial and bilateral. The patella often shows abnormal appearance. Lack of ossification of the patella before the age of 4 makes early diagnosis difficult. Without treatment, flexion, valgus, external rotation deformity of the knee develops. Early surgery is beneficial (Fig. 19.42).

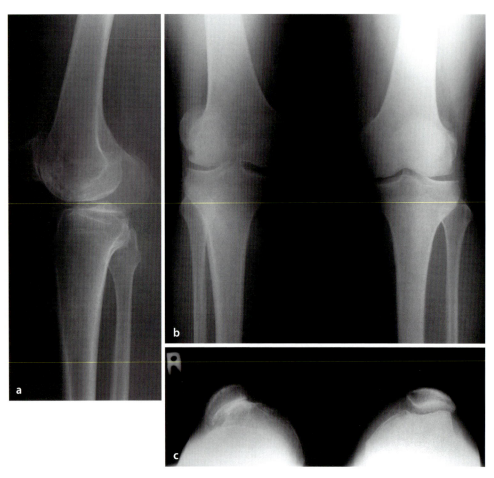

Fig. 19.42 a–c Congenital luxation of patella at the right side in a middle aged patient: lateral radiograph (**a**), and antero–posterior radiograph present a laterally displaced patella (**b**). Axial radiograph (**c**) shows the right patella dislocated laterally from the intercondylar fossa of the femur

19.6.2 Habitual Dislocation of Patella

The term is used when every knee flexion results in lateral dislocation of the patella. This condition becomes apparent usually in early childhood. Habitual dislocation of the patella is the result of quadriceps muscle contracture, very often as a consequence of intramuscular injections. Clinical findings include painless limitation of knee flexion, abnormal skin creases over the knees, dimple over the area of fibrosis. Without treatment, the normal development of the knee might become impaired, leading to flat femoral condyles, hypoplasia of the patella, genu recurvatum and other severe degenerative changes (Fig. 19.43).

19.6.3 Recurrent Dislocation of the Patella

The initial dislocation of the patella can be a result of a more or less severe trauma, but underlying anatomical abnormalities predisposes the kneecap to further dislocation or subluxation. As the pull of the quadriceps mechanism is lateral compared to the axis of the patellar tendon (Q- angle), static and dynamic factors need to stabilize the patella to maintain normal tracking. Thus, impaired function of the vastus medialis oblique muscle (dynamic stabilizer), under-development (lateral flattening) of the lateral femoral condyle, hypoplasia of the patella, shallow intercondylar groove, patella alta, general ligamentous laxity and weak medial capsule predispose the patella to recurrent dislocation (Figs. 19.44–19.49).

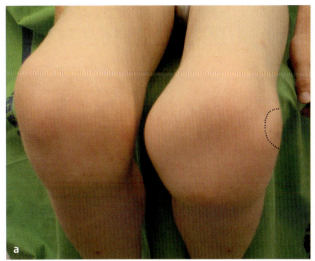

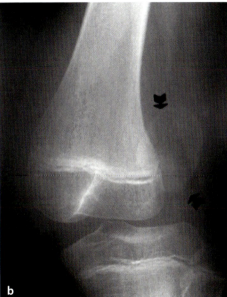

Fig. 19.43 a, b Knee flexion results in the lateral dislocation of the patella in a patient with habitual dislocation of the patella, as presented in the patient's photo (*dotted line* outlines the patella) (a), and radiograph (b, *arrows*)

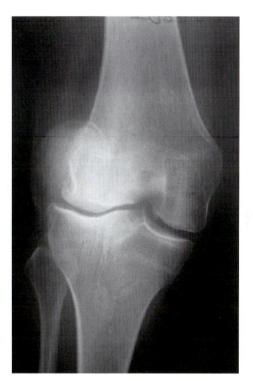

Fig. 19.44 Picture of the dislocated patella with moderate arthritis at the lateral compartment of the right knee

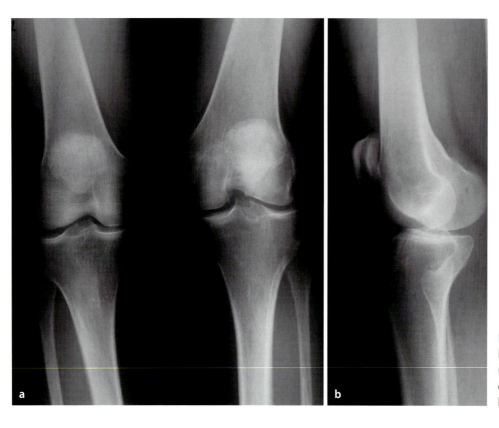

Fig. 19.45 a, b Abnormally high position of the patella (patella alta) with lateral displacement reflects a ligamentous laxity

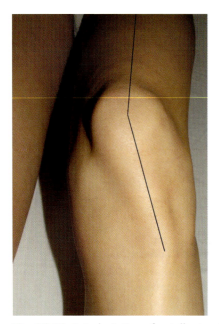

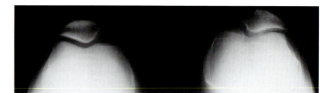

Fig. 19.47 Shallow patellofemoral articular groove and laterally displaced patella on the left side

Fig. 19.46 Axis deviation of patellar tendon due to the laterally displaced tibial tuberositas

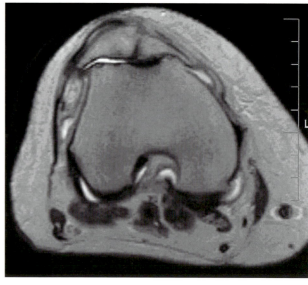

Fig. 19.48 MRI picture reveals the hypoplasia of femoral condyles and patella bipartita

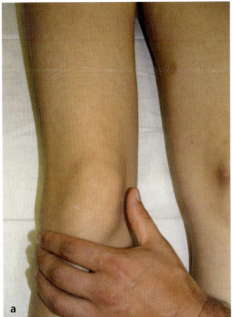

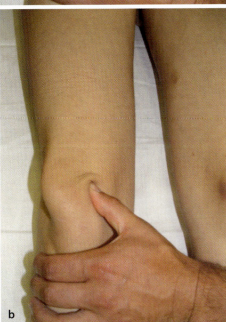

Fig. 19.49 a, b Ligamentous laxity with weak medial capsule predisposes the patella to recurrent dislocation

19.7 Rupture and Insufficiency of Ligaments

19.7.1 Rupture of the Anterior Cruciate Ligament

The anterior cruciate ligament (ACL) plays an immensely important role in the stabilization of the knee restraining the anterior translation of the tibia, preventing hyperextension of the knee, stabilizing the knee against valgus forces and restraining tibial rotation. Besides the aforementioned mechanical functions, the ACL is also very important in terms of giving proprioceptive feedback to the knee.

Most commonly patients presented with a torn ACL have a history of a twisting or hyper- extensive traumatic force during sport activity (soccer, skiing, football, etc.), usually followed by immediate pain and swelling of the joint. It is widely accepted, that ACL rupture is frequently accompanied by meniscal tears, and in the most severe cases ACL tears along with the medial collateral ligament and the medial meniscus bringing on the so called "unhappy triad" (Figs. 19.50–19.53).

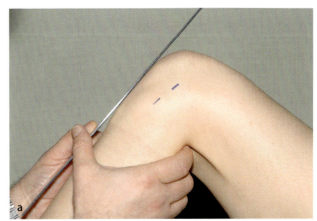

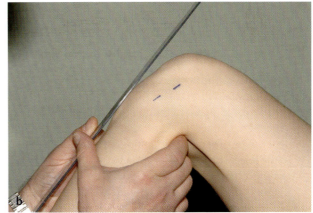

Fig. 19.50 a, b Positive anterior drawer test of a patient with rupture of the ACL. There is no abnormality seen with the knee in flexion at rest (**a**). Anterior translation of the tibia can be observed (positive drawer sign) when the ACL is ruptured (**b**)

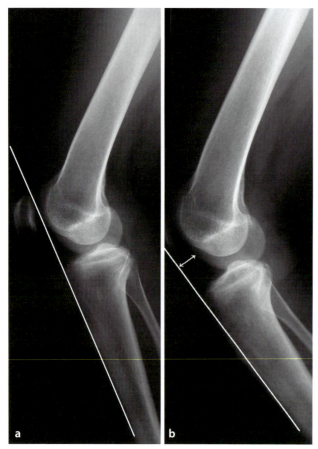

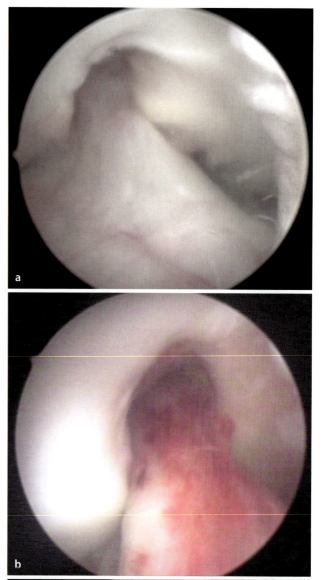

Fig. 19.51 a, b Lateral view radiograph of a patient with complete ACL rupture. The white line represents the anterior border of the tibia: normal position at rest (**a**) and excessive anterior translation (**b**) refers to the ACL rupture

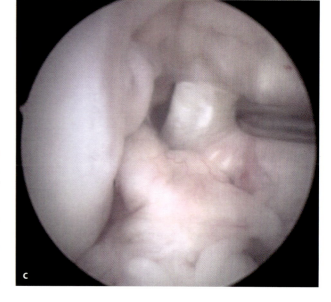

Fig. 19.52 a–c The normal appearance of an intact ACL at arthroscopy (**a**). Acute partial ACL tear is demonstrated on this arthroscopic picture: although the synovial envelope of the ligament is intact, haematoma and thinning of the ligament can be observed at its femoral attachment referring to the injury (**b**). Arthroscopic view of a chronic total ACL tear: the intercondylar notch is empty, only the thickened torn end of the ACL can be seen at its tibial origin. The arthroscopic hook shows the intact PCL (**c**)

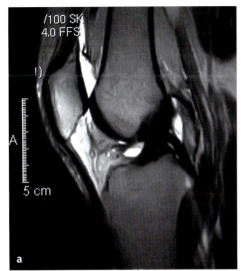

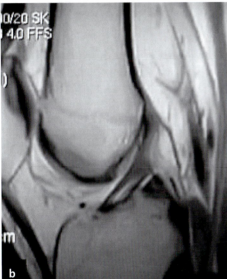

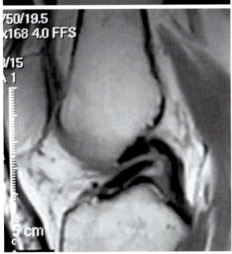

Fig. 19.53 a–c Sagittal MRI picture of the normal ACL (**a**). The oval bright area at the tibial origin of ACL refers to a partial tear (**b**). At a fresh and complete rupture the detachment of the femoral origin of the ACL is seen (**c**)

19.7.2 Chronic Collateral Ligament Insufficiency

The most common cause of chronic collateral ligament instability is a previous sport injury, however osteoarthritis, inflammatory arthritis or infections can also end up in ligament insufficiency. As the stabilizing structures of the knee form a complex structure, isolated medial or lateral collateral deficiencies are rare. The medial collateral ligament tends to get damaged together with the anterior cruciate ligament and the medial meniscus ("unhappy triad") or even with the medial capsule in the most severe cases. The lateral collateral ligament is usually hurt along with the posterolateral complex, the posterior cruciate ligament or in association with the anterior and the posterior cruciate ligament. Neuromuscular diseases like poliomyelitis in childhood can also lead to ligament insufficiency and secondary deformities in the knee (Figs. 19.54 and 19.55).

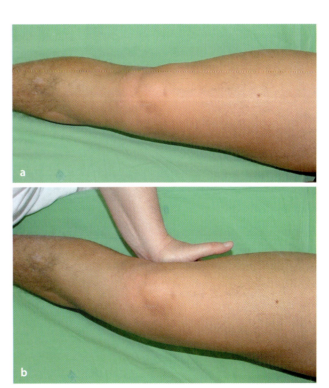

Fig. 19.54 a, b Medial collateral insufficiency due to a previous sport injury. In relaxed position the alignment of the knee is normal (**a**), lateral forces however "open" the knee joint (**b**)

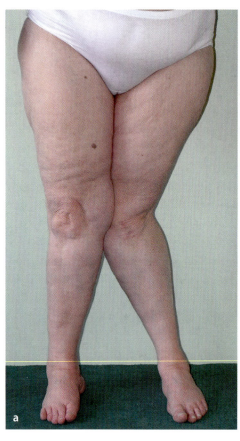

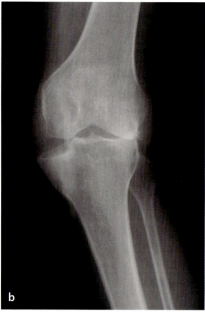

Fig. 19.55 a, b Triple deformity of the knee is seen as a consequence of muscle imbalance in a patient with Heine–Medin disease on the left side. The three deformities are severe valgus, posterior subluxation and external rotation. Requisites for these severe deformities are the laxity of the medial collateral ligament, weakening of the medial and posteromedial part of the joint capsule and the anterior and posterior cruciate ligaments (**a**). AP radiograph of the same patient showing opening of the medial tibiofemoral compartment (**b**)

19.8 Patellofemoral Disorders

Anterior knee pain commonly originates from the patellofemoral joint. Cartilage diseases (chondropathy, osteochondritis dissecans), anatomical variations (patella alta, patella baja, increased Q-angle), maltracking of the patella (subluxation, dislocation), patellar hyperpression or patellofemoral osteoarthritis can all be associated with almost the same symptoms (Figs. 19.56–19.59).

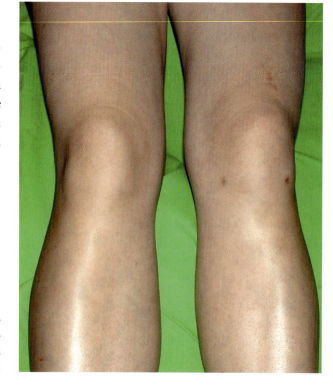

Fig. 19.56 The patient has patellar hyperpression syndrome on the left side, which caused patellar chondropathy. The muscles on the affected thigh are atrophized, the patella is lateralized

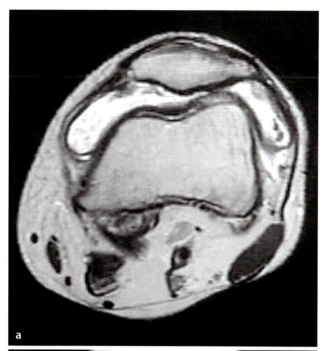

a

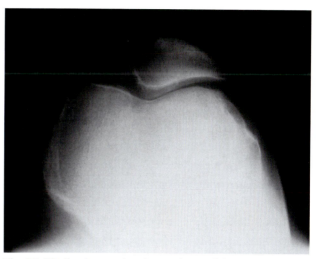

Fig. 19.58 On the sunrise view radiograph laterally tilted patella can be observed with a narrowed joint space between the lateral facet and the femoral groove due to patellar hypertension

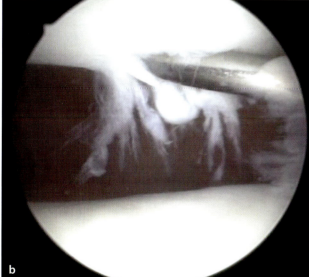

b

Fig. 19.57 a, b MRI presents patellar chondropathy (Outerbridge grade 2) with excessive amount of synovial fluid in the parapatellar pouch (**a**) On arthroscopic examination fibrous changes are visible on the cartilage surface and the arthroscopic probe can be placed into the fissures of the damaged cartilage. (**b**)

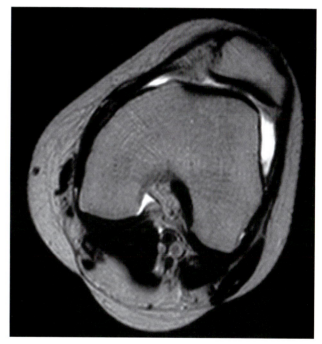

Fig. 19.59 MRI image of the same patient showing the laterally subluxated patella due to shrinkage of the lateral capsule (hyperpression). The increased amount of synovial fluid in the parapatellar pouches refers to the disorder

19.9 Primary Osteoarthritis of the Knee

Knee osteoarthritis is one of the most common disorders among the degenerative diseases of the large weight-bearing joints. Osteoarthritis deteriorates along with the changes of cartilage, the bone and the synovial membrane, furthermore the disease affects the capsule the adjacent muscles and tendons as well. At the end stage of the disorder the typical radiological appearance consists of serious narrowing of the joint space, massive osteophyte and osteoarthritic cyst formation, axis deviation, subchondral sclerosis, osteoporosis due to inactivity and incongruent articular surfaces. From the functional point of view painfully decreased range of movement, contractures, muscle atrophy, stiffness, joint effusion and crepitation dominate the disorder (Figs. 19.60–19.69).

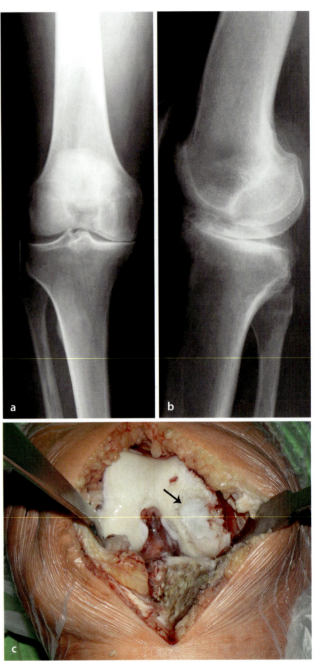

Fig. 19.61 a–c Unicompartmental osteoarthritis of the knee affecting the medial side. (**a**) The lateral and patellofemoral compartments (**b**) are intact. Due to joint space narrowing on the medial side varus deformity of the knee can be observed. Absence of hyaline cartilage on the medial femoral condyle (*black arrow*) (**c**). The lateral and patellofemoral compartments have an almost intact cartilage coverage

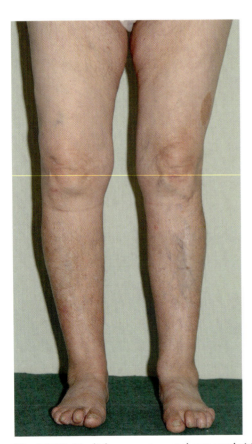

Fig. 19.60 Medial compartmental osteoarthritis of the knee on the right side results in swelling of the affected knee. Due to medial cartilage destruction slight varus deformity can be observed

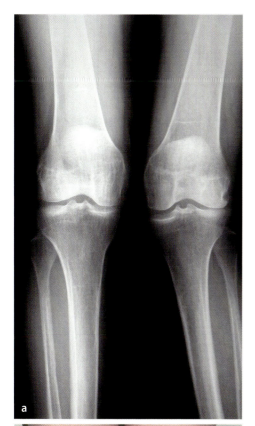

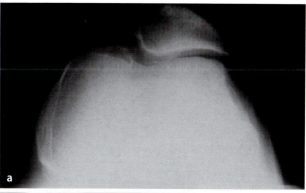

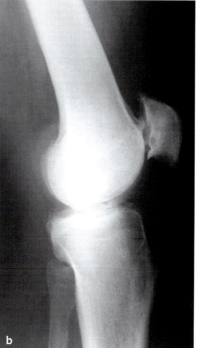

Fig. 19.63 a, b Narrowed joint space with bony spurs refers to osteoarthritic patellofemoral changes on the sunrise view (**a**) and on the lateral view (**b**) radiograph

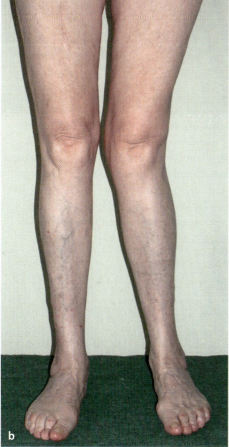

Fig. 19.62 a, b Osteoarthrosis of the lateral compartment of the left knee (**a**). Due to the unicompartmental degenerative process, notable valgus deformity is observed (**b**)

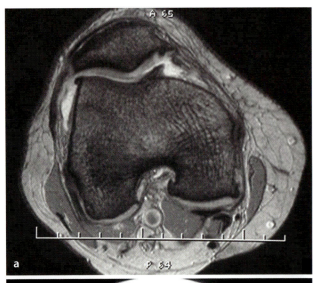

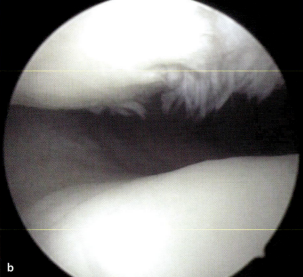

Fig. 19.64 a, b Osteoarthritis of the patellofemoral joint with osteophyte formation is seen on MR picture (**a**). The arthroscopic view reveals absence of hyaline cartilage on the patellar articular surface (**b**)

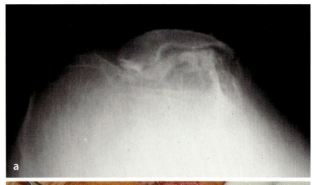

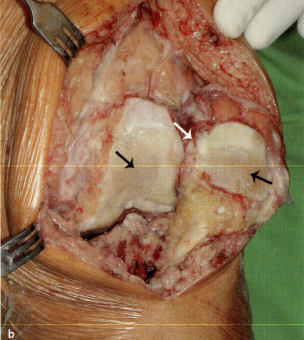

Fig. 19.65 a ,b Severe patellofemoral osteoarthritis: the joint space disappears, subchondral sclerosis and osteophytes can be observed along with irregularity of the articular surface (**a**).Intraoperative picture: remnants of normal cartilage is present on the upper part of patella and femoral intercondylar surface. More distally the hyaline cartilage is destroyed (*black arrows*). Osteophyte formation can be observed on the patella (*white arrow*, **b**)

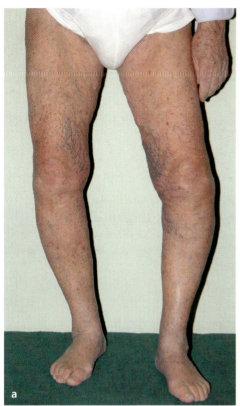

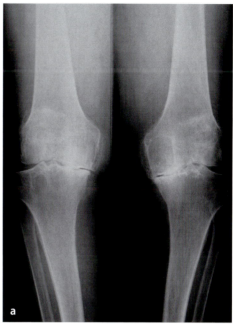

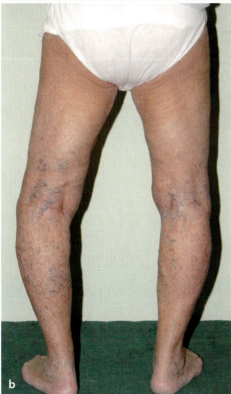

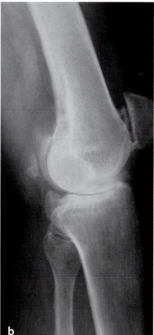

Fig. 19.67 a, b AP and lateral view radiographs of the knee of the previous patient. The joint has a varus deformity (**a**). Massive osteophyte formation can be observed both on the medial end lateral tibiofemoral, and both in the patellofemoral joint (**b**). The joint space on the medial side is seriously narrowed

Fig. 19.66 a, b Patient presented with primary osteoarthrosis of the knee. Swelling of the knee along with varus deformity can be observed referring to a seriously affected medial tibiofemoral compartment

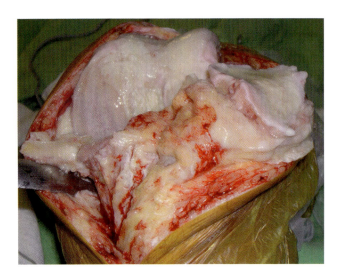

Fig. 19.68 Intraoperative picture of a severe knee osteo-arthritis: seriously damaged patellar surface with massive osteophytes and complete absence of the cartilage. Heavy osteoarthritis of the femoral condyles can be observed as well

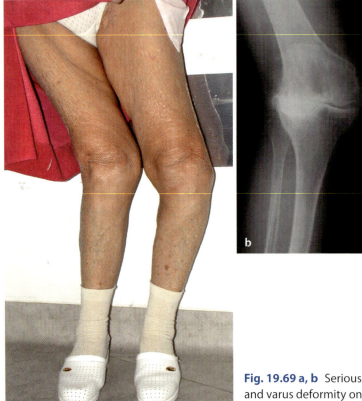

Fig. 19.69 a, b Seriously deformed knees: valgus deformity on the right side and varus deformity on the left side (**a**). Severe osteoarthritis of the knees can be observed on the radiograph taken during weight-bearing (**b**)

19.10 Secondary Osteoarthritis of the Knee

Osteoarthritis often develops as a primary disease, however there are known factors associated to facilitate early degeneration, such as previous meniscectomy, instability, trauma, osteochondritis dissecans, hemophilia, inflammatory arthritis, infections, etc. At the end stage it can be difficult or sometimes impossible to find out the reason of the osteoarthritis (Figs. 19.70–19.73).

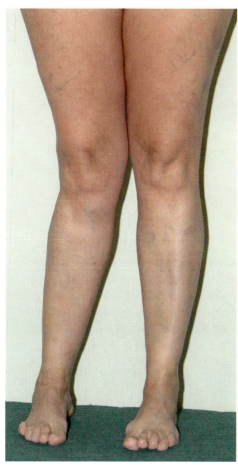

Fig. 19.70 Secondary knee osteoarthritis: the valgus deformity of the right knee is due to lateral compartmental osteoarthritis provoked by a previous lateral meniscectomy. The affected knee is slightly swollen

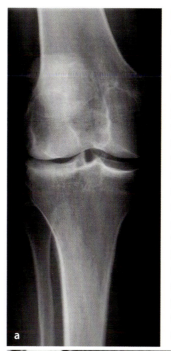

a

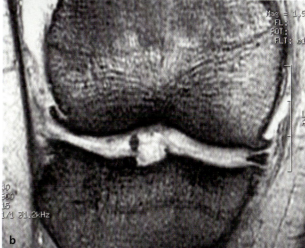

b

Fig. 19.71 a–c radiograph of the previous patient shows narrowing of the joint space and minor degenerative changes on the lateral side (**a**), while on the MR (**b**) picture osteophyte formation can be seen on both sides. Note the absence of the lateral meniscus due to the antecedent total meniscectomy. Arthroscopic picture (**c**) reveals the absence of hyaline cartilage on the tibial plateau 15 years after total meniscectomy. Behind the hook the remnants of the removed meniscus is visible, while the probe points to the damaged articular surface

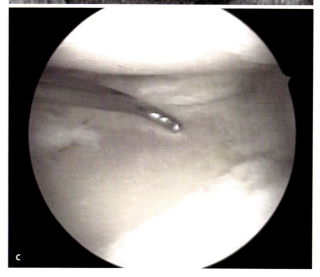

c

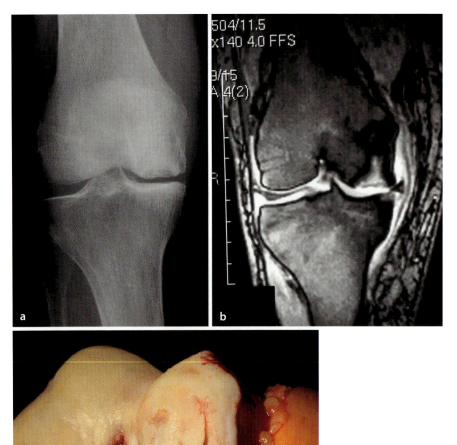

Fig. 19.72 a–c Secondary osteoarthritis: the AP radiograph shows the osteonecrosis of the medial femoral condyle (Albäck's disease) of the right knee (**a**). The extent of the necrosis can be better evaluated on the MRI image (**b**). Intraoperative picture: peeling cartilage surface above the necrotized subchondral bone. The lateral compartment is intact (**c**)

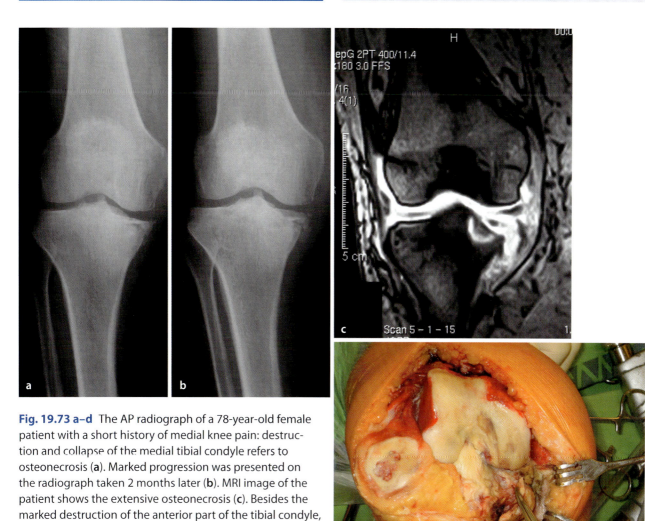

Fig. 19.73 a–d The AP radiograph of a 78-year-old female patient with a short history of medial knee pain: destruction and collapse of the medial tibial condyle refers to osteonecrosis (**a**). Marked progression was presented on the radiograph taken 2 months later (**b**). MRI image of the patient shows the extensive osteonecrosis (**c**). Besides the marked destruction of the anterior part of the tibial condyle, a consecutive injury of the hyaline cartilage of the adjacent femoral condyle and chondropathy of the patella can also be observed (**d**) on the intraoperative photograph

Chapter 20

Ankle and Foot

Contents

20.1 Congenital and Developmental Disorders

20.1.1 Pes Calcaneovalgus

Pes calcaneovalgus, called also flatfoot or pes planus or planovalgus, is less frequent in congenital form than that which appears in adults. This constitutional type of flat-foot in the majority of cases is not pathologic. All infants have flat feet for a year or two after they begin to stand. Later on, this regress spontaneously till the age 8–10. Only a few cases need more aggressive treatment than wearing sole inlay. There are, however, cases where the deformation of the feet is so expressed that an operative correction is necessary (Figs. 20.1 and 20.2).

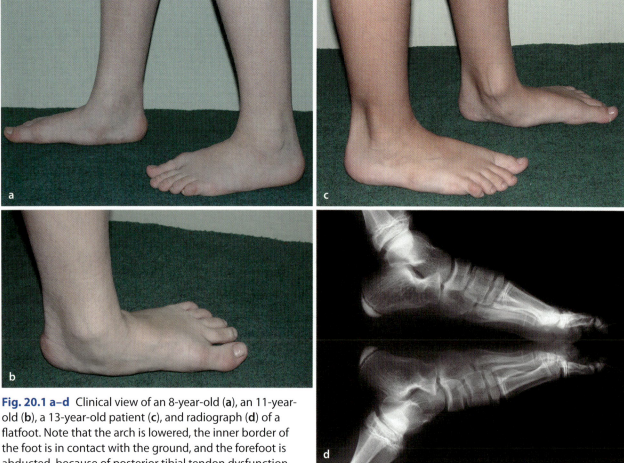

Fig. 20.1 a–d Clinical view of an 8-year-old (**a**), an 11-year-old (**b**), a 13-year-old patient (**c**), and radiograph (**d**) of a flatfoot. Note that the arch is lowered, the inner border of the foot is in contact with the ground, and the forefoot is abducted, because of posterior tibial tendon dysfunction

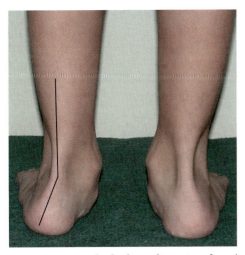

Fig. 20.2 View of a flatfoot of a patient from behind. The test to confirm forefoot abduction and heel valgus: the toes visible lateral to the heel. The posterior tibiocalcaneal angle is increased in the cases of significant heel valgus

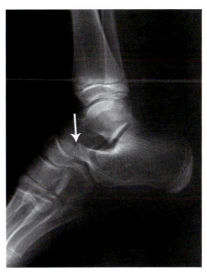

Fig. 20.3 Partial coalition between the navicular and calcaneal bones. The processus anterius calcanei is elongated, and just a thin radiolucent line appears between this two bones (*arrow*), which indicates the fibrous bridge over them

20.1.2 Tarsal Coalitions

The most common types of coalitions are between the calcaneus and either the talus or the navicular bones, but any two or more joined bones in the midfoot or hindfoot are considered to this group of disorders. The incidence of talocalcaneal coalitions is approximately 1%. Patients with tarsal coalition usually present during the second decade of life or adulthood, with mild pain deep in the subtalar joint and limitation of range of motion by prolonged or heavy activity. This disease usually presents as recurrent sprains, and pain in the midfoot and has been associated with peroneal spastic flatfoot, fixed flatfoot, and other abnormalities of the foot. Loss of subtalar motion and valgus position of the hindfoot becomes more apparent as the coalition ossifies, leading to the appearance of pes planus. The coalitions begin to ossify in different ages: talonavicular coalitions at the age of 3–5 years; calcaneonavicular coalitions at the age of 8–12 years; and talocalcaneal coalitions at the age of 12–16 years (Figs. 20.3–20.5).

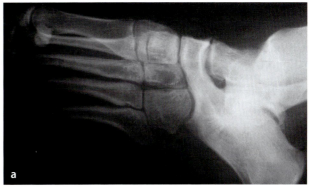

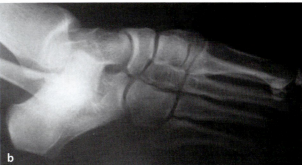

Fig. 20.4 a, b Total coalition between the navicular and calcanel bones on right side (**a**), and normal tarsal joints on left side (**b**). Because of the coalition, there is no motion in subtalar joint. The foot is mobile just in ankle joint, so it is also called pes planus fixatus

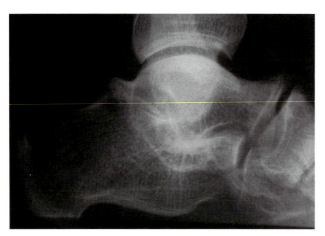

Fig. 20.5 Talocalcaneal synostosis without any movement in subtalar joint. The other tarsal joints are overloaded, leading them to early arthrosis. The walk on broken ground causes pain

20.1.3 Congenital Short Metatarsus, Brachymetatarsia

Brachymetatarsia (congenital short metatarsus) is an uncommon condition and when present, it is usually asymptomatic. As in case of oligodactyly, the lateral rays of the foot are more frequently attached. Brachymetatarsia usually accompanies other syndromes of developmental diseases (Figs. 20.6 and 20.7).

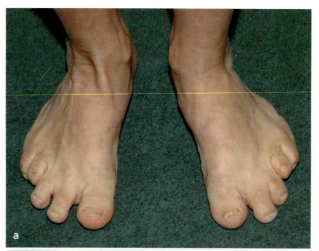

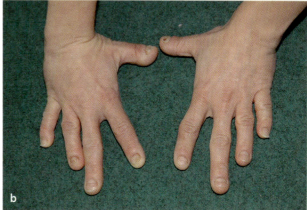

Fig. 20.7 a, b Symmetrical case of brachymetatarsia in severity (**a**), with associated shortening of the metacarpals (**b**) of the fourth and fifth rays, of a 32-year-old woman

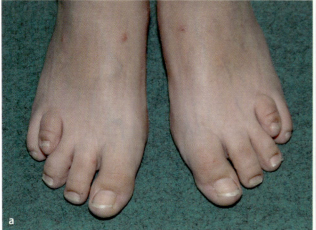

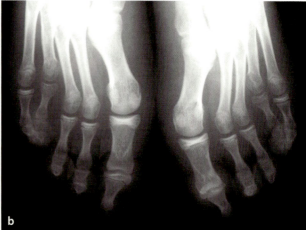

Fig. 20.6 a, b Clinical view (**a**) and radiograph (**b**) of a bilateral case of congenital short metatarsus. The shortening of the fourth metatarsus at the left side is more severe both in clinical and radiological point of view

20.1.4 Ectrodactyly

Ectrodactyly (split-hand or split-foot malformation, also called SHFM) is a clinically variable and genetically heterogeneous group of limb malformations. Forelimb defects, including postaxial ectrodactyly, metacarpal, and ulnar deficiencies, can occur at ethanol-exposed fetuses (Figs. 20.8 and 20.9).

20.1.5 Polydactyly of the Foot

Polydactyly is a relatively common congenital disorder of the foot, which can associate with other anomalies, especially with polydactyly of the hand, or it can present as an isolated malformation. This disorder generally involves the lateral side of the foot, and just rarely presents at the tibial side. The intermetatarsal angle increased where the extra finger is presented. It can impair shoe-fitting, but generally does not cause pain. Familial occurrence is observed (Figs. 20.10–20.12).

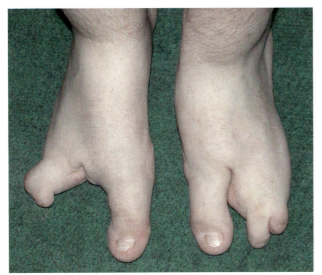

Fig. 20.8 Bilateral oligodactyly of a 20-year-old male, with typical lateral involvemen, and syndactyly of the fingers on lateral side

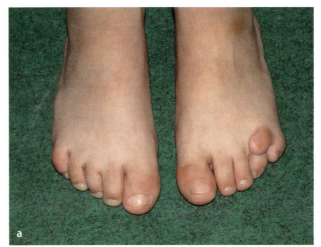

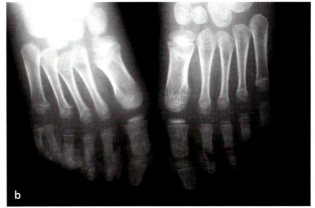

Fig. 20.10 a, b Clinical view (**a**) and radiograph (**b**) of polydactyly at the left side, with extra phalanx of the 5th ray. The disorder involves the lateral side of the left foot. As the metatarsals are not involved, the intermetatarsal angle is normal

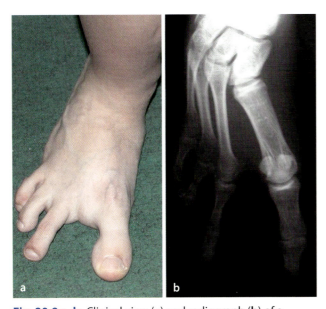

Fig. 20.9 a, b Clinical view (**a**) and radiograph (**b**) of a young woman with ectro- and oligodactyly on the right side

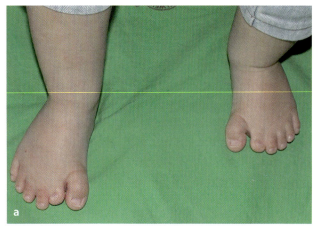

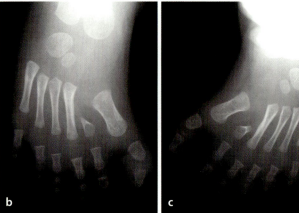

Fig. 20.11 a–c A rare case of polydactyly with bilateral involvement at the tibial side. Extra phalanx present with a partially developed extra metatarsus. Clinical view (**a**) and radiographs (**b,c**). Owing to metatarsal involvement, the intermetatarsal angle is increased between the affected 1st and 2nd ray

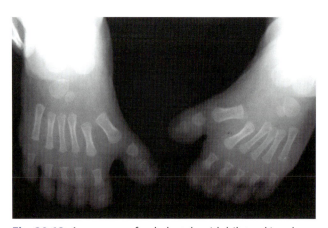

Fig. 20.12 A rare case of polydactyly with bilateral involvement at the tibial side. Radiograph of the foot of a 4-month-old boy, with completely developed extra metatarsus and phalanx between the first two rays. Increased intermetatarsal angle are also present

20.1.6 Oligodactyly

Oligodactyly is a relatively less common congenital disorder of the foot than polydactyly, but it can also associate with other anomalies, especially with oligodactyly of the hand, or it can present as an isolated malformation. This disorder generally involve the lateral side of the foot, and the hallux is just rarely attached. This disorder can impair shoe-fitting, but generally does not cause pain. Familial occurrence is observed (Figs. 20.13 and 20.14).

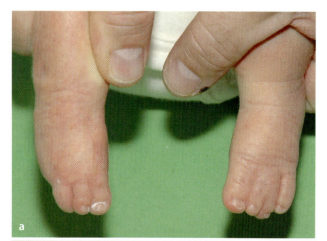

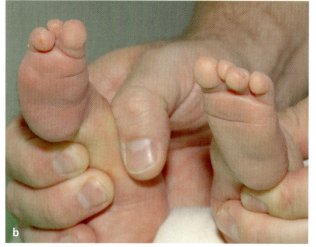

Fig. 20.13 a, b Oligodactyly associated with syndactyly of a 6-month-old boy; dorsal (**a**) and plantar (**b**) clinical view. Three fingers of the foot are present on the right side, and four fingers on the left side

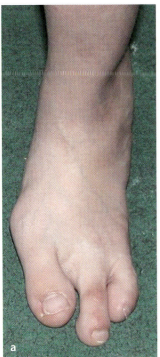

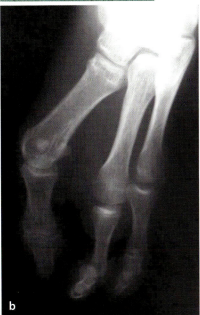

Fig. 20.14 a, b Clinical view (**a**) and radiograph (**b**) of a 11-year-old girl with oligodactyly on left side. This case is in association with fibular aplasia

20.1.7 Syndactyly of the Foot

Syndactyly is a failure of differentiation in which the fingers fail to separate into individual appendages. Simple syndactyly is a cosmetic problem without any function limit and pain or shoe-fitting problem, characterized by disorder of the skin and soft tissues of the toes. When complex syndactyly presents with involvement of bony structures, than angular deformity of toes can develop with pain and impair shoe-fitting (Fig. 20.15).

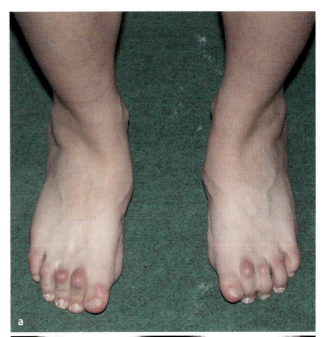

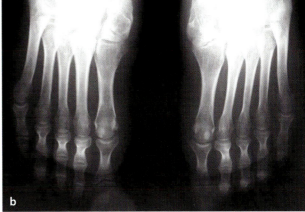

Fig. 20.15 a, b Clinical view of simple cutan bilateral syndactyly of the foot, involving the first, second and third ray. Radiograph of the patient (**b**) without any abnormalities

20.1.8 Macrodactylia (Isolated Overgrowth of the Toes)

Macrodactylia (isolated overgrowth of a toe or more than one ray) is a rare malformation of a digit with unknown etiology, characterized by the increased size of the constituents as phalanges, tendons, vessels and nerves, and subcutaneous fat and skin. It can impair shoe-fitting, and can cause pain. Two forms are known (according to Barsky):

· Static type: enlargement from birth, proportional to the patient's growth.
· Progressive form: disproportionate over growth of a digit (Figs. 20.16 and 20.17).

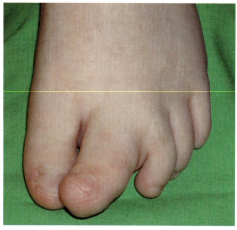

Fig. 20.17 Isolated overgrowth of the second ray of the left feet

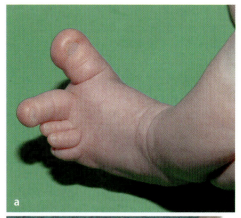

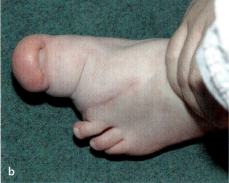

Fig. 20.16 a, b Macrodactyly of a boy, at the first and second finger of the left foot at the age of one (**a**). The same patient at the age of three, after the resection of the second digit (**b**)

20.1.9 Os Tibiale Externum

Os tibiale externum called also accessory navicular bone, which localized medially to the navicular bone, is the only tarsal accessory bone that is frequently responsible for symptoms. It causes painful and palpable prominence at the inner border of the foot, and it can cause shoe wearing difficulties. In case of total coalition, it is called "os naviculare cornutum" as it forms on radiograph a horn (Figs. 20.18 and 20.19).

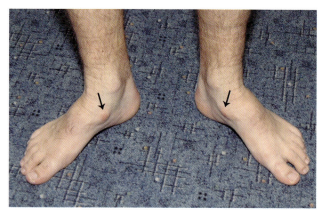

Fig. 20.18 Clinical view of a patient with os tibiale externum. Note the prominence distally to the medial malleolus. The skin rash due to the pressure of the shoes indicates (arrows) the os tibiale externum

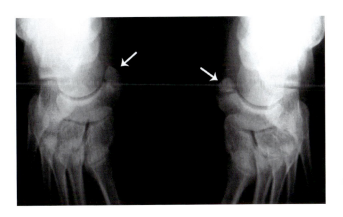

Fig. 20.19 Radiograph of foot: bilateral accessory bones, medially to the navicular bones (arrows)

20.2 Disorders of the Hallux

20.2.1 Hallux Valgus (acquired)

Hallux valgus is diagnosed when the axis of the hallux is deviated laterally. It develops gradually along with the drop of transverse arch. The capsule of the first metatarsophalangeal (MP) joint shrinks laterally and expands medially. The tendons, the plantar side of capsule dislocate laterally and dorsally along with the sesamoid bones. Metatarsal head osteophytes develop, medially bigger and laterally smaller. The hallux is pronated and subluxed in the metatarsophalangeal joint. The angle between the first and second metatarsals increases.

The severity of the acquired hallux valgus is characterized by the following three values:

· Angle of hallux valgus: the angle observed between the axis of the first metatarsal and base phalanx. (HV)
· Intermetatarsal angle: the angle measured between the axis of the first and second metatarsals.
· Lateral displacement of the medial sesamoid in percent (Figs. 20.20–20.22).

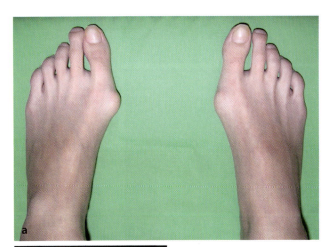
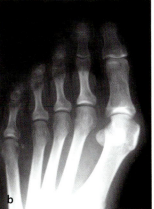

Fig. 20.20 a, b Mild case of hallux valgus (HV < 30°; IM < 9°; sesamoid < 25%)

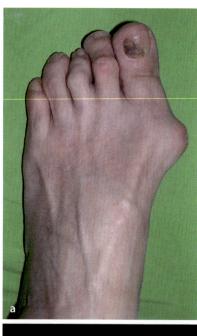

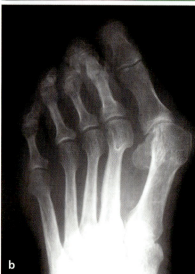

Fig. 20.21 a, b Moderate case, (HV, 30–45°; sesamoid, 25–50%)

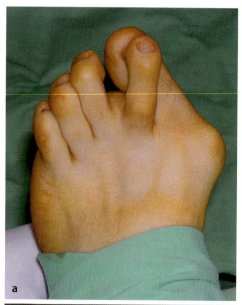

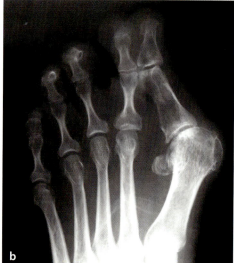

Fig. 20.22 a, b Severe case, (HV > 45°; IM > 16°; sesamoid, 50–100%)

20.2.2 Juvenile Hallux Valgus

Severely deformed first metatarsal joint surface. Lateral deviation of hallux developing in childhood or in teenage. Its etiology is the maldevelopment of the distal joint surface of the 1st metatarsal.

The axis of the base of joint surface (distal metatarsal articular angle = DMAA) and axis of the diaphysis of the 1st metatarsal is less than 90°. The joint is intact anyway, the metatarsal head is protruding medially, but no osteophyte is seen (Fig. 20.23).

20.2.3 Interphalangeal Hallux Valgus

The proximal and distal joint surfaces of the base phalanx of the hallux are not parallel, they have an angle opening medially. Therefore, the end phalanx is positioned in valgus. It is often combined with acquired or juvenile hallux valgus (Fig. 20.24).

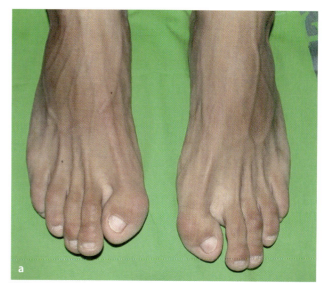

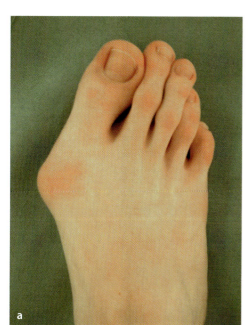

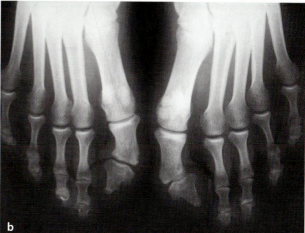

Fig. 20.24 a, b Photograph (**a**) and radiograph (**b**) taken from a 30-year-old male patient with bilateral congenital interphalangeal hallux valgus deformity. The end phalanxes are in valgus, the proximal and distal joint surfaces are not parallel

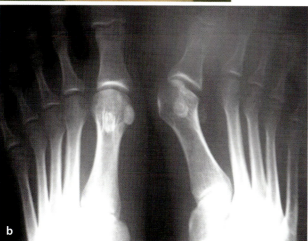

Fig. 20.23 a, b Juvenile hallux valgus and radiograph

20.2.4 Hallux Varus

The hallux is deviated medially (varus) in the metatarso-phalangeal joint. Primary hallux varus is rare, usually it is a consequence of paresis or trauma. It can be associated with other developmental abnormality. This deformity is often seen following clubfoot treatment (Figs. 20.25 and 20.26).

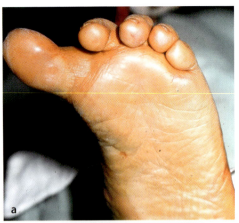

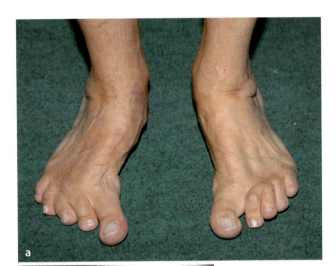

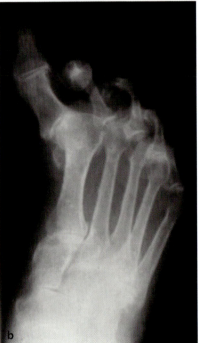

Fig. 20.26 a, b Hallux varus in the MP joint (congenital form)

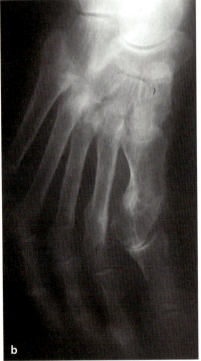

Fig. 20.25 a, b Hallux varus deformity is seen following clubfoot treatment on the photograph (**a**) and radiograph (**b**)

20.2.5 Hallux Flexus

This is the deformity of the base and end phalanges. The metatarsophalangeal (MP) or interphalangel (IP) joint

of hallux is fixed in flexion because of various reasons. Callosities develop on the skin in pressure areas. This deformity usually develops following paresis, often at spina bifida or myelodysplasia (Figs. 20.27 and 20.28).

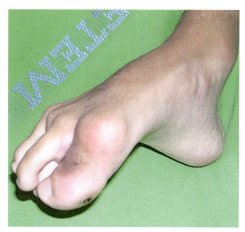

Fig. 20.27 Hallux flexus of a spastic patient; MP joint is in flexion and valgus

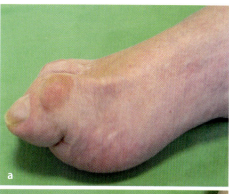

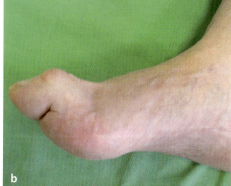

Fig. 20.28 a, b Hallux malleus, base phalanx in extension, the interphalangeal joint is in flexion

20.2.6 Hallux (limitus) Rigidus

In this condition, the range of motion of the metatarsophalangeal joint is limited (hallux limitus) or missing (hallux rigidus). Contributing factors are contracture of the capsule, tension of the plantar flexor muscles, and osteoarthritis or inflammation (gout). In the beginning, no

bony changes are detected and only the upper part of the joint space is narrow. Later, osteophytes appear reaching considerable size, hindering the motion.

The gait is impaired, the forefoot is painful while the patient walks fast or steps a longer step, and the ankle and foot turn supinated, resulting in pain in the lateral ankle (Figs. 20.29–20.32).

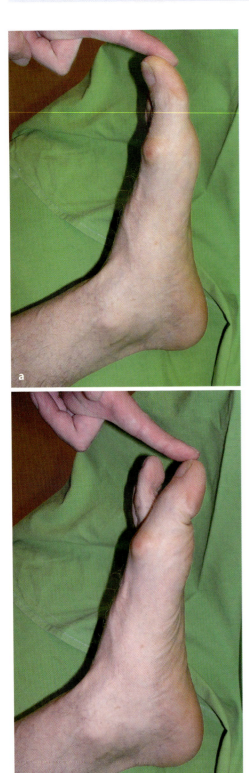

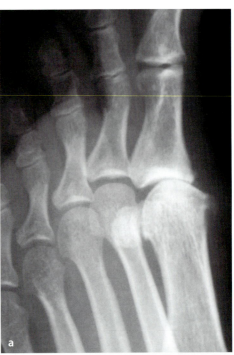

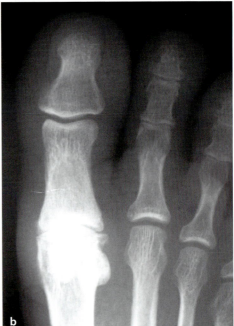

Fig. 20.30 a, b Hallux limitus. Radiograph: Mild degenerative changes and dorsal osteophyte are present in the first MP

Fig. 20.29 a, b Especially the dorsalextension but also the plantarflexion of the hallux are reduced (hallux limitus)

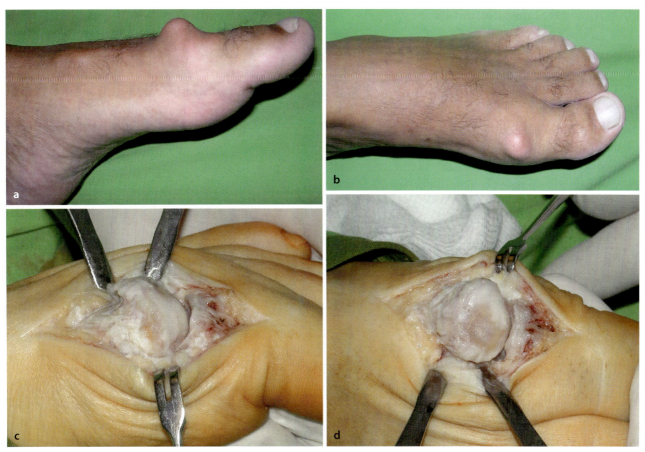

Fig. 20.31 a–d Severe rigid hallux with loss of motion. Patient's photos demonstrate the pronaunced bonunions on the dorsomedial (**a**, **b**) site of the first MP joint. Intraoperative pictures show the collar-like osteophytes around the metatarsal head (**c**) and the extensive degenerative changes - chondropathy - on the joint surface (**d**)

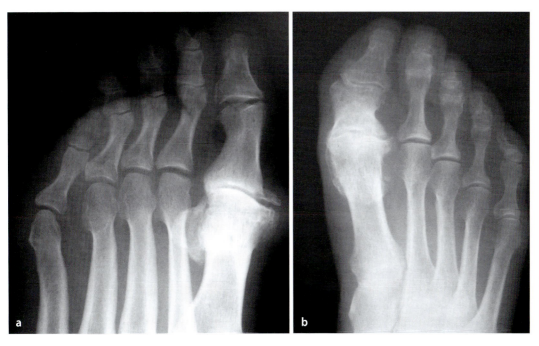

Fig. 20.32 a, b Hallux rigidus with large dorsal osteophyte

20.3 Disorders and Deformities of the Lesser Toes

20.3.1 Flexible Hammer Toe

Drop of longitudinal and transverse arch results in gradual balance disturbance of the muscles. The proximal interphalangeal (PIP) joint is in flexion, the MP joint is in extension. This position is correctable both actively and passively, but the hammer position recurs (Fig. 20.33).

20.3.2 Rigid Hammer Toe

Deformities, flexion contracture in PIP and/or DIP of the small toes, are not fully correctable either actively or passively. Painful skin callosities develop because of the rubbing by the shoe. These are usually associated with hallux valgus (Fig. 20.34).

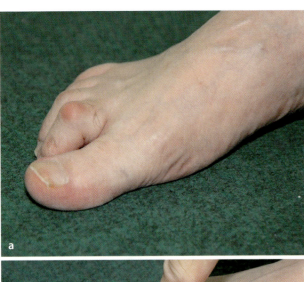

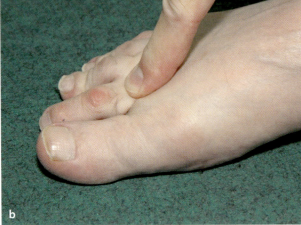

Fig. 20.33 a, b Mild hammer toe II, small redness over the PIP. The position of the toe is reducible

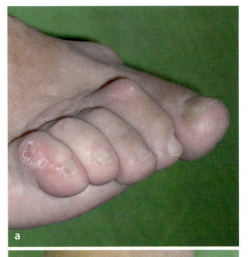

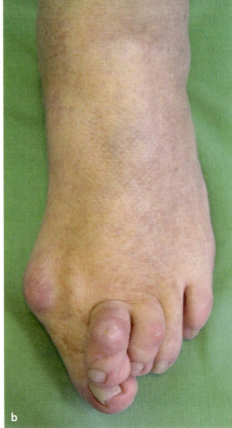

Fig. 20.34 a, b Hammer toes, callosity on II. toe (**a**). Hallux valgus with hammer toes. Callosity over the PIP joints (**b**)

20.3.3 Overlapping Fifth Toe

The fifth toe is positioned over the other toes because of various reasons. The 5th metatarsus is usually shorter, and the extensor tendon and the capsule of the metatarsophalangeal joint are shorter medially. Shoe rubs the toe; callosity often occurs (Fig. 20.35).

20.4 Neurovascular Diseases of the Foot

20.4.1 Diabetic Foot

Metabolic changes of diabetes results in narrowing the blood vessels. The changes in circulation causes malnutrition of peripheral nerves, their function impairs. These factors cause specific changes on the feet, called diabetic foot syndrome. This syndrome consists of inflammation, sensory changes, bone necrosis, and ulceration (Figs. 20.36–20.38).

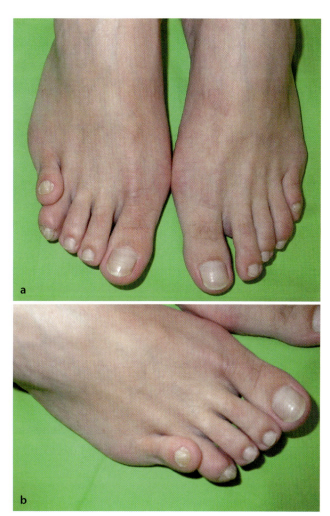

Fig. 20.35 a, b Unilateral overlapping fifth toe on the right side

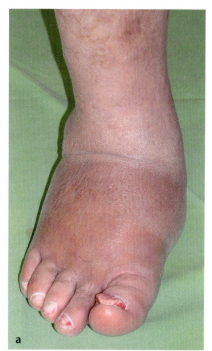

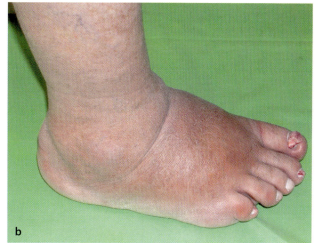

Fig. 20.36 a, b Swollen diabetic foot

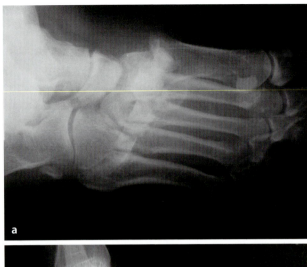

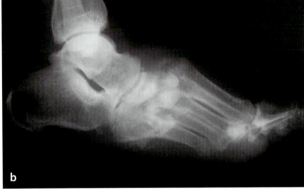

Fig. 20.37 a, b Radiograph of diabetic neuropathy caused osteonecrosis. Note the serious deterioration and subluxation of the Lisfranc's joint

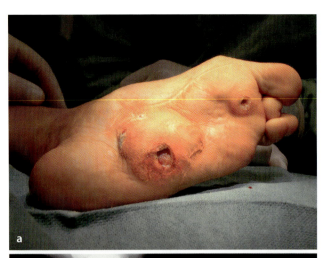

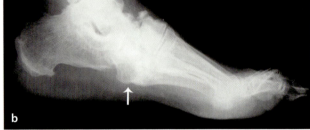

Fig. 20.38 a, b Plantar ulcer of diabetic foot (**a**). Radiograph of the same foot. Behind the ulcer is the deformed Lisfranc's joint and partially necrotized distal tarsal bones (cuboid and cuneiforms) (**b**). The arrow points to the plantar dislocated bony fragment which caused the plantar ulceration of the skin due to its pressure

20.5 Compressive Neuropathies of the Foot and Ankle

Peripheral nerves can get compressed while running through narrowed anatomical strictures, causing pathological symptoms on their supplied area. Muscles get weaker; hyper- and hypesthesia occur. Tibial and foot dorsal cutan nerve compression often develops on calf. Regarding digital nerves, the common branch of the 3rd and 4th is the source of complaints.

20.5.1 Tarsal Tunnel Syndrome

Tibial nerve run through the tarsal tunnel behind the medial ankle. Inflammation, trauma of this area, or other factors can cause compression. Symptoms are hypoesthesia on the sole and weakening of plantar muscles (Fig. 20.39).

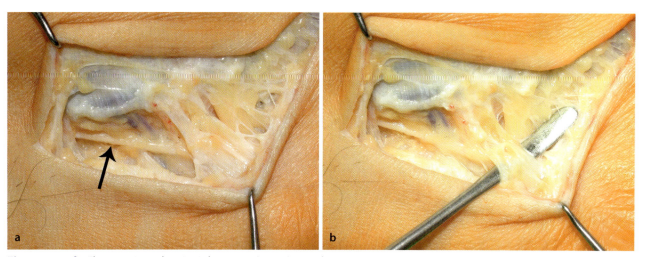

Fig. 20.39 a, b Flexor retinaculum is tight, nerve (*arrow*) is under compression

20.5.2 Morton Neuroma

The common branch of 3rd and 4th toe digital nerves get compressed under the intermetatarsal ligament connecting the two metatarsal heads, a painful nodule (neuroma) appears on the nerve over the compressed area. Clinical symptom is spontaneous electrical pain that is also elicited while pressing the metatarsals against each other or by direct pressure (Figs. 20.40–20.42).

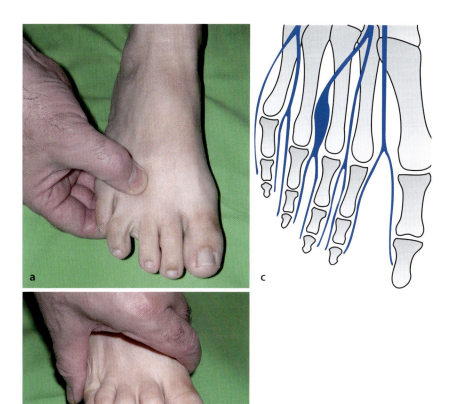

Fig. 20.40 a–c Clinical symptoms of Morton neuroma. Direct pressure (**a**) and pressing the metatarsals against each other (**b**) causes pain. Sketch: Location of Morton neuroma (**c**)

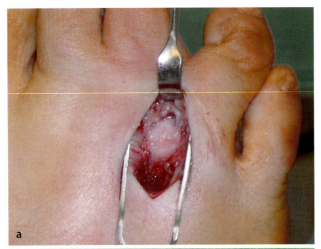

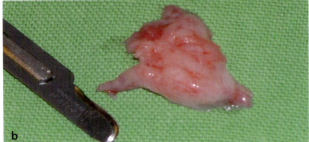

Fig. 20.41 a, b Intraoperative picture of Morton neuroma (**a**) and excised neuroma (**b**, extent of the cutting edge of the knife is 1 cm)

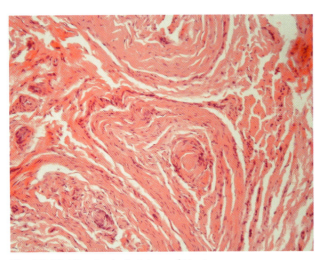

Fig. 20.42 Histological picture of Morton neuroma

20.6 Plantar Heel Pain

Plantar heel pain has various etiology. In most cases, the drop of the longitudinal arch causes increased traction forces on the plantar surface of the heel bone inducing enthesopathia – periostitis. Apart from pain, no other physical changes are detected.

20.6.1 Superficial Plantar Fibromatosis (Ledderhose's disease)

Firm nodules in the subcutan area appear on the sole. The plantar aponeurosis is infiltrated by aggressive growing connective tissue elements, immature fibroblats. In case it involves the weight bearing surfaces hindering the gait, surgical removal is advised. It is often associated with Dupuytren's contracture of the hand (Figs. 20.43–20.45).

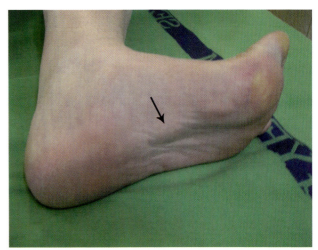

Fig. 20.43 Medial side of the sole: nodules are seen in plantar fascia (*arrow*)

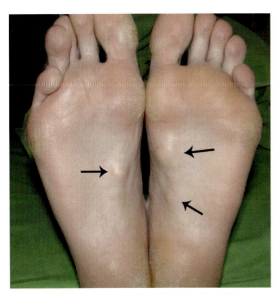

Fig. 20.44 Medial side of both soles: firm fibrotic nodules shrinking the plantar aponeurosis and involving the skin (*arrows*)

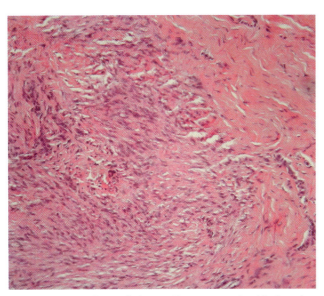

Fig. 20.45 Histology of plantar fibromatosis (Ledderhose's disease). Cellular proliferation of plump, immature appearing spindled cells which infiltrates the tendo-aponeurotic fibrous tissue of the foot

20.6.2 High Arch Foot (pes cavus)

When the longitudinal arch is higher, regardless of the etiology, the condition is called pes cavus. The axis of the heel is higher in sagittal plane, and the dorsum of the foot is steeper; often associated with equinus ankles on claw toes. Etiology is mostly muscle balance disturbance, palsy (myelodysplasia, spina bifida occulta or other neuromuscular disturbance) (Fig. 20.46).

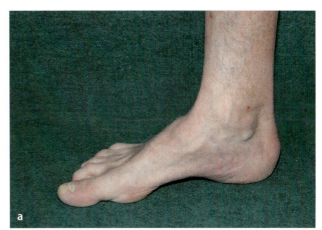

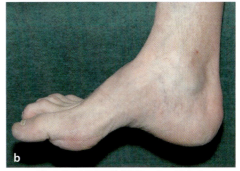

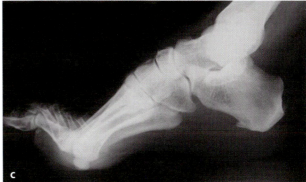

Fig. 20.46 a–c Photograph taken from a foot with pes cavus deformity in loaded (**a**) and unloaded (**b**) position. Radiograph: the longitudinal arch is higher, decreased hind foot – forefoot longitudinal axis (**c**)

20.6.3 Flatfoot (pes planus, pes planovalgus), Traumatic Flatfoot

In this condition, the longitudional arch of the foot is reduced. On standing position, the medial border of the foot is closed to, or in contact with the ground. It is frequently associated with some degree of twisting outwards of the foot on its longitudinal axis.

Pes planovalgus: It is a combination of drop of transverse and longitudinal arches, and valgus displacement of the heel. The medial edge of the foot usually completely sinks. It is observed in cases of long-lasting pes planus. The reason is that the deep flexor musculature, which is to hold the foot in normal position, is unable to do so.

Traumatic flatfoot: This deformity is characterized by rapidly developing, usually unilateral flatfoot.

The longitudinal arch drops, and the medial edge of the plant reaches the ground. The heel turns into valgus. The patient is unable to stand tiptoe.

The reason of this deformity is the insufficiency of the tibialis posterior muscle. It occurs usually in middle-aged females. The fibers of the tibialis posterior tendon degenerate, and suddenly split without any injury.

It may occur, however, following trauma. Injury hits the tibialis posterior tendon in the majority of cases at the medial malleolar area. (At the demonstrated case, the injury was caused by an axe). The cut tendon fails to fulfill its function (Figs. 20.47–20.51).

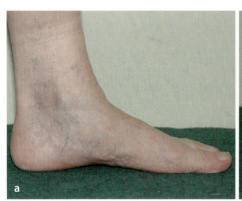 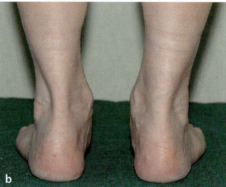

Fig. 20.47 a, b The transverse and longitudinal arches dropped (**a**).The calcaneus is slightly in valgus position (**b**)

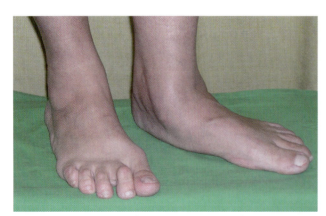

Fig. 20.48 Severe pes planus, medial edge of the sole dropped and touches the ground

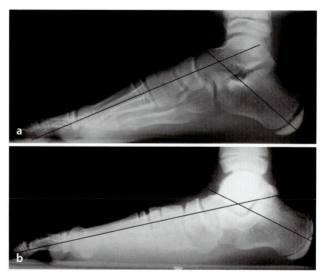

Fig. 20.49 a, b Radiograph of pes planus. The angle between the axis of the heel and the ground is 45°. (normal foot) (**a**). Because of the dropped arch, the angle is around 10° (**b**)

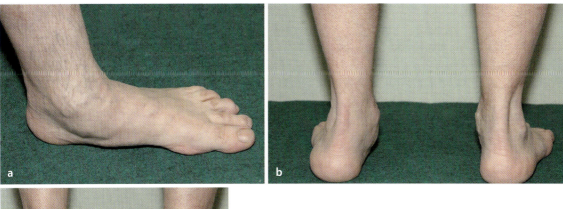

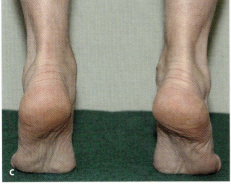

Fig. 20.50 a–c The medial edge of the foot usually completely dropped to the gound (**a**). The heel is in marked valgus (**b**). Walking tiptoe (**c**), the heel returns to its midposition; its normal position shows that the tibialis posterior muscle is intact

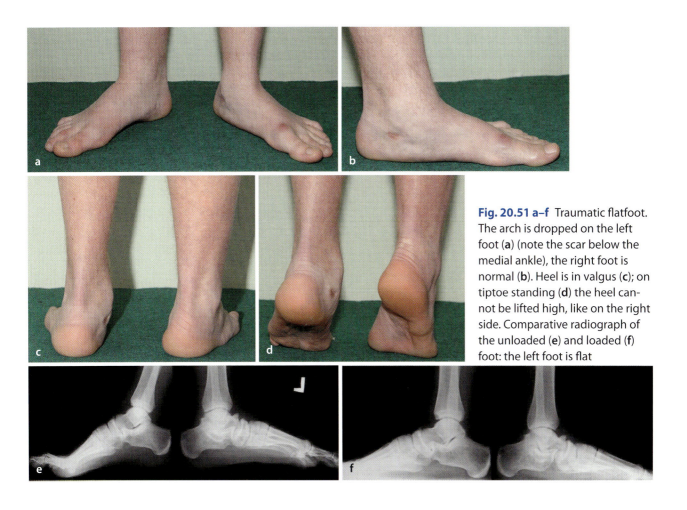

Fig. 20.51 a–f Traumatic flatfoot. The arch is dropped on the left foot (**a**) (note the scar below the medial ankle), the right foot is normal (**b**). Heel is in valgus (**c**); on tiptoe standing (**d**) the heel cannot be lifted high, like on the right side. Comparative radiograph of the unloaded (**e**) and loaded (**f**) foot: the left foot is flat

20.6.4 Metatarsalgia

As a result of the drop of transverse arch, during walking in the rolling phase, the load is transferred to the heads of 2nd and 3rd metatarsals. The drop of transverse arch creates muscle imbalance, the base phalanges are displaced to the dorsal side of the joints and they get subluxed –

pulling with them the joint plantar plate. The metatarsal heads are positioned directly under the skin of the sole. The forefoot is widened. Metatarsalgia is usually associated with hallux valgus. The overload distributed to small areas creates painful callosities on the sole. The transverse arch is usually stiff, impossible to lift even passively (Figs. 20.52 and 20.53).

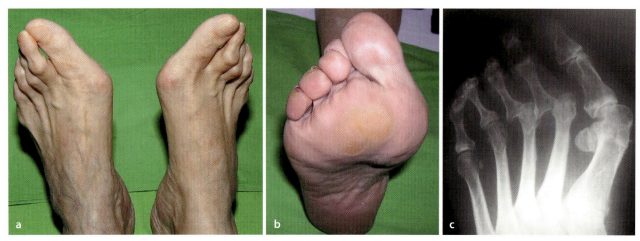

Fig. 20.52 a–c Severely deformed foot is demonstrated with flattening and excavation of the transversal arch (**a**) and callosity on the load-bearing surface (**b**). Radiograph: the 2nd and 3rd MP joint are luxated (**c**)

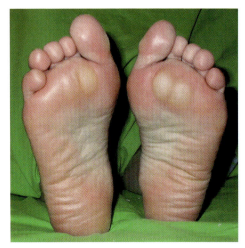

Fig. 20.53 Metatarsalgia creating heavy pain. Inflammated and hyperkeratotic areas under the metatarsals develop because of the enhanced pressure of the sunk metatarsal heads

20.6.5 Calcaneal Spur (cornu calcanei)

The short plantar flexor muscles and plantar aponeurosis have their origin on the calcanear tuber. Irritation or overuse in this region can lead to a painful periostitis which can be associated – but not necessarily– with the formation of a bony spur. Weight bearing, and walking is very painful (Fig. 20.54).

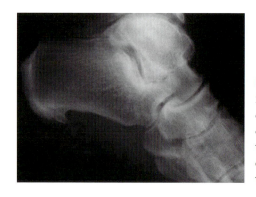

Fig. 20.54 Spur-shaped osteophyte on the plantar surface of calcaneal tuber

20.7 Inflammatory Tendon Diseases of the Foot

Noninfected inflammations are related to degenerative processes, or to rheumatologic diseases (rheumatoid arthritis, gout, etc.) They present as arthritis, tendinitis or tenosynovitis.

Tenosynovitis of tibialis anterior tendon. Tenosynovitis of tibialis anterior tendon is usually a symptom of rheumatoid arthritis or overload; the surrounding tissues swell up (Fig. 20.55).

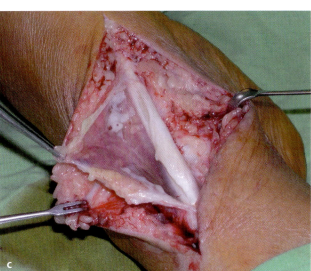

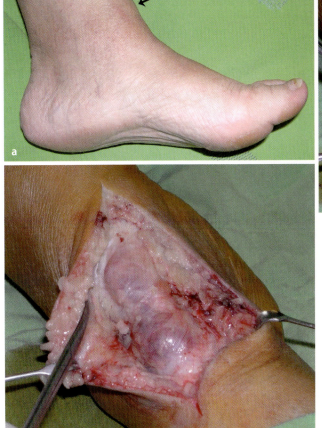

Fig. 20.55 a–c Swelling over tibialis anterior tendon (**a**, *arrow*). Intraoperative pictures: the tendon sheath around the tibialis anterior tendon is filled with fluid (**b**). The inflamated tendon sheath incised above the tibialis anterior (**c**)

20.8 Cysts Around the Foot

20.8.1 Foot Ganglion

These are elastic cysts filled with gelatinous material, connected to joints or tendon sheaths of the foot. The liner of cyst shows evidence of aseptic inflammation. Characteristic of foot ganglion is that the ganglion may change its size, opposed to that of tumors (Figs. 20.56 and 20.57).

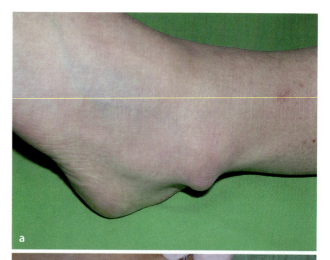

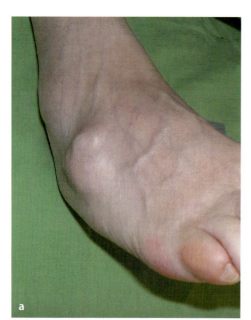

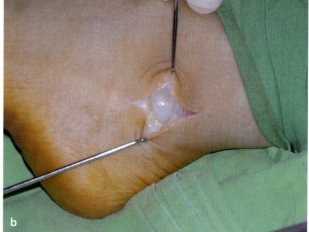

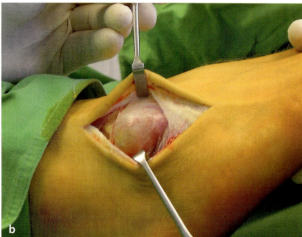

Fig. 20.56 a, b Large ganglion protrudes the skin above the lateral side of the right ankle (**a**). Intraoperative picture (**b**) of the cyst filled with transparent gelatinous material

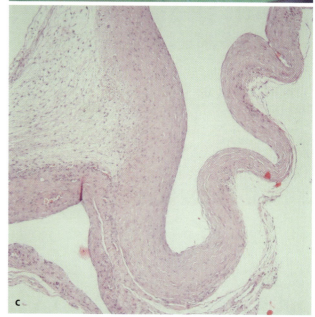

Fig. 20.57 a–c Ganglion behind the ankle connected to the peroneus tendon sheath (**a**), intraoperative picture (**b**) and the histological appearance: simple cyst wall consisted of connective tissue (**c**)

20.8.2 Toe Hygroma

Cutan cysts are filled with fluid on the toes, associated to arthrotic, degenerative joints (Fig. 20.58)

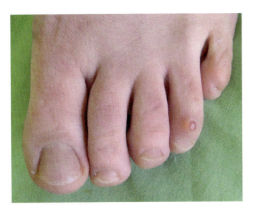

Fig. 20.58 Hygroma over the 4th DIP joint

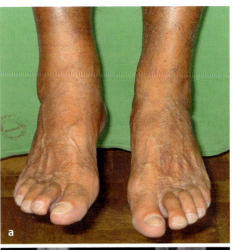

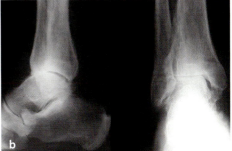

20.9 Osteoarthritis (OA) of the Foot and Ankle Joints

20.9.1 Osteoarthritis of the Tibiotalar Joint

Degenerative changes involving the ankle joint are almost always the consequence of injuries. Fractures with joint involvement or repeated sprains causes damage to the cartilage and end up in arthrosis.

Inflammatory disease, rheumatoid arthritis also gradually destroys the joint. OA, however, may appear because of unknown origin or following postural deformities (Figs. 20.59 and 20.60).

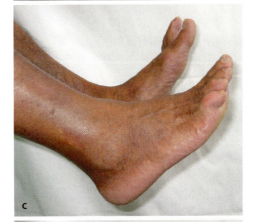

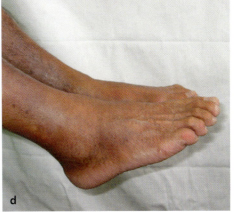

Fig. 20.59 a–d Arthritis of the ankle. Note the markedly swollen right ankle region (**a**). Radiograph: the joint space is narrowed, the adjacent bones are sclerotic and osteophytes are visible at the rim (**b**). The range of movement in the talar joint – especially the extension in this case- is severely restricted (**c**). No major loss in flexion (**d**)

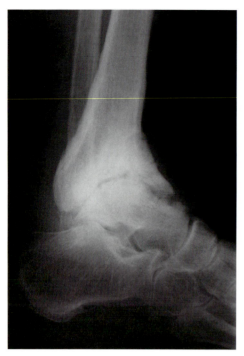

Fig. 20.60 Severe posttraumatic osteoarthritis

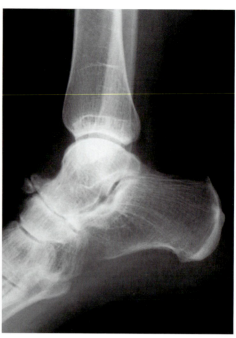

Fig. 20.61 Osteoarthritis of the talonavicular joint, osteophyte and loose body formation. Joint spaces are narrow

20.9.2 Osteoarthritis (OA) of the Subtalar and Chopart's Joints

OA of the subtalar and Chopart's joints is a common condition of hindfoot; often follows heel fractures and subtalar dislocations. The condition may involve the entire hindfoot, but there are cases, where only one joint is damaged. Symptom is the restriction or total loss of the tarsal motion (Figs. 20.61 and 20.62).

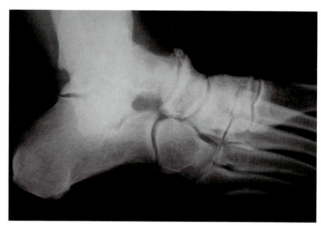

Fig. 20.62 Osteoarthritis of the subtalar and talonavicular joint

20.9.3 Arthritis of the Metatarsophalangeal Joints

Osteoarthritic (OA) changes often involve the metatarsophalangeal joints, especially the 1st MP joint, resulting restriction of motion. On the 2nd to 4th toe is occasion-ally damaged by osteochondritis (Köhler–Freiberg's), predisposing deforming Osteoarthritis (OA). In various phases of rigid hallux, typical OA changes are detected. Rheumatoid arthritis is often accompanied by OA of all the MP joints (Figs. 20.63 and 20.64).

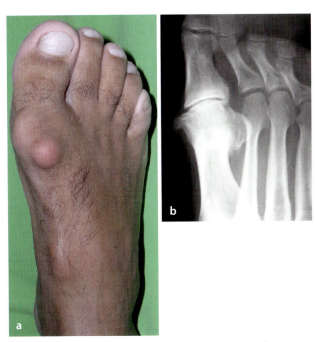

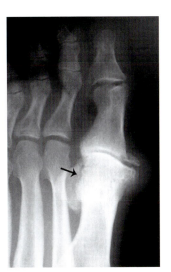

Fig. 20.64 Osteoarthritis of the metatarso–sesamoid joints. OA does not damage the metatarso–sesamoid joint isolated; it may occur in static foot diseases, with severe hallux valgus or rigidus. The thin cartilage may disappear from the joint surface of the sesamoid bone. Severe pain may be elicited by weight bearing or by extending the big toe

Fig. 20.63 a, b Clinical picture presents the bulky first metatarsophalangeal joint. Inflammated and hyperkeratotic skin above the protruding "collar" osteophyte of the metatarsal head (**a**). Radiograph reveals the advanced OA of 1st MP joint, with osteophytes and narrowed joint space (**b**)

20.10 Disorders of the Achilles Tendon, Ligaments, and Retrocalcaneal Region

20.10.1 Achilles Tendinitis-Non Insertional

Achilles tendon swells up 3–4 cm over the heel, gets tender, and is painful. Etiology is the inflammation and scarring of the surrounding peritenon. Similar is the tendinosis Achillei, caused by degenerative areas appearing in the substance of the tendon. The cause is usually due to overload and excessive bodyweight. This is often seen in sportsmen (Fig. 20.65).

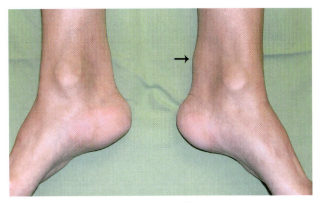

Fig. 20.65 Painful swelling of Achilles tendon 3–4 cm over the heel

20.10.2 Achilles Tendinitis-Insertional

Achilles tendinitis-insertional is caused by inflammation of the loose tissue and enthesopathic changes occur on the calcaneus. It is characterized by swelling on both sides of the tendon and tenderness over the calcaneal tuber. Both overload and degenerative changes may contribute to this. Reactive osteophytosis may develop on the calcaneal tuber (Fig. 20.66).

20.10.3 Closed Rupture of the Achilles Tendon

Part of the Achilles tendon 4–6 cm above the calcaneal tuber has relatively weak blood supply, so it is disposed to degenerative changes. Rupture happens at day-to-day movements with heavy calf pain and weakness of the ankle movement. The fibers of the tendon get torn at various heights. Palpating the tendon, deep impression is detected over the calcaneal tuber (Figs. 20.67 and 20.68).

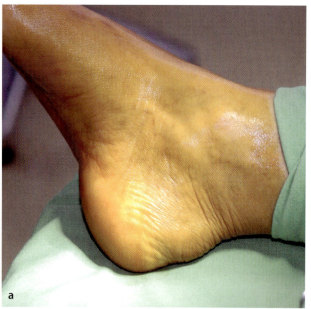

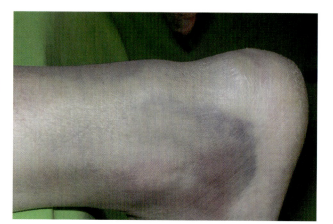

Fig. 20.67 Acute rupture of Achilles tendon. Deep impression is detected over the calcaneal tuber, suffusion, bluish discoloration

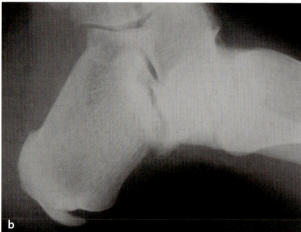

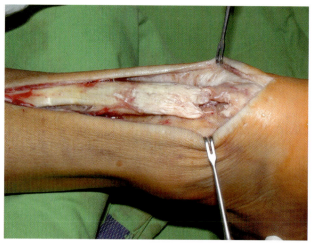

Fig. 20.66 a, b Attachment of the Achilles tendon is swollen (**a**). Radiograph reveals a large osteophyte at the attachment of the Achilles tendon (**b**)

Fig. 20.68 Closed rupture of the Achilles tendon. Intraoperative picture shows the ruptured tendon

20.10.4 Periostitis Calcanei (exostosis calcanei) Haglund's Heel

Protrusion is detected at the lateral side of the heel, near to the Achilles attachment. It is considered as a developmental variation which is completed at the end of growth. It may extend over the tendon separated from the attachment. The bulky heel may cause trouble while wearing shoe. Shoe often rubs against the skin of the heel causing blisters and later callosities (Figs. 20.69 and 20.70).

20.10.5 Chronic Unstable Ankle Joint

In many cases, the violence of the trauma is insufficient to rupture the lateral ligaments of the ankle, though the ligaments may be strained and later a chronic instability of the ankle can be developed. The patient feels instability of the ankle; pain and swelling can be present but not necessarily. Dorsal and plantar flexion of the joint is not decreased but attempted adduction provokes the pain (Fig. 20.71).

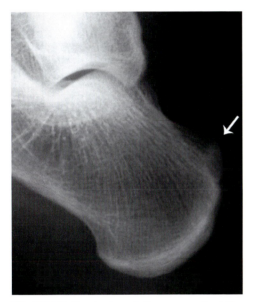

Fig. 20.69 Exostosis pointing upwards at the calcaneal tuber

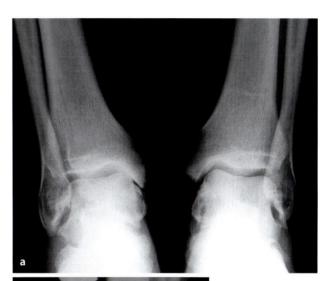

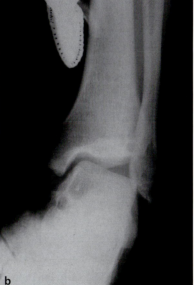

Fig. 20.71 a, b At rest, the ankle joint has a normal position (**a**); in case of attempted adduction stresses, the affected ankle joint can be "opened" (**b**)

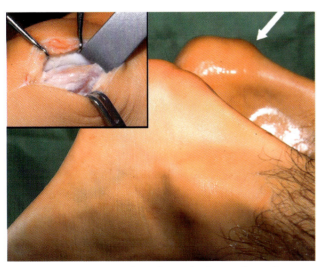

Fig. 20.70 Exostosis at the calcaneal tuber making shoe wearing difficult. Excision relieves the symptoms

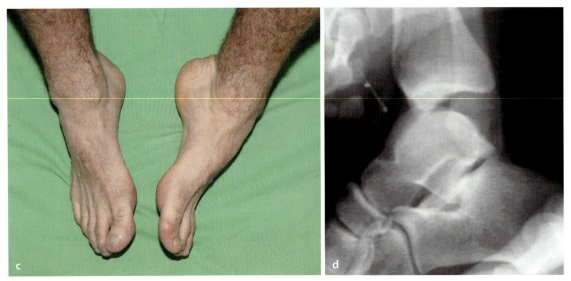

Fig. 20.71 c, d The photograph reveals the difference range of motion in adduction at the ankles (**c**). The lateral view radiograph demonstrates the sagittal anterior instability of the ankle joint (**d**)

20.11 Subungual Exostosis

Exostoses is deforming the toenails,which protrude from the processus unguicularis of the distal phalanx. They could be confused with fungous infections deforming the nail. Subunqual exostosis can be seen under any nail, most often under the nail of hallux (Fig. 20.72).

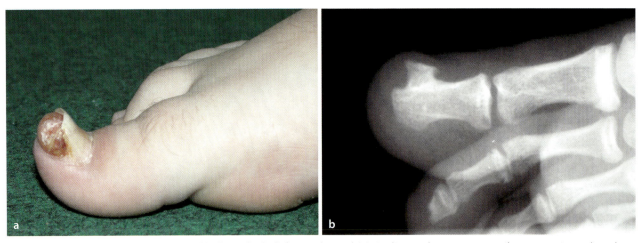

Fig. 20.72 a, b Subungual exostosis of hallux which deforms the nail (**a**). Radiograph presents a spiky exostosis on dorsal side of the distal phalanx

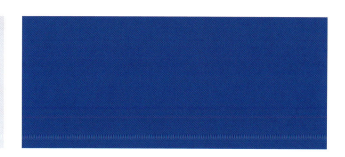

Suggested Reading

1. Adams A, Lehman TJA (2005) Update on the pathogenesis and treatment of systemic onset juvenile rheumatoid arthritis. Curr Opin Rheumatol 17:612–616

2. Adelani MA, Wupperman RM, Holt GE (2008) Benign synovial disorders. J Am Acad Orthop Surg 16(5):268–75

3. Avivi E, Arzi H, Paz L, Caspi I, Chechik A (2008) Skeletal manifestations of Marfan syndrome. Isr Med Assoc J 10:186–188

4. Azouz EM, Teebi AS, Chen MF, Lemyre E, Glanc P (1999) Achondroplasia, hypochondroplasia and thanatophoric dysplasia: review and update. Can Assoc Radiol J 50:185–192

5. Bancroft LW (2007) MR imaging of infectious processes of the knee. Radiol Clin North Am 45(6):931–41

6. Baujat G, Le Merrer M (2007) Ellis-Van Creveld syndrome. Orphanet J Rare Dis 2:27–32

7. Beighton P (1992) McKusick's heritable disorders of connective tissue. Mosby Year Book, St. Louis

8. Benard MA (2000) Congenital vertical talus. Clin Podiatr Med Surg 17(3):471–480

9. Bennell KL, Bruckner PD (1997) Epidemiology and site specificity of stress fractures. Clin Sports Med 16:179–187

10. Berger FH, de Jonge MC, Maas M (2007) Stress fractures in the lower extremity. The importance of increasing awareness amongst radiologists. Eur J Radiol 62:16–26

11. Bogduk N (2001) Complex regional pain syndrome. Curr Opin Anaesthesiol 14:541–546

12. Bovée J (2008) Multiple osteochondromas. Orphanet J Rare Dis 3:3–10

13. Brady RA, Leid JG, Calhoun JH, Costerton JW, Shirtliff ME (2008) Osteomyelitis and the role of biofilms in chronic infection. Immunol Med Microbiol 52(1):13–22

14. Brukner P, Bradshaw C, Khan KM, White S, Crossley K (1996) Stress fractures: a review of 180 cases. Clin J Sports Med 6:85

15. Bukulmez H, Colbert RA (2002) Juvenile spondylopathies and related arthritis. Curr Opin Rheumatol 14:531–535

16. Carter EM, Davies JG, Raggio C (2007) Advances in understanding etiology of achondroplasia and review of management. Orthopaedics 19(1):32–37

17. Cho TJ, Choi IH, Chung CY, Hwang JK (2000) The Sprengel deformity. Morphometric analysis using 3D-CT and its clinical relevance. J Bone Joint Surg Br 82(5):711–718

18. Colina M, Lo Monaco A, Khodeir M, Trotta F (2007) Propionibacterium acnes and SAPHO syndrome: a case report and literature review. Clin Exp Rheumatol 25(3):457–60

19. Crawford AJ, Hamblen DL (1992) Outline of fractures. 10th edition. Churchill Livingstone, Oxford, UK

20. Crawford Adams J, Hamblen DL (1995) Outline of orthopaedics. 12th edn. Churchill Livingstone, Oxford, UK.

21. Crawford AH, Schorry EK (2006) Neurofibromatosis update. J Pediatr Orthop 26:413–423

22. Cushner FD, Scott WN, Scuderi GR (2005) Surgical techniques for the knee. Thieme, New York

23. Damron TA, Sim FH (1997) Soft-tissue tumors about the knee. J Am Acad Orthop Surg 5(3) 141–152

24. Devas MB (1975) Stress fractures. Churchill Livingston, Edinburgh

25. Diduch DR, Insall JN, Scott WN, Scuderi GR, Font-Rodriguez D (1997) Total knee replacement in young, active patients. Long-term follow-up and functional outcome. J Bone Joint Surg Am 79:575–582

26. Do T (2002) Orthopedic management of the muscular dystrophies. Curr Opin Pediatr 14(1):50–53

27. Egol KA, Jazrawi LM, DeWal H, Su E, Leslie MP, Di Cesare PE (2001) Orthopaedic manifestations of systemic lupus erythematosus. Bull Hosp Jt Dis 60(1):29–34

28. Ellman MH, Becker MA (2006) Crystal-induced arthropathies: recent investigative advances. Curr Opin Rheumatol 18:249–255

29. Feldman BM, Rider LG, Reed AM, Pachman LM (2008) Juvenile dermatomyositis and other idiopathic inflammatory myopathies of childhood. Lancet 371:2201–2212

30. Freyschmidt J (2001) Melorheostosis: a review of 23 cases. Eur Radiol 11:474–487

31. Gembun Y, Nakayama Y, Shirai Y, Miyamoto M, Sawaizumi T, Kitamura S (2001) A case report of spondyloepiphyseal dysplasia congenita. J Nippon Med Sch 68:186–189

32. Gholve PA, Scher DM, Khakharia S, Widmann RF, Green DW (2007) Osgood Schlatter syndrome. Curr Opin Pediatr 19(1): 44–50

33. Gibbs CP, Weber K, Scarborough MT (2001) Malignant bone tumors. J. Bone Joint Surg Am 83:1728–1745

34. Gitelis S, Wilkins R, Conrad EU (1995) Benign bone tumors. J Bone Joint Surg Am 77:1756–1782

35. Glorieux FH (2008) Osteogenesis imperfecta. Best Pract Res Clin Rheumatol 22:85–100

36. Goodwin RW, O'Donnel P, Saifuddin A (2007) MRI appearance of benign soft tissue tumors. Clin Radiol 62(9):843–53

37. Guidera KJ, Satterwhite Y, Ogden JA, Pugh L, Ganey T (1991) Nail-patella syndrome. A review of 44 orthopaedic patients. J Pediatr Orthop 11:737–742

38. Gunther KP, Puhl W, Brenner H, Sturmer T (2002) Clinical epidemiology of hip and knee osteoarthritis: the Ulm osteoarthritis study. Z Rheumatol 61(3):244–249

39. Hall JG (1997) Arthrogryposis multiplex congenita: etiology, genetics, classification, diagnostic approach, and general aspects. J Pediatr Orthop B 6(3):159–166

40. Healy PJ, Helliwell PS (2005) Classification of the spondyloarthropathies. Curr Opin Rheumatol 17:395–399

41. Hedequist D, Emans J (2007) Congenital scoliosis: a review and update. J Pediatr Orthop 27(1):106–116

42. Helpert C et al (2004) Differential diagnosis of tumors and tumor-like lesions of the infrapatellar fat pad: pictorial review with an emphasis on MR imaging. Eur Radiol 14:2337–2346

43. Hernandez C, Cetner AS, Jordan JE, Puangsuvan SN, Robinson JK (2008) Tuberculosis in the age of biologic therapy. J Am Acad Dermatol 59(3):363–380

44. Herring JA (2001) Tachdjian's pediatric orthopaedics. Elsevier, Amsterdam

45. Herring JA, Kim HT, Browne R (2004) Legg-Calve-Perthes disease. Part I: classification of radiographs with use of the modified lateral pillar and Stulberg classifications. J Bone Joint Surg Am 86(10):2103–2120

46. Hesse B, Kohler G (2003) Does it always have to be Perthes' disease? What is epiphyseal dysplasia? Clin Orthop 414:219–227

47. Holick MF (2007) Vitamin D deficiency. NEJM 357:266–281

48. Honeyman A, Friedman H, Bendinelli M (2001) Staphylococcus aureus. Infection and disease. Series: infectious agents and pathogenesis. Springer, Berlin

49. Hosalkar HS et al (2006) Desmoid tumors and current ctatus of management. Orthop Clin North Am 37:53–63

50. Ilaslan H, Sundaram M (2006) Advances in musculoskeletal tumor imaging. Orthop Clin North Am 37: 375–91

51. Insall JN, Scott WN (2001) Surgery of the knee, 3rd edn. Churchill Livingstone, Oxford, UK

52. Janssens K, Vanhoenacker F, Bonduelle M et al (2006) Camurati-Engelmann disease: review of the clinical, radiological, and molecular data of 24 families and implications for diagnosis and treatment. J Med Genet 43:1–11

53. Jordan KM, Arden NK, Doherty M et al (2003) EULAR recommendations: an evidence based approach to the management of knee osteoarthritis. Ann Rheum Dis 62(12):1145–1155

54. Kanis JA, Burlet N, Cooper C, Delmas PD, Reginster JY, Borgstrom F, Rizzoli R (2008) European guidance for the diagnosis and management of osteoporosis in postmenopausal women. Osteoporos Int 19(4):399–428

55. Kaplan FS, Xu M, Glaser DL, Collins F, Connor M, Kitterman J, Sillence D, Zackai E, Ravitsky V, Zasloff M, Ganguly A, Shore EM (2008) Early diagnosis of fibrodysplasia ossificans progressiva. Pediatrics 121(5):1295–300

56. Kessel L (1980) A colour atlas of clinical orthopaedics. Wolfe Medical, Holland

57. Kilpatrick SE, Wenger DE, Gilchrist GS et al (1995) Langerhans' cell histiocytosis (histiocytosis x) of bone. A clinicopathologic analysis of 263 pediatric and adult cases. Cancer 76(12):2471–2484

58. Kim TH, Uhm WS, Inman RD (2005) Pathogenesis of ankylosing spondylitis and reactive arthritis. Curr Opin Rheumatol 17:400–405

59. Kitaoka HB (2002) The foot and ankle, 2nd edn. Lippincott Williams and Wilkins, Philadelphia

60. Laville JM, Lakermance P, Limouzy F (1994) Larsen's syndrome: review of the literature and analysis of thirty-eight cases. J Pediatr Orthop 14:63–73

61. Lee SH, Baek JR, Han SB, Park SW (2005) Stress fractures of the femoral diaphysis in children. A report of 5 cases and review of literature. J Pediatr Orthop 25:734–738

62. Levesque J, Marx RG, Bell RS, Wunder JS et al (1998) A clinical guide to primary bone tumors. Lippincott Williams and Wilkins, Philadelphia

63. Loder RT, Aronsson DD, Weinstein SL, Breur GJ, Ganz R, Leunig M (2008) Slipped capital femoral epiphysis. Instruct Course Lect 57:473–498

64. Lowe TG (2007) Scheuermann's kyphosis. Neurosurg Clin N Am 18(2):305–315

65. Luck JV Jr, Silva M, Rodriguez-Merchan C, Ghalambor N, Zahiri CA, Finn RS (2004) Hemophilic Arthropathy. J Am Acad Orthop Surg 12:234–245

66. Makitie O, Sulisalo T, de la Chapelle A, Kaitila I (1995) Cartilage-hair hypoplasia. I Med Genet 32:39–43

67. Mankin HJ, Hornicek FJ (2005) Aneurysmal bone cyst. A review of 150 patients. J Clin Oncol 23:6756–6762

68. Mease PJ (2004) Recent advances in the management of psoriatic arthritis. Curr Opin Rheumatol 16:366–370

69. Mik G, Gholve PA, Scher DM, Widmann RF, Green DW (2008) Down syndrome: orthopedic issues. Curr Opin Pediatr 20: 30–36

70. Milgram JW (1977) Synovial osteochondromatosis: a histological study of thirty cases. J Bone Joint Surg Am 59(6):792–801

71. Morrissy RT (1996) Lovell and Winter's Pediatric Orthopaedics. Lippincott Williams and Wilkins, Philadelphia

72. Nattiv A, Armsey TD Jr (1997) Stress injury to bone in the female athlete. Clin Sports Med 16:197

73. Neonakis IK, Alexandrakis MG, Gitti Z, Tsirakis G, Krambovitis E, Spandidos DA (2008) Miliary tuberculosis with no pulmonary involvement in myelodysplastic syndromes: a curable, yet rarely diagnosed, disease: case report and review of the literature. Ann Clin Microbiol Antimicrob 13:70–78

74. Parekh SG, Donthineni-Rao R, Ricchetti E, Lackman RD (2004) Fibrous dysplasia. J Am Acad Orthop Surg 12:305–313

75. Peris P (2003) Stress fracture. Best practice and research. Clin Rheumatol 17(6):1043–1061

76. Potts JT (2005) Parathyroid hormone: past and present. J Endocrinol 187:311–325

77. Raja SN, Grabow TS (2002) Complex regional pain syndrome I (reflex sympathetic dystrophy). Anaesthesiology 96:1254–1260

78. Riad J, Haglund-Akerlind Y, Miller F (2007) Classification of spastic hemiplegic cerebral palsy in children. J Pediatr Orthop 27(7):758–764

79. Rockwood CA Jr, Matsen FA III, Wirth MA, Lippitt SB (2004) The shoulder, vol. 1, 3rd edn. Saunders, NC, USA

80. Rodriguez Merchan EC (2003) The haemophilic joints. New perspectives. Blackwell, Oxford

81. Roodman GD, Windle JJ (2005) Paget disease of bone. Clin Invest 115(2): 200–208

82. Roos H, Lauren M, Adalberth et al. (1998) Knee osteoarthritis after meniscectomy. Prevalence and radiographic changes after twenty-one years compared with matched controls. Arthritis Rheum 41:687–693

83. Rosero VM, Kiss S, Terebessy T, Köllö K, Szöke G (2007) Dysplasia epiphysealis hemimelica (Trevor's disease): 7 of our own cases and a review of the literature. Acta Orthop 78:856–861

84. Rubin P (1964) Dynamic classification of bone dysplasias. Year Book Medical, Chicago, USA

85. Scarpa R, Mathieu A (2000) Psoriatic arthritis: evolving concepts. Curr Opin Rheumatol 12:274–280

86. Schmidt H, Ullrich K, Von Lengerke HJ (1987) Radiological findings in patients with mucopolysaccharidosis I. Pediatr Radiol 17:409–414

87. Sheldon PJ, Forrester DM, Learch TJ (2005) Imaging of intraarticular masses. Radiographics 25:105–119

88. Shetty AK, Kumar A (2007) Osteomyelitis in adolescents. Adolesc Med State Art Rev 18(1):79–94

89. Shipman SA, Helfand M, Moyer VA, Yawn BP (2006) Screening for developmental dysplasia of the hip: a systematic literature review for the US Preventive Services Task Force. Pediatrics 117(3):557–576

90. Siapkara A, Duncan R (2007) Congenital talipes equinovarus: a review of current management. J Bone Joint Surg Br 89(8):995–1000

91. Silve C, Jüppner H (2006) Ollier disease. Orphanet J Rare Dis 1:37–43

92. Sim FH, Frassica FJ, Frassica DA (1994) Soft-tissue tumors: diagnosis, evaluation, and management. J Am Acad Orthop Surg 2:202–211

93. Spranger JW, Brill PW, Poznanski AK (2001) Bone dysplasias: An atlas of genetic disorders of skeletal development. 2nd edition. Oxford University Press, Oxford

94. Staheli LT (2007) Fundamentals of pediatric orthopaedics. 4th edition. Lippincott Williams and Wilkins, Philadelphia

95. Stanitski DF, Nadjarian R, Stanitski CL, Bawle E, Tsipouras P (2000) Orthopaedic manifestations of Ehlers-Danlos syndrome. Clin Orthop Relat Res 376:213–221

96. Sundaram M, McLeod RA (1990) MR imaging of tumor and tumorlike lesions of bone and soft tissue. Am J Roentgenol 155:817–824

97. Szendrői M, Deodhar A (2000) Synovial neoformations and tumours. Baillieres Clin Rheumatol 14(2):363–383

98. Tatli B, Aydinli N, Caliskan M, Ozmen M, Bilir F, Acar G (2006) Congenital muscular torticollis: evaluation and classification. Pediatr Neurol 34(1):41–44

99. Taybi H (1998) Handbook of syndromes and metabolic disorders: Radiologic and clinical manifestations. Mosby, St Louis

100. Temple HTT et al (2002) Benign bone tumors. AAOS Instruct Course Lect 51:429–439

101. Trampuz A, Zimmerli W (2008) Diagnosis and treatment of implant-associated septic arthritis and osteomyelitis. Curr Infect Dis Rep 10(5):394–403

102. Treble NJ, Jensen FO, Bankier A, Rogers JG, Cole WG (1990) Development of the hip in multiple epiphyseal dysplasia. J Bone Joint Surg Br 72:1061–104

103. Tse SML, Laxer RM (2003) Juvenile spondyloarthropathy. Curr Opin Rheumatol 15:374–379

104. Underwood M (2006) Diagnosis and management of gout. BMJ 332:1315–1319

105. Unni KK, Dahlin (1996) Dahlin's bone tumors: General aspects and data on 11,087 cases. 5th edition. Lippincott Williams and Wilkins, Philadelphia

106. van der Linden S, van der Heijde D (2000) Clinical aspects, outcome assessment, and management of ankylosing spondylitis and postenteric reactive arthritis. Curr Opin Rheumatol 12:263–268

107. Weinstein SL, Dolan LA, Cheng JC, Danielsson A, Morcuende JA (2008) Adolescent idiopathic scoliosis. Lancet 371(9623):1527–1537

108. Weiss SW, Goldblum JR (2008) Soft tissue tumors. Mosby, St Louis

109. Wilkins RM (2000) Unicameral bone cysts. J Am Acad Orthop Surg 8(4):217–224

110. Wynne-Davies R, Gormley J (1985) The prevalence of skeletal dysplasias. J Bone Joint Surg Br 67:133–137

111. Zhang W, Doherty M, Pascual E et al (2006) EULAR evidence based recommendations for gout. Part I: diagnosis. Ann Rheum Dis 65(10):1301–1311

112. Zhang W, Doherty M, Bardin et al (2006) EULAR evidence based recommendations for gout. Part II: management. Ann Rheum Dis 65(10):1312–1324

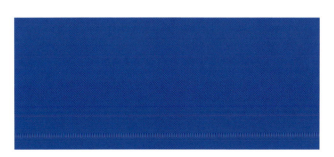

Subject Index

Printing and Binding: Stürtz GmbH, Würzburg